T0259392

Clinical Trials in Surgical Oncology

Editor

ELIN R. SIGURDSON

SURGICAL ONCOLOGY CLINICS OF NORTH AMERICA

www.surgonc.theclinics.com

Consulting Editor
NICHOLAS J. PETRELLI

October 2017 • Volume 26 • Number 4

ELSEVIER

1600 John F. Kennedy Boulevard • Suite 1800 • Philadelphia, Pennsylvania, 19103-2899

http://www.theclinics.com

SURGICAL ONCOLOGY CLINICS OF NORTH AMERICA Volume 26, Number 4
October 2017 ISSN 1055-3207, ISBN-13: 978-0-323-54692-8

Editor: John Vassallo (j.vassallo@elsevier.com)
Developmental Editor: Meredith Madeira

Surgical Oncology Clinics of North America (ISSN 1055-3207) is published quarterly by Elsevier Inc., 360 Park Avenue South, New York, NY 10010-1710. Months of publication are January, April, July, and October. Business and Editorial Offices: 1600 John F. Kennedy Blvd., Ste. 1800, Philadelphia, PA 19103-2899. Customer Service Office: 3251 Riverport Lane, Maryland Heights, MO 63043. Periodicals postage paid at New York, NY and additional mailing offices. Subscription prices are $296.00 per year (US individuals), $490.00 (US institutions) $100.00 (US student/resident), $337.00 (Canadian individuals), $620.00 (Canadian institutions), $205.00 (Canadian student/resident), $418.00 (foreign individuals), $620.00 (foreign institutions), and $205.00 (foreign student/resident). Foreign air speed delivery is included in all *Clinics* subscription prices. All prices are subject to change without notice. **POSTMASTER**: Send address changes to *Surgical Oncology Clinics of North America,* Elsevier Health Science Division, Subscription Customer Service, 3251 Riverport Lane, Maryland Heights, MO 63043. **Customer Service: 1-800-654-2452 (US and Canada). 314-447-8871 (outside US and Canada). Fax: 314-447-8029. E-mail: journalscustomerservice-usa@elsevier.com (for print support); journalsonline support-usa@elsevier.com (for online support).**

Reprints. For copies of 100 or more, of articles in this publication, please contact the Commercial Reprints Department, Elsevier Inc., 360 Park Avenue South, New York, New York 10010-1710. Tel. 212-633-3874; Fax: 212-633-3820; E-mail: reprints@elsevier.com.

Surgical Oncology Clinics of North America is covered in *MEDLINE/PubMed (Index Medicus)* and *EMBASE/ Excerpta Medica, Current Contents/Clinical Medicine, and ISI/BIOMED.*

Contributors

CONSULTING EDITOR

NICHOLAS J. PETRELLI, MD, FACS
Helen F. Graham Cancer Center & Research Institute, Christiana Care Health System, Newark, Delaware, USA

EDITOR

ELIN R. SIGURDSON, MD, PhD, FACS
Chief, Division of General Surgery, Fox Chase Cancer Center, Philadelphia, Pennsylvania, USA

AUTHORS

CHARLOTTE ARIYAN, MD, PhD
Associate Attending, Department of Surgery, Memorial Sloan Kettering Cancer Center, New York, New York, USA

IGOR ASTSATUROV, MD, PhD
Associate Professor, Department of Hematology and Oncology, Fox Chase Cancer Center, Philadelphia, Pennsylvania, USA

KAYLA BARNARD, MD
Fellow in Breast Surgical Oncology, UAMS Winthrop P. Rockefeller Cancer Institute, Little Rock, Arkansas, USA

GEORGE CHANG, MD, MS
The University of Texas MD Anderson Cancer Center, Houston, Texas, USA

YANA CHERTOCK, MA
Department of Clinical Genetics, Fox Chase Cancer Center, Philadelphia, Pennsylvania, USA

JOHN M. DALY, MD, FACS, FRCSI (Hon), FRCSG (Hon)
Dean Emeritus, Harry C Donahoo Professor of Surgery, Lewis Katz School of Medicine, Temple University, Fox Chase Cancer Center, Philadelphia, Pennsylvania, USA

LAURA A. DAWSON, MD, FRCPC
Radiation Medicine Program, Princess Margaret Cancer Centre, University Health Network, Toronto, Ontario, Canada

EFRAT DOTAN, MD
Assistant Professor, Department of Medical Oncology, Fox Chase Cancer Center, Philadelphia, Pennsylvania, USA

THOMAS J. GEORGE, MD, FACP
Associate Professor & GI Oncology Program Director, Department of Medicine, University of Florida, Gainesville, Florida, USA

NEHA GOEL, MD
Department of Surgical Oncology, Fox Chase Cancer Center, Philadelphia, Pennsylvania, USA

ABHA GUPTA, MD, MSc
Associate Professor, Department of Hematology/Oncology, The Hospital for Sick Children, Department of Medical Oncology, Princess Margaret Cancer Centre, University Health Network, Toronto, Ontario, Canada

MICHAEL J. HALL, MD, MS
Department of Clinical Genetics, Fox Chase Cancer Center, Philadelphia, Pennsylvania, USA

NARUHIKO IKOMA, MD
The University of Texas MD Anderson Cancer Center, Houston, Texas, USA

ATIF IQBAL, MD
Assistant Professor, Department of Surgery, University of Florida, Gainesville, Florida, USA

LISA A. KACHNIC, MD
Professor and Chair, Department of Radiation Oncology, Vanderbilt University Medical Center, Nashville, Tennessee, USA

GIORGOS KARAKOUSIS, MD
Assistant Attending, Department of Surgery, Hospital of the University of Pennsylvania, Philadelphia, Pennsylvania, USA

V. SUZANNE KLIMBERG, MD, PhD
Professor of Surgery and Pathology, Chief of Breast and Surgical Oncology, UAMS Winthrop P. Rockefeller Cancer Institute, Little Rock, Arkansas, USA

JENNIFER KNOX, MD, MSc, FRCPC
Associate Professor, Department of Medical Oncology and Hematology, Princess Margaret Cancer Centre, University Health Network, Toronto, Ontario, Canada

YANG LIU, MD
Fellow, Department of Hematology and Oncology, Fox Chase Cancer Center, Philadelphia, Pennsylvania, USA

ANDREA J. MACNEILL, MD, MSc
Assistant Professor, Division of Surgical Oncology, Department of Surgery, Diamond Health Care Centre, BC Cancer Agency, The University of British Columbia, Vancouver, British Columbia, Canada

JOHN C. McAULIFFE, MD, PhD
Attending Surgeon, Assistant Professor, Department of Surgery, Montefiore-Einstein Center for Cancer Care, Bronx, New York, USA

MAUREEN D. MOORE, MD
Research Fellow and Resident in Surgery, Weil Cornell College of Medicine, New York Presbyterian Hospital, Cornell Medical Center, New York, New York, USA

MITCHELL C. POSNER, MD, FACS
Thomas D. Jones Professor of Surgery, Vice Chairman, Surgical Oncology, Chief, Section of General Surgery, Department of Surgery, Professor, Department of Radiation and Cellular Oncology, Physician-in-Chief, Comprehensive Cancer Center, The University of Chicago Medicine, Chicago, Illinois, USA

KANWAL RAGHAV, MD, MBBS
The University of Texas MD Anderson Cancer Center, Houston, Texas, USA

CHETHAN RAMAMURTHY, MD
Department of Medical Oncology, Fox Chase Cancer Center, Philadelphia, Pennsylvania, USA

SANJAY S. REDDY, MD
Assistant Professor, Department of Surgical Oncology, Fox Chase Cancer Center, Philadelphia, Pennsylvania, USA

HAO-WEN SIM, MBBS (Hons), BMedSci, FRACP
Department of Medical Oncology and Hematology, Princess Margaret Cancer Centre, University Health Network, Toronto, Ontario, Canada

CLAYTON A. SMITH, MD, PhD
Assistant Professor, Division of Radiation Oncology, Mitchell Cancer Institute, University of South Alabama, Mobile, Alabama, USA

CAROL J. SWALLOW, MD, PhD
Professor and Chair, Division of General Surgery, Department of Surgery, University of Toronto, Toronto, Ontario, Canada

JENNIFER TSENG, MD
Surgical Oncology Fellow, Department of Surgery, The University of Chicago Medicine, Chicago, Illinois, USA

MARGARET VON MEHREN, MD
Professor, Department of Hematology and Oncology, Fox Chase Cancer Center, Philadelphia, Pennsylvania, USA

EDWARD M. WOLIN, MD
Director, Professor, Neuroendocrine Tumor Program, Division of Medical Oncology, Department of Medicine, Montefiore-Einstein Center for Cancer Care, Bronx, New York, USA

Contents

Randomized Controlled Trials in Soft Tissue Sarcoma: We Are Getting There!   531

Andrea J. MacNeill, Abha Gupta, and Carol J. Swallow

Soft tissue sarcoma (STS) is a family of malignancies for which individual management decisions can be complex. There is a paucity of level 1 evidence, as the rarity and heterogeneity of STS pose challenges to the design and execution of randomized controlled trials. Radiotherapy (RT) is routinely used to facilitate function-preserving surgery and to improve local control. Delivery of RT in the preoperative setting can decrease chronic toxicities at the cost of increased wound complications in the short term. The role of adjuvant systemic therapies remains controversial in adult STS.

Randomized Clinical Trials in Gastrointestinal Stromal Tumors   545

Yang Liu and Margaret von Mehren

This review explores the current standard of care for the surgical management of gastrointestinal stromal tumors, highlights important studies in the medical management of gastrointestinal stromal tumors, and provides guidance in how these studies changed the standard of care in clinical practice.

An Update on Randomized Clinical Trials in Melanoma   559

Giorgos Karakousis and Charlotte Ariyan

Despite many advances in the treatment of melanoma, it still continues to be a disease that affects many people. Fortunately, there has been a multitude of randomized trials that have refined the treatment of this prevalent disease. From 1975 to 2000, there were 154 prospective randomized trials on the treatment of local, regional, and metastatic melanoma. From 2001 to now, additional randomized trials have focused on the role of surgery, adjuvants to surgery, and treatment of metastatic disease. The results of the practice-changing trials are summarized in this review.

5-fluorouracil with or without oxaliplatin in stage III and possibly high-risk stage II colon cancer is associated with improved survival. Multimodality management of rectal cancer continues to evolve; total mesorectal excision is the cornerstone. Oncologic results do not support the use of laparoscopic resection in rectal cancer. Preoperative short- or long-course radiation for stage II or III rectal cancer is the standard of care. Long course chemoradiation is recommended for bulky tumors.

Clayton A. Smith and Lisa A. Kachnic

Management of anal carcinoma began as abdominoperineal resection and has evolved to combined chemotherapy and radiation. Early randomized trials demonstrated superior clinical outcomes of combined modality therapy over radiotherapy alone. Subsequent trials investigated alterations in the standard backbone of radiotherapy concurrent with 5-fluorouracil and mitomycin C with an intent to maintain clinical outcomes while reducing treatment-related morbidity. The addition of intensity-modulated radiotherapy to radiation planning and delivery has subsequently reduced acute toxicity and detrimental treatment breaks. Ongoing and future trials are aimed at reducing therapy in favorable patient populations to decrease morbidity while intensifying treatment in patients with negative prognostic factors.

Efrat Dotan

The aging of the population worldwide brings a "Tsunami" of older patients to oncology practices. Oncologists are faced with determining the fitness of patients for therapy and tailoring appropriate therapy. Ongoing treatment of this patient population is challenging because of physiologic changes of aging, comorbidities, and various geriatric syndromes. Underrepresentation of older patients in clinical trials results in a gap in knowledge and lack of clear evidence to guide treatment approach. In recent years, some advancements have been made with publication of elderly specific studies. However, much remains to be done by the oncologic community to continue and invest in these research efforts and expand the knowledge base in this arena.

Chethan Ramamurthy, Yana Chertock, and Michael J. Hall

Conducting randomized controlled trials (RCTs) in patients with germline mutations in genes that predispose to adult-onset cancer is hampered by the rarity of these mutations, barriers to their identification, and challenges inherent to randomizing high-risk individuals as part of a clinical trial. Most of the clinically relevant RCTs have been conducted in 3 syndromes in only some of the high-risk genes for which clinical testing is currently available. This article reviews the surgical, screening, and chemoprevention RCTs in each of the syndromes in clinically relevant studies conducted in the past 10 years.

Understanding of neuroendocrine tumors has increased greatly in the last 2 decades. Along with this, the prevalence of neuroendocrine tumors has increased because of the ubiquitous use of cross-sectional imaging, improved endoscopic screening, and the indolent nature of the disease. Up to 35% of patients have symptoms at the time of diagnosis, whereas the others have occult disease. Neuroendocrine tumors are a diverse group of malignancies with unique clinical courses. This article critically reviews the most important randomized controlled trials for neuroendocrine tumors and introduces a few awaiting completion.

The management of pancreatic cancer has grown rapidly in the last decade. The Gastrointestinal Tumor Study Group trial in 1985 supported postoperative chemoradiation, and a more recent study recommended 6 months of adjuvant gemcitabine and capecitabine or monotherapy with gemcitabine or fluorouracil plus folinic acid, in the absence of neoadjuvant therapy. Clinicians are now studying the role of targeted therapy in pancreatic cancer and neoadjuvant chemotherapy in resectable, borderline resectable, and locally advanced pancreatic cancer. This article critically evaluates the evolution of pancreatic cancer management, focusing on level 1a, prospective randomized control trials from 2007 to 2017.

The design of modern oncology clinical trials seeks to match patients' cancer molecular biomarkers with medications that specifically target those biomarkers, a general paradigm shift in cancer care coined *clinical cancer biology*. This approach exploits the synthetic lethality between a specific genetic alteration in the cancer cell and a drug: rapid termination of exaggerated kinase activity exemplifies this phenomenon. Synthetic lethality-based investigations are driven by rapidly evolving technologies for cancer molecular profiling. As these technologies evolve, future clinical trials will test drugs' activity based on the molecular mechanisms rather than by the tumor's appearance under a microscope.

SURGICAL ONCOLOGY CLINICS OF NORTH AMERICA

RELATED INTEREST

Surgical Clinics, June 2017 (Vol. 97, Issue 3)
Advances in Colorectal Neoplasia
Sean J. Langenfeld, *Editor*
Available at: www.surgical.theclinics.com

THE CLINICS ARE AVAILABLE ONLINE!
Access your subscription at:
www.theclinics.com

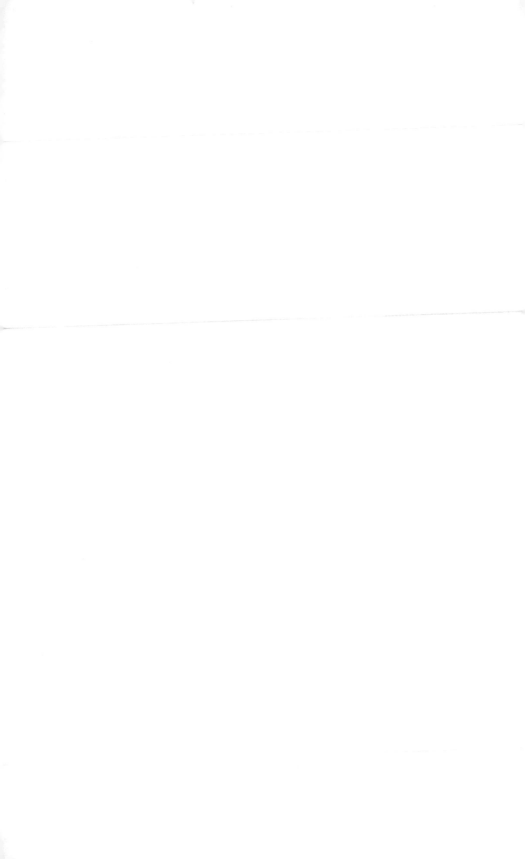

Foreword

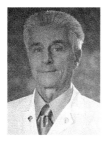

Nicholas J. Petrelli, MD, FACS
Consulting Editor

This issue of the *Surgical Oncology Clinics of North America* is devoted to clinical trials in oncology. The guest editor is Elin R. Sigurdson, MD, PhD, FACS. Dr Sigurdson joined the Surgical Oncology Department at Fox Chase Cancer Center in 1992 as Director of Surgical Research. Her surgical expertise is in the treatment of patients with colorectal and breast cancer. She is also Chief of the Division of General Surgery and the Associate Chief Academic Officer. Dr Sigurdson's career has centered around the development of clinical trials in oncology. She is not only an advocate of clinical trials but also has contributed to the development of several clinical trials throughout her career.

There is no question that progress in the last 40 years in the prevention and treatment of patients with cancer has been in the arena of clinical trials. The gold standard today still remains the randomized phase 3 clinical trial. This issue of the *Surgical Oncology Clinics of North America* spans the gamut of clinical trial development. For example, see Clayton A. Smith, and Lisa A. Kachnic's article, "Randomized Clinical Trials in Localized Anal Cancer," in this issue. See Atif Iqbal and Thomas George's article, "Randomized Clinical Trials in Colon and Rectal Cancer," in this issue discusses issues related to laparoscopic technique in colon and rectal cancer along with the issues related to preoperative radiation for stage II or III rectal cancer versus postoperative treatment. Last, see Chethan Ramamurthy and colleagues' article, "Randomized Controlled Trials in Hereditary Cancer Syndromes," in this issue for a discussion on the challenges in conducting clinical trials in hereditary cancer syndromes because of genetic heterogeneity.

Dr Sigurdson and her colleagues demonstrate that well-constructed and -designed clinical trials in oncology are a key part in developing successful treatment for patients with the diagnosis of cancer. It is imperative that federal funding be increased for the support of clinical trials in oncology so that the time period to success is lessened and the next generation of oncologists can continue to carry the torch in the treatment and prevention of cancer. I would like to thank Dr Sigurdson and her colleagues for an excellent issue of the *Surgical Oncology Clinics of North America* in taking on a topic that is the strong foundation for oncology care.

Surg Oncol Clin N Am 26 (2017) xiii–xiv
http://dx.doi.org/10.1016/j.soc.2017.07.001
1055-3207/17/© 2017 Published by Elsevier Inc.

surgonc.theclinics.com

This is my last Foreword for *Surgical Oncology Clinics of North America*. I want to thank John Vassallo and the Elsevier team for this opportunity. I'd also like to thank my colleagues across the country for all their efforts in making *Surgical Oncology Clinics of North America* a success. I know Dr. Tim Pawlik will do a great job in continuing the success. Lastly, my thanks go to Dr. Blake Cady who, several years ago, recommended me for this position.

Nicholas J. Petrelli, MD, FACS
Helen F. Graham Cancer Center & Research Institute
Christiana Care Health System
4701 Ogletown-Stanton Road, Suite 1233
Newark, DE 19713, USA

E-mail address:
npetrelli@christianacare.org

Preface

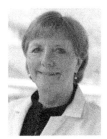

Elin R. Sigurdson, MD, PhD, FACS
Editor

It has been an honor for me to serve as guest editor for *Surgical Oncology Clinics of North America*. This issue addresses the role and results of clinical trials in the surgical and adjuvant treatment of patients with solid tumors. It has been more than a decade since these topics have been reviewed by *Surgical Oncology Clinics of North America*.

In that time, cooperative group randomized controlled clinical trials have demonstrated significant advances for most solid tumor types. Thirty years ago, the early "gold standard" randomized controlled trials were undertaken by organizations such as the GI Tumor Study Group, the National Surgical Adjuvant Breast and Bowel Project, and the North Central Cancer Treatment Group. The studies enrolled 200 to 500 patients. Since then, oncologists became accustomed to phase 3 trials enrolling thousands of patients with diseases such as breast, colon, and prostate cancer. This issue reviews these studies and the many advances made in solid tumor therapy in the past decade.

It also considers significant changes in trial design, increasingly directed to gene abnormalities of the tumor. Precision medicine has become a defining feature of trial design. Tumors undergo screening to ascertain whether their tumors harbor specific abnormalities (actionable mutations) that can be matched to drugs or drug combinations. Many current trials assign patients with an actionable mutation to treatment arms that may result in response to treatment, regardless of their site of origin. One example is the National Cancer Institute (NCI)-sponsored MATCH trial.

In NCI-MATCH, patients are assigned to receive their treatment based upon the genetic changes found in their tumors. Patients whose tumors have genetic changes that correspond to one of the agents in the trial may receive that treatment, if they meet other eligibility criteria. The trial seeks to determine whether treating cancers based upon specific genetic changes is an effective approach. As the profession moves from large phase 3 trials for specific solid tumors to trials based on actionable mutations, the NCI must address the twin challenges of increasing accrual and funding for both types of clinical trials.

In this issue, randomized trials, based upon solid tumor type, are updated. In addition, we try to peer into the future, in an effort to discern what the next decade will deliver in the pursuit of precision medicine.

Surg Oncol Clin N Am 26 (2017) xv–xvi
http://dx.doi.org/10.1016/j.soc.2017.07.002
1055-3207/17/© 2017 Published by Elsevier Inc.

surgonc.theclinics.com

I wish to thank all the authors, who took time from their busy schedules to write these excellent reviews. No work on clinical trials, or the trials themselves, would be complete without the considerable efforts of physicians and surgeons who enroll patients in clinical trials or (of course) the patients who participate in these studies. Their priceless contributions have resulted in major improvements to cancer care. Here you will see these significant advances!

Elin R. Sigurdson, MD, PhD, FACS
Division of General Surgery
Fox Chase Cancer Center
333 Cottman Avenue
Philadelphia, PA 19111, USA

E-mail address:
Elin.Sigurdson@fccc.edu

Introduction

The Evolution of Oncology Clinical Research: Lessons Learned

The purpose of clinical research is to add to medical knowledge using hypothesis-driven scientific methods for the betterment of clinical care and for ultimate improvement in patient outcomes. Over the millennia, development and dissemination of medical knowledge have moved in a nonsequential fashion from observation of individual patients to retrospective and prospective evaluation of institutional, national, and international groups of patients. Randomized controlled clinical trials, whose onset has often been dated to 1948, have usually been based on general drug, device, type of intervention, and patient characteristics.[1] More recently, clinical trials are based on the unique molecular and genetic tumor characteristics in an individual patient.[2] Previously, the discipline of surgery has been severely criticized for the lack of such published studies.[3] But in the last decade, there has been a marked increase in surgery-only randomized trials (laparoscopy vs open interventions for colon and rectal cancer)[4] as well as surgeons both leading and participating in multidisciplinary randomized oncology clinical trials.[5] Of course, while it is generally recognized that properly conducted, randomized clinical trials are the "gold standard," there are many individual and group (institution and large database) observations such as the introduction and evaluation of laparoscopic cholecystectomy that have led to controlled trials and major improvements in clinical outcomes for patients.[6]

Prospective randomized clinical trials do not discover or create new drugs or therapies, but their purpose is to identify true advances in drug therapy, device usage, and technological surgical advances that lead to changes in clinical practice and make outcome improvements for our patients with cancer. Statistical methods such as meta-analysis of randomized trials performed in a uniform way can provide an overall perspective.[7] However, even using strict methodology, meta-analysis techniques and results from them are only as good as the individual trials that are compiled, and complicated statistical techniques cannot make up for improper research methods, lack of blinding of investigators, bias, and too few patient numbers, leading to a lack of observation power and incorrect conclusions.

Major issues impeding progress in the development of new medical knowledge in our current environment are the costs of clinical trials research, the ability to incorporate all segments of our population into randomized trials, the plethora of new drugs and devices that are coming from research laboratories, and the difficulties with patient accrual to such trials. More recently, statistical methods have been used to shorten the time to completion of randomized clinical trials using adaptive randomization within individual studies. These techniques have resulted in more rapid determination of outcome results within phase 2 trials by eliminating therapeutic arms unlikely to demonstrate meaningful results and concentrating on those drug interventions that

Surg Oncol Clin N Am 26 (2017) xvii–xx
http://dx.doi.org/10.1016/j.soc.2017.07.003
1055-3207/17/© 2017 Published by Elsevier Inc.

have a high likelihood of success. For example, the I-SPY 2 trial compares up to 12 experimental therapies with a common control in subgroups of patients with breast cancer.[8,9] The randomization is stratified by tumor HER2 and hormone receptor status and 70 gene signatures. Adaptive randomization increases the likelihood of assignment to a given therapy as evidence accrues that the treatment improves results. Importantly, this trial design is a model for future clinical research as it offers molecular fingerprinting of the tumor for truly personalized experimental intervention and adaptive randomization that reduces the number of subjects required and decreases the time to identify potential candidate drugs for subsequent phase 3 trials.

The development of strict guidelines for the conduct of randomized clinical trials and statistical methods to improve time to trial completion has been an important milestone in clinical research. The ethical advances in human protection have also included several milestones, such as the Nuremberg Code, the Declaration of Helsinki, the Belmont Report, and the International Conference on Harmonization and Good Clinical Practice guidance in 1996. More recently, the National Institutes of Health (NIH) has issued guidance on the required use of a central Institutional Review Board to help speed the initiation of randomized clinical trials among multiple institutions. In addition, in September 2016, the NIH issued a final policy to promote broad and responsible dissemination of information from NIH-funded clinical trials through ClinicalTrials.gov. Under this policy, every clinical trial funded in whole or in part by NIH is expected to be registered on ClinicalTrials.gov and have summary results information submitted and posted in a timely manner. Taken together, all of these actions have decreased the time from drug and device discovery to proper clinical testing through prospective, randomized clinical trials to dissemination of results, both good and bad, leading to new, updated governmental and specialized society guidelines for patients receiving antineoplastic therapy.

This issue of *Surgical Oncology Clinics of North America* brings together the results of recent randomized clinical trials within disease sites, providing new guidelines for clinical care. Several important results are noted herein, but full reading of all the articles should be done.

In their article, Tseng and Posner summarized results of 24 randomized trials in the management of patients with gastric cancer and noted that a D2 lymph node dissection has not been consistently shown to improve overall survival over D1 lymph node dissection and is associated with an increase in perioperative complications and mortality. Neoadjuvant therapy has become a standard approach in many centers for patients with locally advanced gastric cancer (T3, N any) who are fit to tolerate treatment. Over 1000 patients after curative D2 gastrectomy were randomly assigned (Classic Trial) to receive adjuvant chemotherapy or surgery alone. Three-year disease-free survival was 74% in the chemotherapy and surgery group and 59% in the surgery-only group ($P<.0001$), indicating the short-term value of adjuvant chemotherapy. Iqbal and George described more recent trials for patients with colon and rectal cancer, noting that 14 additional randomized controlled trials and meta-analysis on laparoscopic surgery for colon cancer have confirmed the short-term benefits and oncologic noninferiority of the open approach. Sim, Knox, and Dawson in their article noted that use of lamivudine for chronic hepatitis B significantly reduced the rate of hepatocellular carcinoma development from 7% to 4% in a recent randomized trial. McAuliffe and Wolin reported the largest and most important randomized controlled trial evaluating the antiproliferative effects of a somatostatin analogue. Eligible patients were those with somatostatin receptor–positive, locally advanced or metastatic sporadic, nonfunctioning neuroendocrine tumors of well or moderate differentiation with a Ki-67 less than 10% and mitotic index of less than 2 mitoses per 10 high-power fields.

At 24 months, the estimated progression-free survival was 65% in the Lanreotide group and 33% in the placebo group. Finally, in another trial, patients with well-differentiated, somatostatin receptor–positive, metastatic midgut neuroendocrine tumors were treated with ^{177}Lu-Dotatate plus octreotide LAR or octreotide LAR alone. The 20-month progression-free survival was 65.2% for those treated with ^{177}Lu-Dotatate as compared with 10.8% in the control group.

These reports are but a few examples of the major progress to date in patients with a variety of solid tumors treated in a multidisciplinary approach with greater understanding of the biology of cancer. Adaptation of the results of these trials and other trials described in this issue into standards of care for our patients with cancer offers great promise for significant improvement in patient outcomes. Our patients can't wait; we can't wait.

Maureen D. Moore, MD
Weil Cornell College of Medicine
New York Presbyterian Hospital
Cornell Medical Center
New York, NY, USA

John M. Daly, MD, FACS, FRCSI(Hon), FRCSG(Hon)
Lewis Katz School of Medicine
at Temple University
Fox Chase Cancer Center
Philadelphia, PA 19111, USA

E-mail addresses:
mud9014@med.cornell.edu (M.D. Moore)
johndaly@temple.edu (J.M. Daly)

REFERENCES

1. Bothwell LE, Podolsky SH. The emergence of the randomized, controlled trial. N Engl J Med 2016;375(6):501–4.

2. Ahmed N, Brawley VS, Hegde M, et al. Human epidermal growth factor receptor 2 (HER2)—specific chimeric antigen receptor-modified t cells for the immunotherapy of HER2-positive sarcoma. J Clin Oncol 2015;33(15):1688–96.

3. ACS Surgery News—January 2016. Available at: http://www.acssurgerynews-digital.com/acssurgerynews/january_2016?pg=1#pg1. Accessed January 9, 2017.

4. Colon Cancer Laparoscopic or Open Resection Study Group, Buunen M, Veldkamp R, Hop WC, et al. Survival after laparoscopic surgery versus open surgery for colon cancer: long-term outcome of a randomised clinical trial. Lancet Oncol 2009;10(1):44–52.

5. Giuliano AE, Ballman K, McCall L, et al. Locoregional recurrence after sentinel lymph node dissection with or without axillary dissection in patients with sentinel lymph node metastases: long-term follow-up from the American College of Surgeons Oncology Group (Alliance) ACOSOG Z0011 Randomized Trial. Ann Surg 2016;264(3):413–20.

6. Barkun JS, Barkun AN, Sampalis JS, et al. Randomised controlled trial of laparoscopic versus mini cholecystectomy. The McGill Gallstone Treatment Group. Lancet 1992;340(8828):1116–9.

7. Urschel JD, Vasan H. A meta-analysis of randomized controlled trials that compared neoadjuvant chemoradiation and surgery to surgery alone for resectable esophageal cancer. Am J Surg 2003;185(6):538–43.
8. Park JW, Liu MC, Yee D, et al. Adaptive randomization of neratinib in early breast cancer. N Engl J Med 2016;375(1):11–22.
9. Harrington D, Parmigiani G. I-SPY 2—a glimpse of the future of phase 2 drug development? N Engl J Med 2016;375(1):7–9.

Randomized Controlled Trials in Soft Tissue Sarcoma: We Are Getting There!

Andrea J. MacNeill, MD, MSc[a], Abha Gupta, MD, MSc[b,c],
Carol J. Swallow, MD, PhD[d,e],*

KEYWORDS

- Randomized controlled trial • Soft tissue sarcoma • Extremity sarcoma
- Retroperitoneal sarcoma • Preoperative radiotherapy • Chemotherapy

KEY POINTS

- The rarity and heterogeneity of soft tissue sarcoma (STS) pose challenges to the design and conduct of randomized controlled trials (RCTs).
- The only level 1 evidence to guide the surgical management of STS is a small RCT that established the equivalence of limb salvage to amputation for extremity STS.
- Improved local control of extremity STS with radiotherapy (RT) has been demonstrated in 2 landmark RCTs, and the relative advantages of preoperative versus postoperative RT are documented in the NCIC SR2 trial. Level 1 evidence regarding the use of RT in retroperitoneal sarcoma is as yet pending, from the European Organization for Research and Treatment of Cancer–led STRASS trial.
- With the exception of specific histologic subtypes, there is a lack of evidence to support routine neoadjuvant/adjuvant chemotherapy as a standard of care for most adult STS. However, multiple agents have been shown to prolong survival in the metastatic setting.
- Large collaborations in pediatric oncology have generated robust level 1 evidence for the management of pediatric STS.

Disclosure Statement: The authors have nothing to disclose.
[a] Division of Surgical Oncology, Department of Surgery, Diamond Health Care Centre, BC Cancer Agency, University of British Columbia, 5199-2775 Laurel Street, Vancouver, British Columbia V5Z 1M9, Canada; [b] Department of Hematology/Oncology, The Hospital for Sick Children, 555 University Avenue, Toronto, Ontario M5G 1X8, Canada; [c] Department of Medical Oncology, Princess Margaret Cancer Centre, 610 University Avenue, Toronto, Ontario M5G 2M9, Canada; [d] Department of Surgical Oncology, Mount Sinai Hospital/Princess Margaret Cancer Centre, 600 University Avenue, Suite 1225, Toronto, Ontario M5G 1X5, Canada; [e] Department of Surgery, University of Toronto, Stweart Building, 149 College Street, Toronto, Ontario M5T 1P5, Canada
* Corresponding author. Mount Sinai Hospital, 600 University Avenue, Suite 1225, Toronto, Ontario M5G 1X5, Canada.
E-mail address: Carol.Swallow@sinaihealthsystem.ca

Surg Oncol Clin N Am 26 (2017) 531–544
http://dx.doi.org/10.1016/j.soc.2017.05.001

INTRODUCTION

Soft tissue sarcoma (STS) is a family of rare malignant neoplasms with an incidence of 4 to 5 per 100,000. As these are of predominantly mesenchymal origin, they can occur in any anatomic location. This anatomic diversity has important implications for treatment, in particular with respect to operative considerations, such that extremity/trunk and retroperitoneal/intra-abdominal STS are in many ways distinct entities.

More than 70 histologic subtypes of STS are now recognized with widely variable biology and sensitivity to systemic treatments. Increasingly, the discovery of characteristic underlying molecular alterations is facilitating targeted treatment of individual subtypes. For these reasons, it is imperative to conceptualize STS as a family of disparate malignancies requiring treatment strategies tailored to individual patients and disease. The rarity and heterogeneity of STS pose a considerable challenge to the design, conduct, and interpretation of randomized controlled trials (RCTs). The STS literature is, therefore, limited in high-level evidence and in the general applicability of many of the existing RCTs.

Surgery remains the mainstay of curative-intent treatment of STS. The ability to achieve complete excision is the primary determinant of survival and overt local recurrence for most histologies.[1–3] Radiotherapy (RT) is often used to allow preservation of critical structures and to decrease local recurrence, but a survival benefit has not been shown.[4,5] Chemotherapy has an important role in the primary treatment of specific chemosensitive subtypes of STS, including nonpleomorphic rhabdomyosarcoma (RMS) and Ewing sarcoma (ES), but in other subtypes its use is generally reserved for treatment of advanced or metastatic disease. The level 1 evidence available for each of these treatment modalities is discussed below.

SURGERY

Seminal work on the surgical approach to extremity STS was published in 1982 by Rosenberg and his colleagues[6] at the National Institutes of Health (NIH). A total of 43 patients were randomized to either amputation (N = 16) or limb salvage with adjuvant external beam RT (N = 27). All patients received postoperative systemic chemotherapy. There was no significant difference in overall survival (OS) between the two groups, and local control in the limb salvage group was 85%. These results instigated a paradigm shift toward limb preservation that has long remained the standard of care.

The optimal extent of surgery for retroperitoneal sarcoma (RPS) has not been evaluated in a similarly rigorous fashion. The anatomic constraints of the retroperitoneum render microscopic margin negative resection difficult. In contradistinction to extremity/trunk STS, local failure remains a predominant pattern of RPS recurrence, leading to disease-specific mortality that continues to accrue even 20 years postoperatively.[7] Based on retrospective data from multiple institutions, particularly in Europe, there has been an evolution in recent years toward more liberal en bloc resection of adherent but grossly uninvolved organs in an attempt to improve local control in RPS.[8,9] However, this approach has not been compared with more conservative resection using true prospective data collection, even in an observational manner; it is difficult to imagine how a meaningful RCT could be conducted.

RADIATION
Extremity Soft Tissue Sarcoma

As in the limb-sparing approach supported by the landmark work of Rosenberg and colleagues,[6] RT has for several decades been used to facilitate function-preserving surgery by allowing close/microscopically positive margins along critical neurovascular structures. Two randomized trials in the 1990s helped to firmly establish the role of adjuvant RT in improving local control in extremity STS. Following macroscopically complete resection of extremity or superficial trunk STS, Pisters and colleagues[4] randomized 164 patients intraoperatively to receive postoperative brachytherapy (BRT) or no additional treatment. They found a significant benefit to BRT in patients with high-grade tumors (5-year actuarial local control 82% compared with 69% without BRT, $P = .04$) but no benefit in low-grade tumors. There was no difference in OS for high or low grade. Similarly, in a trial involving 141 patients who had undergone complete resection of extremity STS, Yang and colleagues[10] demonstrated significantly improved local control in the group randomized to postoperative external beam RT (XRT) versus no additional therapy; in this trial, a local control benefit was seen for both high- and low-grade tumors. The latter study also examined quality of life; the investigators suggested that, in patients at low risk of recurrence, XRT could likely be safely omitted. As with the Pisters and colleagues'[4] trial, no improvement in OS was seen with adjuvant RT. The magnitude of the improvement in local control observed by Yang and colleagues[10] was interpreted by some as a signal that XRT was perhaps superior to BRT in the adjuvant treatment of STS. Long-term follow-up (median 17.9 years) of the XRT trial has confirmed the durability of improved local control with adjuvant RT, without a corresponding survival benefit.[5]

Sequencing of Radiotherapy and Surgery

The National Cancer Institute of Canada Sarcoma2 (NCIC-SR2) trial compared the delivery of 50 Gy of XRT in the preoperative setting (n = 94) versus 66 Gy XRT postoperatively (n = 96) for extremity STS and found higher rates of significant wound healing complications with preoperative XRT (35% vs 17%, $P = .01$).[11] Local recurrence rates were similar between groups, but, surprisingly and intriguingly, OS was slightly higher in the preoperative XRT group ($P = .048$). Longer follow-up revealed higher rates of late toxicities, such as fibrosis, joint stiffness, and edema after postoperative RT, with significantly lower limb function ratings.[12] Given that the acute wound healing complications seen with preoperative XRT are typically recoverable, whereas the late effects associated with postoperative XRT are more likely to be irreversible, these data supported consideration of preoperative RT for high-risk extremity STS. Other related advantages include more limited, targeted treatment volume.

Modified RT techniques to mitigate the earlier-described toxicities have been investigated in 2 recent nonrandomized trials. Using preoperative image-guided intensity-modulated RT (IG-IMRT) to minimize the dose to uninvolved tissues, O'Sullivan and colleagues[13] compared wound healing in lower extremity STS (n = 70) with that documented in the NCIC's SR2 trial. Significant wound complications were observed in 30.5% (vs 43.0%, $P = .2$) and reoperations for wound complications were necessary in 33.0% (vs 43.0%, $P = .55$). The rate of primary wound closure was 93.2% in the IG-IMRT cohort (vs 71.4% in the SR2 trial, $P = .002$), which was associated with less need for tissue transfer. In another nonrandomized trial (Radiation Therapy Oncology Group [RTOG]-0630), image-guided radiation therapy (IGRT) to a reduced target volume resulted in late toxicity scores of grades 2 or greater in only 10.5% of 79 eligible patients with extremity STS, compared with the NCIC SR2 trial rate of 37% ($P<.001$); notably, there was no apparent increase in marginal-field recurrences, defined as recurrence at the edge of the clinical target volume.[14]

The increased rates of late toxicity observed with postoperative XRT have been attributed, at least in part, to the delivery of a higher biological equivalent dose (the prescribed dose of postoperative XRT was 66 Gy to the wound and tumor bed, as opposed to 50 Gy with the tumor in situ). The need for a higher dose in the postoperative setting has recently been called into question, and an RCT designed to explore this issue is currently enrolling patients at Princess Margaret Cancer Centre, Toronto. The trial randomizes patients to 50 Gy XRT preoperatively or 50 Gy XRT postoperatively (NCT02565498). Deferring the decision about RT administration to the postoperative period allows due consideration of the final histopathologic analysis, including microscopic margin status. It is well accepted that select patients with STS of the extremities that have favorable features (<5 cm and/or low grade) can be appropriately treated with surgery alone.[15] Recent retrospective series have questioned whether the indications for RT can be better tailored to avoid overtreatment of patients who undergo quality surgery.[16,17] In a study that investigates the selection criteria for safe omission of RT, the French Sarcoma Group is currently accruing patients to an RCT (NCT00870701) in which patients who have undergone resection of extremity STS with final pathologic margins of 1 cm or greater are randomized to postoperative XRT versus no further treatment, regardless of tumor size or grade.

Retroperitoneal Sarcoma

Given the anatomic challenges in obtaining a microscopically complete resection of STS in the retroperitoneum, RT is conjectured to be of potential benefit; but there is currently no level I evidence to support its use. Two prospective, nonrandomized trials from Princess Margaret Cancer Centre (PMCC) and MD Anderson Cancer Center (MDACC) evaluated the safety and feasibility of preoperative XRT in RPS.[18] These studies established that preoperative XRT for RPS was well tolerated in terms of acute RTOG toxicity scores. The associated oncologic outcomes seemed to compare favorably with historical controls. Concurrently, a phase I/II trial at PMCC investigated dose escalation in the form of postoperative BRT after preoperative XRT and complete macroscopic resection of RPS.[19,20] Although it is important to note that the treatment groups were not randomized, it was clear that postoperative BRT entailed excessive toxicity without any apparent improvement in disease control.

In 2004, the American College of Surgeons Oncology Group opened a phase III trial (Z9031) of preoperative XRT plus surgery versus surgery alone for primary RPS, but the study closed prematurely because of poor accrual over the first year. Led by Sylvie Bonvalot,[21] the European Organization for Research and Treatment for Cancer (EORTC) has succeeded in carrying out a similarly designed multi-institutional trial that has enrolled patients with primary RPS across Europe and North America, with target accrual completed as of early 2017 (EORTC 62092–22092 STRASS). The recently reported second interim safety analysis showed no statistically significant increase in adverse events with XRT.[21]

A German phase I/II trial is currently underway examining the addition of intraoperative RT (IORT) to preoperative IMRT in primary RPS, with an interim analysis reporting acceptable levels of toxicity and comparable oncologic outcomes with historical and contemporary series.[22]

CHEMORADIATION

The combination of preoperative XRT and perioperative systemic treatment has been prospectively investigated in both extremity and retroperitoneal sarcoma but not in any RCT of which the authors are aware. After an encouraging single-institution pilot study, the RTOG conducted a phase II trial of neoadjuvant mesna, doxorubicin, ifosfamide, and dacarbazine (MAID) interdigitated with 44 Gy of preoperative XRT, followed by resection and 3 cycles of postoperative MAID (RTOG 0514) in patients with high-risk extremity and body wall STS.[23] This regimen proved to have substantial toxicity that precluded further study or use outside of a trial. Long-term follow-up of these patients revealed resolution of treatment-related toxicities within 1 year, with oncologic outcomes that compared favorably with other published series.[24]

In 1996, Pisters and colleagues[4] (MDACC) commenced a phase I trial of low-dose doxorubicin with concurrent preoperative XRT for high-grade RPS. The results were reported as a combined experience with PMCC, whereby 37 high-grade RPS were treated with preoperative XRT ±BRT in a phase I/II trial.[18] Long-term results of the combined use of preoperative chemoradiation (CRT) for RPS at MDACC have not been reported, and the regimen is not currently used at that center. Gronchi and colleagues[25] reported a phase I/II trial of preoperative high-dose prolonged-infusion ifosfamide in combination with 50.4 Gy preoperative XRT for resectable RPS and found that only two-thirds of patients could complete the planned treatment regimen. Given the toxicity and feasibility concerns raised in these preliminary studies, further investigation of combined preoperative CRT for RPS has not been pursued in RCTs.

SYSTEMIC THERAPY

STS demonstrates widely variable sensitivity to cytotoxic chemotherapies. RMS and ES are highly responsive to chemotherapy, which forms a cornerstone of the multidisciplinary management of these diseases. These histologies, however, occur predominantly in children and young adults and are addressed separately below. The focus of the rest of this section is on adult STS.

Adjuvant Chemotherapy

The potential role of adjuvant chemotherapy in STS has been explored in numerous RCTs and 2 meta-analyses. The first meta-analysis summarized 14 trials including 1568 patients evaluating the efficacy of adjuvant doxorubicin-based therapy in localized, resectable STS[26] and demonstrated a significant improvement in recurrence-free survival (RFS) (hazard ratio [HR] 0.75, $P = .0001$) but only a 4% difference in OS at 10 years, which was not significant (HR 0.89, $P = .12$). Within the subgroup of patients with extremity STS, there was a 7% absolute difference in 10-year OS with adjuvant chemotherapy (HR 0.80, $P = .029$), suggesting that this population may derive marginal benefit from systemic treatment. In 2008, an updated meta-analysis considered 4 additional trials of adjuvant chemotherapy, all of which included ifosfamide, for a total of 1747 patients.[27] Small but significant absolute risk reductions again were seen for local (4%, 95% confidence interval [CI] 0%–7%, $P = .04$), distant (9%, 95% CI 5%–14%, $P = .000$), and overall recurrences (10%, 95% CI 5%–15%, $P \leq .001$). With the inclusion of the newer studies, there was also a significant improvement in OS (ARR 6%, 95% CI 2%–11%, $P = .003$). Whether this difference was the result of a larger sample size or the inclusion of ifosfamide remains unclear, but it should be noted that all of the newer trials included ifosfamide-based chemotherapy in contrast to only one study in the Sarcoma Meta-analysis Collaboration (SMAC). When weighed against the toxicity of combination chemotherapy, the marginal improvements noted in this meta-analysis were insufficient to shift practice toward routine administration. More recently, an EORTC phase III trial comparing adjuvant doxorubicin + ifosfamide to surgery alone for resected high-grade sarcomas failed to show a difference in RFS (HR 0.91, 95% CI 0.67–1.22, $P = .51$) or OS (HR 0.94, 95% CI 0.68–1.31).[28]

Neoadjuvant Chemotherapy

The Italian and Spanish Sarcoma groups randomized patients to 3 versus 5 cycles of preoperative epirubicin + ifosfamide.[29] Despite noninferiority of the truncated regimen, subgroup analysis revealed significant differences in outcome between histologic subtypes, prompting a subsequent phase III trial of histology-tailored chemotherapy in high-risk, resected STS (Italian Sarcoma Group-STS-1001). In this trial, patients with high-risk STS of the extremity or body wall were randomized to either 3 cycles of epirubicin + ifosfamide or 3 cycles of a histology-tailored regimen, all given preoperatively: gemcitabine + docetaxel for undifferentiated pleomorphic sarcoma, trabectedin for high-grade myxoid liposarcoma (LPS), high-dose pro-longed-infusion ifosfamide for synovial sarcoma, etoposide + ifosfamide for malignant peripheral nerve sheath tumors, or gemcitabine + dacarbazine for leiomyosarcoma (LMS). The trial was closed early because of superior RFS and OS with the standard epirubicin + ifosfamide regimen compared with a histology-specific approach (RFS 0.62 vs 0.38, P = .004; OS 0.89 vs 0.64, P = .033).[30] Subgroup analysis showed that trabectedin had comparable activity to epirubicin + ifosfamide in myxoid LPS, which is now being further investigated because of the presumed lower toxicity of tra-bectedin compared with conventional chemotherapy.

At present, the role of routine (neoadjuvant/adjuvant) chemotherapy in the treatment of localized, resectable STS remains contentious. Although not standard, major consensus guidelines acknowledge that adjuvant chemotherapy can be considered in high-risk patients (high grade, deep, >5 cm); work is ongoing to better define what patient population may derive the most benefit from this treatment modality.[31]

Regional Techniques

Regional delivery of chemotherapy was explored by the University of California, Los Angeles sarcoma group in the treatment of distal extremity lesions. Doxorubicin was administered intra-arterially in the early experience and later via an intravenous route to the lower extremity before limb-preserving resection of distal STS.

The addition of regional hyperthermia (RHT) was subsequently investigated as a means of augmenting the efficacy of systemic treatment.[32] An EORTC trial (62,961) compared perioperative etoposide + ifosfamide + doxorubicin (EIA) alone or in com-bination with RHT, in addition to best local control (surgery ± RT).[33] Patients with localized, high-risk STS of the extremity (n = 149) or nonextremity sites (trunk, retro-peritoneum, head and neck; n = 192) were eligible, along with both primary and recur-rent disease. The addition of RHT increased response rates, assessed radiologically after induction therapy according to World Health Organization's criteria (28.8% vs 12.7%, P = .002). Disease-Free Survival (DFS) was superior in the RHT group (HR 0.70 with EIA + RHT vs EIA alone, 95% CI 0.54–0.92, P = .011). Although there was no difference in OS with RHT in the intention-to-treat cohort, among those pa-tients who actually completed induction therapy (4 cycles of EIA + 8 cycles of RHT vs 4 cycles of EIA alone; n = 269), OS was better in the combined therapy group (HR 0.66, 95% CI 0.45–0.98, P = .038). Long-term follow-up of the subgroup of pa-tients with macroscopically completely resected (R0/R1) abdominal and retroperito-neal STS revealed significantly improved local progression-free survival (LPFS) and DFS in the group who received combined treatment with RHT (5-year LPFS 56% vs 45%, P = .044; DFS 34% vs 27%, P = .027), but no difference in OS.[34]

Intraperitoneal Chemotherapy

The French Sarcoma Group investigated the role of intraperitoneal (IP) chemotherapy in combination with cytoreductive surgery for peritoneal sarcomatosis.[35] Patients who had undergone cytoreductive surgery were randomized to 5 days of postoper-ative IP doxorubicin and cisplatin or no IP therapy. There was no difference in local or distant RFS or in OS between patients who received IP chemotherapy and those who did not.

Although several groups are using IP chemotherapy in addition to cytoreductive surgery for desmoplastic small round cell tumor, this has not been the subject of an RCT.

Advanced/Metastatic Disease

The management of locally advanced or metastatic STS is complex and requires individually tailored multidisciplinary care by a specialist sarcoma team. Systemic treatment can be administered with multiple possible objectives, including prolongation of life, relief of symptoms, or downsizing for possible resection. The goals of care should be identified at the outset, as decisions regarding type and duration of systemic therapy are contingent thereupon. As in the adjuvant setting, anthracycline-based regimens remain the standard of care for most STS. Multiple recent trials have investigated alternative agents or combinations; however, until very recently, none has demonstrated definitive superiority to single-agent doxorubicin particularly in terms of OS (**Table 1**). The EORTC 62012 trial investigated single-agent doxorubicin versus doxorubicin + ifosfamide for locally advanced, unresectable, or metastatic STS and found significant differences in the objective response rate and progression-free survival (PFS) but no difference in OS.[36] The addition of ifosfamide was advantageous if the goal of treatment was tumor shrinkage; failing this, there was no benefit to intensified treatment of palliation of patients with advanced STS. Similarly, the PICASSO III trial demonstrated that the addition of palifosfamide, an active metabolite of ifosfamide, to doxorubicin compared with doxorubicin alone in adults with metastatic sarcoma failed to improve PFS or OS but increased toxicity in the combination arm.[37] The GeDDIS trial also failed to demonstrate any advantage of gemcitabine + docetaxel over single-agent doxorubicin for locally advanced or metastatic STS but only higher toxicity in the experimental arm.[38] Aldoxorubicin, an albumin-binding prodrug of doxorubicin, was investigated as an alternative to doxorubicin in a phase II study of locally advanced or metastatic STS and found to have superior PFS with no difference in OS. The manageable side effect profile and lack of cardiotoxicity with aldoxorubicin warrants further investigation.[39]

Gemcitabine in combination with docetaxel has been shown to be superior to single-agent gemcitabine but at the cost of increased toxicity.[40] LMS, especially of the uterus, has specific sensitivity to these regimens; both gemcitabine alone and in combination with docetaxel are reasonable options in women with advanced disease.[41] The combination of gemcitabine and dacarbazine is better tolerated, and the addition of dacarbazine has been shown to improve PFS and OS compared with gemcitabine alone in adults with all STS.[42] Trabectedin has recently been approved as second-line therapy, having demonstrated superior activity to dacarbazine in the treatment of adults with metastatic LMS and LPS.[43]

In recent years, a variety of targeted therapies have been investigated in the treatment of advanced or metastatic STS. The phase III PALETTE trial demonstrated that pazopanib, a multi-agent tyrosine kinase inhibitor, offered significant improvement in PFS in patients with metastatic STS of nonadipogenic origin compared with placebo, permitting its registration as an approved drug for STS.[44] Eribulin was compared with dacarbazine in patients with metastatic LMS and LPS, with a small but significant improvement in OS in the eribulin group.[45] Finally, Tap and colleagues[46] compared single-agent doxorubicin to combination with olaratumab; the combination was associated with a highly significant 11.8-month survival benefit. Although this was only a phase II study, the remarkable benefit in OS facilitated rapid approval of olaratumab for STS.

Table 1
Randomized trials investigating the use of systemic therapy in the treatment of locally advanced or metastatic soft tissue sarcoma

Trial	Study Design	N	Objective Response Rate	Progression-Free Survival	OS	Conclusions
Maki et al,[40] 2007	Phase II: Gemcitabine + docetaxel vs gemcitabine	122	16% vs 8%	6.2 mo vs 3.0 mo	18 mo vs 12 mo	Combination superior but has increased toxicity (prohibitive of long-term use)
Garcia-Del-Muro et al,[42] 2011	Phase II: Gemcitabine + dacarbazine vs gemcitabine	113	49% vs 25% $P = .009$	4.2 mo vs 2.0 mo $P = .005$	16.8 mo vs 8.2 mo $P = .014$	Combination superior and well tolerated, no increased toxicity
PALETTE Van der Graaf et al,[44] 2012	Phase III: Pazopanib vs placebo in nonadipocytic STS	369	6% vs 0%	4.6 mo vs 1.6 mo $P<.0001$	12.5 mo vs 10.7 mo $P = .25$	Superior disease control with pazopanib, acceptable toxicity
EORTC 62012 Judson et al,[36] 2014	Phase III: Doxorubicin + ifosfamide vs doxorubicin	455	26% vs 14% $P<.0006$	7.4 mo vs 4.6 mo $P = .03$	14.3 mo vs 12.8 mo $P = .076$	No benefit to combination for palliation of advanced STS unless the goal of treatment is tumor shrinkage
GeDDiS Seddon et al,[38] 2015 (abstract only)	Phase III: Gemcitabine + docetaxel vs doxorubicin	257	N/A	5.5 mo vs 5.4 mo $P = .07$	14.5 mo vs 16.4 mo $P = .67$	Increased toxicity with combination with no difference in disease control
Chawla et al,[39] 2015	Phase II: Aldoxorubicin vs doxorubicin	123	25% vs 0%	5.6 mo vs 2.7 mo $P = .02$	15.8 mo vs 14.3 mo $P = .21$	Superior disease control with aldoxorubicin with manageable adverse effects and no cardiotoxicity
Demetri et al,[43] 2016	Phase III: Trabectedin vs dacarbazine in LPS and LMS	518	9.9% vs 6.9% $P = .33$	4.2 mo vs 1.5 mo $P<.0001$	12.4 mo vs 12.9 mo $P = .37$	Superior disease control with trabectedin; led to FDA approval
PICASSO III Ryan et al,[37] 2016	Phase III: Doxorubicin + Palifosfamide vs Doxorubicin	447	28.3% vs 19.9%	6.0 mo vs 5.2 mo $P = 0.19$	15.9 mo vs 16.9 mo $P = 0.74$	Increased toxicity with combination with no difference in oncologic outcomes
Tap et al,[46] 2016	Phase II: Doxorubicin + olaratumab vs doxorubicin	133	18.2% vs 11.9% $P = 0.3421$	6.6 mo vs 4.1 mo $P = .06$	26.5 mo vs 14.7 mo $P = .0003$	Highly significant 11.8-mo survival benefit with olaratumab
Schoffski et al,[45] 2016	Phase III: Eribulin vs dacarbazine in LPS and LMS	452	4% vs 5% $P = .62$	2.6 mo vs 2.6 mo $P = .229$	13.5 mo vs 11.5 mo $P = .0169$	Survival benefit with eribulin in LPS and LMS

Abbreviation: FDA, Food and Drug Administration N/A, Not Accessed.

CHEMOSENSITIVE SOFT TISSUE SARCOMAS: RHABDOMYOSARCOMA AND EWING SARCOMA

RMS and ES belong to the family of small, round, blue cell tumors characterized by much higher sensitivity to chemotherapy than most STS. Both are typically treated with multimodal therapy consisting of chemotherapy plus surgery and/or RT. Although these subtypes of STS occur predominantly in children and young adults, they are discussed here because of the considerable body of level 1 evidence available to guide their treatment. This large body of evidence is the result of international and multidisciplinary collaboration between large cooperative pediatric oncology groups, which could serve as an exemplar for the adult STS academic community seeking to generate a similarly robust literature.

Ewing's Sarcoma

Standard chemotherapy for ES in North America consists of vincristine, doxorubicin, and cyclophosphamide (VDC) alternating with ifosfamide and etoposide (IE). This standard stems from the Intergroup-0091 trial, which showed significantly better 5-year RFS with the addition of IE to the standard regimen of VDC and dactinomycin in patients with localized ES.[47] Cyclophosphamide and ifosfamide were shown to be equally effective in the treatment of patients with standard-risk ES in the EICESS-92 study.[48] This study also suggested some benefit to the addition of etoposide in the treatment of high-risk ES. A Children's Oncology Group (COG) study investigated interval compression of standard chemotherapy and showed that VDC/IE delivered every 2 weeks was more effective than when given at 3-week intervals, with no increased toxicity.[49] It has been difficult to recapitulate this practice in older patients in the practical setting. The Euro-EWING99 study is a large international trial carried out by multiple cooperative groups consisting of three randomizations based on a backbone of vincristine, ifosfamide, doxorubicin, and etoposide. The Euro-EWING99-R1 trial showed that cyclophosphamide may be able to replace ifosfamide in consolidation treatment of standard-risk localized ES.[50] Euro-EWING99-R2 demonstrated improved outcomes with busulfan + melphalan chemotherapy in patients with localized ES with a poor histologic response to chemotherapy or with a large tumor volume.[51] Euro-EWING99-R3 identified no benefit to busulfan + melphalan chemotherapy in patients with ES with lung or pleural metastases compared with conventional chemotherapy combined with lung irradiation.[52]

Rhabdomyosarcoma

A series of RCTs carried out by the Intergroup Rhabdomyosarcoma Study Group (IRS) over the past 4 decades has compared various protocols of multi-agent chemotherapy, with or without surgery/RT, permitting refinement according to risk category.[53–56] This evolution in RMS management is reflected in an improvement in OS for patients with localized RMS from 55% in IRS-I to 71% in IRS-IV. However, standard RMS chemotherapy has remained largely unchanged since the 1970s consisting of vincristine, actinomycin, and cyclophosphamide (VAC). Since IRS-IV, the COG, which has subsumed the IRS, has carried out 2 RCTs investigating modifications to standard RMS chemotherapy in intermediate-risk RMS. D9803 found no benefit to the introduction of topotecan into standard chemotherapeutic regimens.[57] In ARST0331, a regimen of alternating VAC with vincristine plus irinotecan (VI) was found to be as effective as standard chemotherapy but less toxic.[58] Ongoing trials within COG are continuing to investigate modifications to VAC/VI with the addition of novel, targeted agents in the treatment of RMS.

DISCUSSION

The evolution of STS care has been punctuated by a small number of practice-changing RCTs. Rosenberg and colleagues'[6] early demonstration of the feasibility of limb salvage in a very small cohort enabled further study of function-preserving techniques that have long since supplanted amputation as the standard of care for extremity STS.[6] Pisters and colleagues[4] and Yang and colleagues[10] established the role of RT in enhancing local control; O'Sullivan and colleagues'[11] comparison of preoperative versus postoperative RT shifted the default approach to RT in STS, thereby altering the late effects profile of this patient population. Numerous negative trials of adjuvant chemotherapy brought an end to the practice of routine administration of chemotherapy for all STS in many centers.[26,27] However, there remain many outstanding questions in the multidisciplinary management of STS; as our understanding of this family of diseases deepens, it becomes increasingly apparent that the RCT paradigm may be prohibitive. The challenge of conducting RCTs in a disease with only 12,000 new diagnoses per year is compounded by the fact that the many histologic subtypes of STS can exhibit markedly different biological behavior and differential sensitivity to chemotherapy or RT and that even single subtypes can behave differently based on anatomic location. Acknowledgment of these limitations should inform future inquiry in several ways.

RCTs concerning systemic therapies should increasingly be tailored to individual or similar subtypes of STS. Recent evidence has elucidated subtype-specific behavior, such as the lack of efficacy of pazopanib in adipogenic STS and the relative resistance of LMS to ifosfamide, calling into question the generalizability of older trials including all STS and raising the possibility that adjuvant chemotherapy may in fact be beneficial in certain subtypes. The recent multicenter European RCT comparing standard chemotherapy to histology-driven regimens is evidence of a shift toward a more nuanced approach to systemic therapy in STS.[30] The pediatric sarcomas provide a model of the robust literature that can emerge from this type of subtype-specific focus.

Similarly, extremity/trunk and retroperitoneal STS should be differentiated in the design of future RCTs. The optimal extent of surgery and potential benefit of RT, for example, cannot be reasonably extrapolated from extremity data to an anatomic location in which local failure is the primary cause of disease-specific mortality. The EORTC STRASS trial represents a laudable international effort to overcome the barriers to level 1 evidence in RPS and provide disease-specific data in an area where there has long been clinical equipoise and considerable variability in institutional practice.

Recognizing the impracticality of RCTs in addressing many of the knowledge gaps in adult STS, it is worthwhile to acknowledge the value of high-quality observational data and the pivotal role they can play in informing the management of a rare disease. Most of the surgical literature in adult STS consists, at present, of single- or multi-institution series. In 2013, the Transatlantic RPS Working Group (TARPSWG) was convened to overcome the challenges of a rare disease and generate prospective, observational data to provide quality evidence surrounding the management of RPS. To date, the TARPSWG has published the largest reported retrospective experience of RPS[59,60]; a prospective registry has been initiated, capturing data from more than 35 institutions in multiple countries. The potential of this type of large-scale collaboration has been demonstrated by the 4 decades of high-level evidence generated by the IRS/COG, which has directed a thoughtful, cohesive body of research in RMS. This model of multidisciplinary, international collaboration is vital to the creation of meaningful, reliable evidence to guide the complex management of STS.

REFERENCES

1. Lewis JJ, Leung D, Woodruff JM, et al. Retroperitoneal soft-tissue sarcoma: analysis of 500 patients treated and followed at a single institution. Ann Surg 1998; 228(3):355–65.

2. Heslin MJ, Lewis JJ, Nadler E, et al. Prognostic factors associated with long-term survival for retroperitoneal sarcoma: implications for management. J Clin Oncol 1997;15(8):2832–9.

3. Stojadinovic A, Leung DHY, Allen P, et al. Primary adult soft tissue sarcoma: time-dependent influence of prognostic variables. J Clin Oncol 2002;20(21):4344–52.

4. Pisters PW, Harrison LB, Leung DH, et al. Long-term results of a prospective randomized trial of adjuvant brachytherapy in soft tissue sarcoma. J Clin Oncol 1996;14(3):859–68.

5. Beane JD, Yang JC, White D, et al. Efficacy of adjuvant radiation therapy in the treatment of soft tissue sarcoma of the extremity: 20-year follow-up of a randomized prospective trial. Ann Surg Oncol 2014;21(8):2484–9.

6. Rosenberg SA, Tepper J, Glatstein E, et al. The treatment of soft-tissue sarcomas of the extremities: prospective randomized evaluations of limb-sparing surgery plus radiation therapy compared with amputation and the role of adjuvant chemotherapy. Ann Surg 1982;196(3):305–15.

7. Tan MCB, Brennan MF, Kuk D, et al. Histology-based classification predicts pattern of recurrence and improves risk stratification in primary retroperitoneal sarcoma. Ann Surg 2015;263(3):593–600.

8. Gronchi A, Lo Vullo S, Fiore M, et al. Aggressive surgical policies in a retrospectively reviewed single-institution case series of retroperitoneal soft tissue sarcoma patients. J Clin Oncol 2008;27(1):24–30.

9. Bonvalot S, Rivoire M, Castaing M, et al. Primary retroperitoneal sarcomas: a multivariate analysis of surgical factors associated with local control. J Clin Oncol 2008;27(1):31–7.

10. Yang JC, Chang AE, Baker AR, et al. Randomized prospective study of the benefit of adjuvant radiation therapy in the treatment of soft tissue sarcomas of the extremity. J Clin Oncol 1998;16(1):197–203.

11. O'Sullivan B, Davis AM, Turcotte R, et al. Preoperative versus postoperative radiotherapy in soft-tissue sarcoma of the limbs: a randomised trial. Lancet 2002;359(9325):2235–41.

12. Davis A, O'Sullivan B, Turcotte R, et al. Late radiation morbidity following randomization to preoperative versus postoperative radiotherapy in extremity soft tissue sarcoma. Radiother Oncol 2005;75(1):48.

13. O'Sullivan B, Griffin AM, Dickie CI, et al. Phase 2 study of preoperative image-guided intensity-modulated radiation therapy to reduce wound and combined modality morbidities in lower extremity soft tissue sarcoma. Cancer 2013; 119(10):1878–84.

14. Wang D, Zhang Q, Eisenberg BL, et al. Significant reduction of late toxicities in patients with extremity sarcoma treated with image-guided radiation therapy to a reduced target volume: results of Radiation Therapy Oncology Group RTOG-0630 Trial. J Clin Oncol 2015;33(20):2231–8.

15. Pisters PWT, Pollock RE, Lewis VO, et al. Long-term results of prospective trial of surgery alone with selective use of radiation for patients with T1 extremity and trunk soft tissue sarcomas. Ann Surg 2007;246(4):675–81.

16. Cahlon O, Brennan MF, Jia X, et al. A postoperative nomogram for local recurrence risk in extremity soft tissue sarcomas after limb-sparing surgery without adjuvant radiation. Ann Surg 2011;255(2):343–7.

17. Gronchi A. Individualizing the use/non-use of radiation therapy (RT) in soft tissue sarcoma (STS): when abstention is better than care. J Surg Oncol 2014;111(2): 133–4.

18. Pawlik TM, Pisters PWT, Mikula L, et al. Long-term results of two prospective trials of preoperative external beam radiotherapy for localized intermediate- or high-grade retroperitoneal soft tissue sarcoma. Ann Surg Oncol 2006;13(4):508–17.

19. Jones JJ, Catton CN, O'Sullivan B, et al. Initial results of a trial of preoperative external-beam radiation therapy and postoperative brachytherapy for retroperitoneal sarcoma. Ann Surg Oncol 2002;9(4):346–54.

20. Ridgway PF, Catton CN, Cannell AJ, et al. Combined management of retroperitoneal sarcoma with dose intensification radiotherapy and resection: long-term results of a prospective trial. Radiother Oncol 2014;110(1):165–71.

21. Bonvalot S, Raut CP, Pollock RE, et al. Technical considerations in surgery for retroperitoneal sarcomas: position paper from E-Surge, a master class in sarcoma surgery, and EORTC-STBSG. Ann Surg Oncol 2012;19(9):2981–91.

22. Roeder F, Ulrich A, Habl G, et al. Clinical phase I/II trial to investigate preoperative dose-escalated intensity-modulated radiation therapy (IMRT) and intraoperative radiation therapy (IORT) in patients with retroperitoneal soft tissue sarcoma: interim analysis. BMC Cancer 2014;14:617.

23. Kraybill WG, Harris J, Spiro IJ, et al. Phase II study of neoadjuvant chemotherapy and radiation therapy in the management of high-risk, high-grade, soft tissue sarcomas of the extremities and body wall: radiation therapy oncology group trial 9514. J Clin Oncol 2006;24(4):619–25.

24. Kraybill WG, Harris J, Spiro IJ, et al. Long-term results of a phase 2 study of neoadjuvant chemotherapy and radiotherapy in the management of high-risk, high-grade, soft tissue sarcomas of the extremities and body wall. Cancer 2010; 116(19):4613.

25. Gronchi A, De Paoli A, Dani C, et al. Preoperative chemo-radiation therapy for localised retroperitoneal sarcoma: a phase I-II study from the Italian Sarcoma Group. Eur J Cancer 2013;50(4):784–92.

26. Adjuvant chemotherapy for localised resectable soft-tissue sarcoma of adults: meta-analysis of individual data. Sarcoma Meta-analysis Collaboration. Lancet 1997;350(9092):1647–54.

27. Pervaiz N, Colterjohn N, Farrokhyar F, et al. A systematic meta-analysis of randomized controlled trials of adjuvant chemotherapy for localized resectable soft-tissue sarcoma. Cancer 2008;113(3):573–81.

28. Woll PJ, Reichardt P, Le Cesne A, et al. Adjuvant chemotherapy with doxorubicin, ifosfamide, and lenograstim for resected soft-tissue sarcoma (EORTC 62931): a multicentre randomised controlled trial. Lancet Oncol 2012;13(10):1045.

29. Gronchi A, Frustaci S, Mercuri M, et al. Short, full-dose adjuvant chemotherapy in high-risk adult soft tissue sarcomas: a randomized clinical trial from the Italian Sarcoma Group and the Spanish Sarcoma Group. J Clin Oncol 2012;30(8):850–6.

30. Gronchi A, Ferrari S, Quagliuolo V, et al. Full-dose neoadjuvant anthracycline + ifosfamide chemotherapy is associated with a relapse free survival (RFS) and overall survival (OS) benefit in localized high-risk adult soft tissue sarcomas (STS) of the extremities and trunk wall: interim analysis of a prospective randomized trial. Proceedings of the European Society for Medical Oncology. Copenhagen, Denmark, October 7–11, 2016.

31. The ESMO/European Sarcoma Network Working Group. Soft tissue and visceral sarcomas: ESMO clinical practice guidelines for diagnosis, treatment and follow-up. Ann Surg Oncol 2014;25(Suppl 3):102–12.
32. Selch MT, Kopald KH, Ferreiro GA, et al. Limb salvage therapy for soft tissue sarcomas of the foot. Int J Radiat Oncol Biol Phys 1990;19(1):41–8.
33. Issels RD, Lindner LH, Verweij J, et al. Neo-adjuvant chemotherapy alone or with regional hyperthermia for localised high-risk soft-tissue sarcoma: a randomised phase 3 multicentre study. Lancet Oncol 2010;11(6):561.
34. Angele MK, Albertsmeier M, Prix NJ, et al. Effectiveness of regional hyperthermia with chemotherapy for high-risk retroperitoneal and abdominal soft-tissue sarcoma after complete surgical resection. Ann Surg 2014;260(5):749.
35. Bonvalot S, Cavalcanti A, Le Péchoux C, et al. Randomized trial of cytoreduction followed by intraperitoneal chemotherapy versus cytoreduction alone in patients with peritoneal sarcomatosis. Eur J Surg Oncol 2005;31(8):917–23.
36. Judson I, Verweij J, Gelderblom H, et al. Doxorubicin alone versus intensified doxorubicin plus ifosfamide for first-line treatment of advanced or metastatic soft-tissue sarcoma: a randomised controlled phase 3 trial. Lancet Oncol 2014; 15(4):415–23.
37. Ryan CW, Merimsky O, Agulnik M, et al. PICASSO III: a phase III, placebo-controlled study of doxorubicin with or without palifosfamide in patients with metastatic soft tissue sarcoma. J Clin Oncol 2016;34(32):3898–905.
38. Seddon B, Whelan J, Strauss S, et al. GeDDiS: a prospective randomised controlled phase III trial of gemcitabine and docetaxel compared with doxorubicin as first-line treatment in previously untreated advanced unresectable or metastatic soft tissue sarcomas (EudraCT 2009-014907-29). J Clin Oncol 2015; 33(suppl) [abstract: 10500].
39. Chawla SP, Papai Z, Mukhametshina G, et al. First-line aldoxorubicin vs doxorubicin in metastatic or locally advanced unresectable soft-tissue sarcoma: a phase 2b randomized clinical trial. JAMA Oncol 2015;1(9):1272–80.
40. Maki RG, Wathen JK, Patel SR, et al. Randomized phase II study of gemcitabine and docetaxel compared with gemcitabine alone in patients with metastatic soft tissue sarcomas: results of Sarcoma Alliance for Research Through Collaboration Study 002. J Clin Oncol 2007;25(19):2755.
41. Gupta AA, Yao X, Verma S, et al. Chemotherapy (gemcitabine, docetaxel plus gemcitabine, doxorubicin, or trabectedin) in inoperable, locally advanced, recurrent, or metastatic uterine leiomyosarcoma: a clinical practice guideline. Curr Oncol 2013;20(5):e448–54.
42. García-Del-Muro X, Lopez-Pousa A, Maurel J, et al. Randomized phase II study comparing gemcitabine plus dacarbazine versus dacarbazine alone in patients with previously treated soft tissue sarcoma: a Spanish Group for Research on Sarcomas study. J Clin Oncol 2011;29(18):2528–33.
43. Demetri GD, Mehren von M, Jones RL, et al. Efficacy and safety of trabectedin or dacarbazine for metastatic liposarcoma or leiomyosarcoma after failure of conventional chemotherapy: results of a phase III randomized multicenter clinical trial. J Clin Oncol 2015;34(8):786–93.
44. van der Graaf WT, Blay JY, Chawla SP, et al. Pazopanib for metastatic soft-tissue sarcoma (PALETTE): a randomised, double-blind, placebo-controlled phase 3 trial. Lancet 2012;379(9829):1879–86.
45. Schöffski P, Chawla S, Maki RG, et al. Eribulin versus dacarbazine in previously treated patients with advanced liposarcoma or leiomyosarcoma: a randomised, open-label, multicentre, phase 3 trial. Lancet 2016;387(10028):1629–37.

46. Tap WD, Jones RL, Van Tine BA, et al. Olaratumab and doxorubicin versus doxorubicin alone for treatment of soft-tissue sarcoma: an open-label phase 1b and randomised phase 2 trial. Lancet 2016;388(10043):488.

47. Grier HE, Krailo MD, Tarbell NJ, et al. Addition of ifosfamide and etoposide to standard chemotherapy for Ewing's sarcoma and primitive neuroectodermal tumor of bone. N Engl J Med 2003;348(8):694–701.

48. Paulussen M, Craft AW, Lewis I, et al. Results of the EICESS-92 Study: two randomized trials of Ewing's sarcoma treatment–cyclophosphamide compared with ifosfamide in standard-risk patients and assessment of benefit of etoposide added to standard treatment in high-risk patients. J Clin Oncol 2008;26(27): 4385–93.

49. Womer RB, West DC, Krailo MD, et al. Randomized controlled trial of interval-compressed chemotherapy for the treatment of localized Ewing sarcoma: a report from the Children's Oncology Group. J Clin Oncol 2012;30(33):4148–54.

50. Le Deley M-C, Paulussen M, Lewis I, et al. Cyclophosphamide compared with ifosfamide in consolidation treatment of standard-risk Ewing sarcoma: results of the randomized noninferiority Euro-EWING99-R1 trial. J Clin Oncol 2014;32(23): 2440–8.

51. Whelan J, Le Deley MC, Dirksen U, et al. Efficacy of busulfan-melphalan high dose chemotherapy consolidation (BuMel) in localized high-risk Ewing sarcoma (ES): results of EURO-EWING 99-R2 randomized trial (EE99R2Loc). J Clin Oncol 2016;36(suppl) [abstract: 11000].

52. Dirksen U, Le Deley MC, Brennan B, et al. Efficacy of busulfan-melphalan high dose chemotherapy consolidation (BuMel) compared to conventional chemotherapy combined with lung irradiation in Ewing sarcoma (ES) with primary lung metastases: results of EURO-EWING 99-R2pulm randomized trial (EE99R2-pul). J Clin Oncol 2016;34(suppl) [abstract: 11001].

53. Maurer HM, Beltangady M, Gehan EA, et al. The intergroup rhabdomyosarcoma study-I. A final report. Cancer 1988;61(2):209–20.

54. Maurer HM, Gehan EA, Beltangady M, et al. The Intergroup Rhabdomyosarcoma Study-II. Cancer 1993;71(5):1904–22.

55. Crist W, Gehan EA, Ragab AH, et al. The Third Intergroup Rhabdomyosarcoma Study. J Clin Oncol 1995;13(3):610–30.

56. Crist WM, Anderson JR, Meza JL, et al. Intergroup Rhabdomyosarcoma Study-IV: results for patients with nonmetastatic disease. J Clin Oncol 2001;19(12):3091–102.

57. Arndt CAS, Stoner JA, Hawkins DS, et al. Vincristine, actinomycin, and cyclophosphamide compared with vincristine, actinomycin, and cyclophosphamide alternating with vincristine, topotecan, and cyclophosphamide for intermediate-risk rhabdomyosarcoma: children's oncology group study D9803. J Clin Oncol 2009;27(31):5182–8.

58. Hawkins D, Anderson J, Mascarenhas L, et al. Vincristine, dactinomycin, cyclophosphamide (VAC) versus VAC/V plus irinotecan (VI) for intermediate-risk rhabdomyosarcoma (IRRMS): a report from the Children's Oncology Group Soft Tissue Sarcoma Committee. J Clin Oncol 2014;32(5 suppl) [abstract: 10004].

59. Gronchi A, Strauss DC, Miceli R, et al. Variability in patterns of recurrence after resection of primary retroperitoneal sarcoma (RPS): a report on 1007 patients from the multi-institutional collaborative RPS working group. Ann Surg 2016; 263:1002–9.

60. MacNeill AJ, Miceli R, Strauss DC, et al. Post-relapse outcomes after primary extended resection of retroperitoneal sarcoma: a report from the Trans-Atlantic RPS Working Group. Cancer 2017. http://dx.doi.org/10.1002/cncr.30572.

Randomized Clinical Trials in Gastrointestinal Stromal Tumors

Yang Liu, MD, Margaret von Mehren, MD*

KEYWORDS

- Gastrointestinal stromal tumors • Imatinib • Tyrosine kinase inhibitors

KEY POINTS

- In limited stage disease, complete surgical resection remains the standard of care.
- There is a role for surgical resection in metastatic disease in the setting of limited disease progression, and for tumors that have experienced significant clinical response to neoadjuvant imatinib.
- The current standard of care in the adjuvant setting is 3 years of adjuvant imatinib therapy in patients with features putting them at high risk of disease recurrence; the benefit and tolerability of 5 years of adjuvant imatinib is currently being investigated.
- In patients with metastatic disease, imatinib is continued indefinitely until disease progression or side-effect intolerance. Rechallenge with imatinib after progression off of therapy or after progression on imatinib and sunitinib has been associated with clinical response.
- Both regorafenib and nilotinib are novel tyrosine kinase inhibitors that have been investigated in the management of advanced metastatic gastrointestinal stromal tumors, with regorafenib receiving US Food and Drug Administration approval in 2013; masitinib is a potentially promising tyrosine kinase inhibitor that is being investigated in metastatic gastrointestinal stromal tumors.

Gastrointestinal stromal tumors (GISTs) are mesenchymal or stromal tumors involving the gastrointestinal tract, originating most commonly in the stomach and the small intestine. They are rare tumors and make up approximately 1% of all of gastrointestinal cancers. The true incidence of GIST is unknown, with studies

Disclosure: Dr Y. Liu has no relationships to disclose. Dr M. von Mehren served as an investigator for the GRID trial and the nilotinib randomized trial in the advanced disease setting. She has served as a paid consultant to Bayer and Novartis in the past.
Department of Hematology/Oncology, Fox Chase Cancer Center, 333 Cottman Avenue, Philadelphia, PA 19111, USA
* Corresponding author.
E-mail address: Margaret.vonMehren@fccc.edu

suggesting approximately 4000 to 6000 new cases each year. Although most cases are sporadic, some are associated with familial autosomal dominant syndromes, including neurofibromatosis 1, primary familial GIST syndrome, and Carney-Stratakis syndrome. GISTs are primarily characterized by activating mutations in *KIT* (85%) or platelet-derived growth factor-α *(PDGFRA*; 5%), whereas a small percentage are wild-type in both genes and require further characterization. Mutations in *KIT* lead to constitutive activation of the KIT receptor tyrosine kinase; 75% of *KIT* mutations involve exon 11, which encodes the intracellular juxtamembrane domain resulting in spontaneous ligand-independent dimerization and activation. Mutations in exon 11 generally confer response to imatinib mesylate, a tyrosine kinase inhibitor (TKI) that inhibits activation induced by *KIT* and *PDGFRA* mutations; imatinib has been the backbone of therapy in both the adjuvant and metastatic setting for most GIST tumors.

This review focuses on therapeutic advances in the management of GIST, with an emphasis on randomized clinical trials (RCTS) performed between 2010 to 2016 related to medical management; there are no recent RCTs in the literature that have changed the surgical approach to this disease. The consensus among the surgical community is to pursue complete surgical resection with histologically negative margins, with careful attention to maintain the integrity of the tumor pseudocapsule because of its friable nature to avoid tumor spillage. Per the National Comprehensive Cancer Network guidelines, resection of adjacent lymph nodes is not indicated because of the low rate of metastases. Furthermore, re-resection is generally not indicated for microscopic positive margins on final pathology. In general, there is a limited role for surgical resection in metastatic disease, unless there is disease progression in a limited area and for tumors that have experienced significant clinical benefit from imatinib or other TKIs.[1]

Between 2010 and 2016, several key RCTs were published that changed the management of patients with GIST. These studies evaluated the optimal duration of adjuvant imatinib after R0 or R1 resections in high-risk disease, made further explorations into the optimal duration of imatinib treatment in metastatic disease, and explored the efficacy and safety of novel TKIs in the metastatic setting.

THE ROLE OF IMATINIB IN ADJUVANT THERAPY

Before 2010, the American College of Surgical Oncology Z9001 study established imatinib as standard adjuvant treatment after resected GIST. In a large phase III study, 713 patients with localized primary GIST who had received complete gross resection were randomly assigned to receive either imatinib, 400 mg daily, or placebo for 1 year after surgical resection. The study found that at a median follow-up of 19.7 months, imatinib significantly improved recurrence-free survival at 1 year compared with placebo (98%; 95% confidence interval [CI], 96–100 vs 83%; 95% CI, 78–88; hazard ratio [HR], 0.35; $P<.0001$). This study established adjuvant imatinib as a safe, tolerable, and effective therapy after resection. However, further follow-up found an increase in disease recurrence around 18 months after surgery, raising questions regarding the optimal duration of imatinib therapy.[2] Factors associated with lower rates of recurrence-free survival included large tumor size, small bowel location, and high mitotic rate.

The SSG XVIII trial from the Scandinavian Sarcoma Group established 3 years of adjuvant imatinib as the standard of care in resected GIST with a high risk of recurrence.[3]

# Patients Randomized	Inclusion Criteria	Study Groups	Stratification	Significance Demonstrated	% Change Identified in Trial
N = 400	1. Histological-ly diagnosed surgically resectable GIST, CD117 (KIT) positive 2. High esti-mated risk of recur-rence per NIH Consensus Criteria 3. ECOG per-formance status ≤2	Adjuvant imatinib, 400 mg daily × 12 mo (n = 200) Adjuvant imatinib, 400 mg daily × 36 mo (n = 200)	Local disease (R0 resection and no tumor spillage) R1 resection or tumor rupture (intra-abdominal disease)	5-y RFS and OS longer in patients receiving adjuvant imatinib × 36 mo compared with 12 mo	5-y RFS 65.6% vs 47.9% (HR, 0.46; 95% CI, 0.32–0.65) P<.001 5-y OS 92.% vs 81.7% (HR, 0.45; 95% CI, 0.22–0.89; P = .02)

Abbreviation: ECOG, Eastern Cooperative Oncology Group.

In this prospective phase III, multicenter open-label RCT, patients 18 years or older with histologically diagnosed, surgically resected GIST harboring KIT (CD117) by immunohistochemistry and an estimated high risk of recurrence were randomly assigned to receive either 36 months (n = 200) or 12 months (n = 200) of adjuvant imatinib. High risk of recurrence was consistent with the 2002 National Institutes of Health (NIH) Consensus Criteria: (1) tumor greater than 10 cm in diameter, (2) greater than 10 mitoses per 50 high-power fields, (3) tumor diameter greater than 5.0 cm and mitotic count greater than 5 but also included tumor rupture before or at the time of surgery. The primary endpoint was recurrence-free survival (RFS) by intention-to-treat analysis. At a median duration of follow-up of 54 months, RFS was higher in the 36-month group compared with the 12-month group (65.6% vs 47.9%; HR, 0.46; 95% CI, 0.32–0.65; $P<.001$) as was overall survival (5-year survival, 92% vs 81.7%; HR, 0.45; 95% CI, 0.22–0.89; $P = .02$).

Exploratory subgroup analysis found that the benefit in RFS was observed in patients with *KIT* exon 11 mutation but not in those with the *KIT* exon 9, *PDGFRA*, or those without *KIT/PDGFRA* mutations; however, the number of patients with these tumor characteristics were small and may have limited the ability to discern a difference. Alternatively, the known resistance to imatinib therapy in tumors with *PDGFRA* D842V and requirement for higher dose therapy in tumors with exon 9 mutations may be the explanation for the lack of observed benefit in those 2 groups. Lastly, the assessment of mutations was only limited to *KIT* and *PDGFRA*; it is likely that other known drivers, including SDH deficiencies, *NF-1* mutations, or *RAF/RAS* mutations were included in the wild-type cohort, many of which have shown little response to imatinib.

The benefit of adjuvant therapy was confirmed in the interim analysis of a larger, phase III, open-label, international multicenter study from the European Organisation for Research and Treatment of Cancer.[4]

# Patients Randomized	Inclusion Criteria	Study Groups	Stratification	Significance Demonstrated	% Change Identified in Trial
N = 908	1. Histologically diagnosed primary resected GIST with positive immunostaining for KIT (CD117) 2. High estimated risk of recurrence per NIH Consensus Criteria 3. ECOG performance status ≤2	Adjuvant imatinib, 400 mg daily × 2 y (n = 454) Observation (n = 454)	1. Treatment center 2. Risk category (high vs intermediate) 3. Tumor site (gastric vs other) 4. Resection level (R0 vs R1)	5-y IFFS not significantly different between the 2 groups 3- and 5-y RFS improved in adjuvant imatinib arm	5-y IFFS 87% vs 84% (HR, 0.79; 98.5% CI, 0.50–1.25; P = .21) 3-y RFS (84 vs 66% at 3 y, 69 vs 63% at 5 y)

Abbreviation: ECOG, Eastern Cooperative Oncology Group.

Similar to the Scandinavian Sarcoma Group study, the study population included patients with histologically confirmed GIST with positive immunostaining for KIT and high risk of recurrence per the 2002 NIH consensus criteria. Patients were randomly assigned to either 2 years of adjuvant imatinib versus observation beginning 2 weeks to 2 months after an R0 or R1 resection (R1 resection included intraoperative rupture). The primary endpoint, initially overall survival, was changed to imatinib failure-free survival (IFFS) because of improvement in survival in patients with GIST receiving TKI therapies for recurrent disease. IFFS was defined as the time from randomization to the start of new systemic treatment other than imatinib or time to death; the study allowed for patients treated with 2 years of adjuvant therapy to reinitiate treatment with imatinib at the time of recurrence at the discretion of the treating physician. At a median follow-up of 4.7 years, there was no difference in the 5-year IFFS 87% versus 84% in the adjuvant imatinib versus the observation group, respectively (HR, 0.79; 98.5% CI, 0.5–1.25; P = .21). However, as in the SSG XVIII study, 3- and 5-year RFS rates were significantly higher in the adjuvant arm (84% vs 66% at 3 years and 69 vs 63% at 5 years; log-rank P<.001). There was no difference in 5-year overall survival reported, with more than 90% of patients still remaining alive. The role of adjuvant therapy is confirmed by this study given the benefit in RFS. It does, however, raise the questions as to the best way to utilize imatinib for disease control, directly in the adjuvant setting or at the time of disease relapse. It also suggests that a duration of 2 years of therapy is not sufficient for adjuvant therapy and is the reason for lack of overall survival benefit and IFFS.

An ongoing RCT (NCT02413736) is investigating the benefit of 5 years of adjuvant treatment compared with 3 years. In addition, another phase II nonrandomized trial of 5 years of imatinib in the adjuvant setting (NCT00867113) will provide additional information on the optimal duration of treatment, safety, and whether it provides improved disease control.

THE ROLE OF IMATINIB IN UNRESECTABLE OR METASTATIC DISEASE

Since 2010, investigators have completed RCTs investigating the duration of imatinib in unresectable and metastatic GIST and the effect of imatinib interruption and rechallenge. There are also randomized studies investigating novel targeted therapeutics as either first-line treatment or after failure of imatinib and sunitinib.

Before 2010, GIST investigators defined the efficacy, safety, and appropriate dosing of imatinib in metastatic GIST. A seminal phase II RCT, published in 2002,[5] found an unprecedented clinical response rate (complete response [CR], partial response [PR] and stable disease [SD]) of 81.6% in patients with metastatic GIST to imatinib therapy either at 400 mg daily or 300 mg twice daily. This study was followed up by 2 phase III clinical trials that randomly assigned patients to 400 mg daily or 400 mg twice daily. The US intergroup trial randomly assigned 746 patients with metastatic GIST.[6] The study showed no significant difference in progression-free survival (PFS) or overall survival (OS) between the 2 dose levels, establishing 400 mg daily as the standard starting dose in the metastatic setting. Of 117 patients who crossed over to the higher dose of 400 mg twice daily after progressing on 400 mg daily, 31% (3% PR and 28% SD) achieved additional disease control on the higher dose of therapy. A further international intergroup study randomly assigned 946 patients to 400 mg imatinib daily or twice daily and found a slightly increased PFS in the imatinib, 400-mg twice daily, group.[7] At a median follow-up of 760 days, 56% of patients taking imatinib, 400 mg daily, had progressed compared with 50% in the imatinib twice-daily group (HR, 0.82; 95% CI, 0.69–0.98; P = .026). However, the twice-daily group had more dose reductions and treatment interruptions. Interestingly, subgroup analysis suggested that the benefit of higher-dose therapy was largely seen in patients with the *KIT* exon 9 mutation.[8]

Before 2010, there were also efforts to define the optimal duration of imatinib therapy in the metastatic setting. In 2007, the French Sarcoma Group published early results from their BFR14 phase III clinical trial, in which they hypothesized that patients with advanced or metastatic GIST would have improved PFS with continuous imatinib compared with treatment interruption after 1 year.[9] Within a larger cohort of 182 patients, the study investigators identified 98 patients with tumor response or stable disease after 1 year of treatment with imatinib and randomly assigned them to either treatment interruption or continuous imatinib. At the time of evaluation, median PFS was significantly increased in the group receiving continuous imatinib. Because cross-over was allowed and 81% of patients in the interruption group crossed over, there was no measurable benefit in OS. However, the study investigators noted that 92% of patients who crossed over responded to reintroduction of therapy.

To further investigate the optimal duration of imatinib in unresectable or metastatic GIST, the French Sarcoma Group continued to follow up with patients in the BFR14 trial with advanced but controlled disease (defined as CR, PR, or SD) on imatinib, 400 mg daily, and evaluated treatment continuation versus interruption after 3 years.[10]

# Patients in Cohort	Inclusion Criteria	Study Groups	Stratification	Significance Demonstrated	% Change Identified in Trial
N = 434	1. Histologically proven metastatic GIST with c-kit (CD117) expression 2. ECOG performance status 0–3 3. Received imatinib for 3 y with nonprogressive disease	Interruption vs continued imatinib after 3 y (n = 25 each)	1. Participating center 2. Presence or absence of residual disease on CT scan	2-y PFS greater in group continuing imatinib	80% (95% CI, 58%–91%) vs 16% (95% CI, 5%–33%), P<.0001

Abbreviations: CT, computed tomography; ECOG, Eastern Cooperative Oncology Group.

Patients were 18 years and older with histologically proven metastatic GIST with positive immunostaining for KIT (CD 117). The study randomly assigned patients to continued therapy or to treatment interruption after 3 years of imatinib therapy with nonprogressive disease; patients were rechallenged with imatinib at the time of Response Evaluation Criteria In Solid Tumors (RECIST)-defined progression. In the report on the patients randomly selected after 3 years of imatinib, there were 36% in CR in both cohorts, 52% and 48% in PR, and 12% and 14% with SD in the interruption and continuation groups, respectively. The primary endpoint was PFS. Randomization was stopped early because of high rates of progression in the treatment interruption group. At a median follow-up of 35 months, the 2-year PFS was 80% (95% CI, 58–91) in the continuation group compared with 16% (95% CI, 5–33) in the interruption group (P<.0001).

The BFR14 study investigators also randomly assigned patients with nonprogressive disease to treatment interruption after 5 years of imatinib versus continuation of imatinib. They observed 45% of patients relapsing within 1 year of drug interruption.[11] These findings suggest that even in patients with CR after 5 years of therapy, there is micrometastatic disease present that will regrow after treatment interruption. These findings have established the standard of care to continue imatinib in unresectable or metastatic disease until intolerable side effects or progression of disease.

The BRF14 trial investigators then used this same study cohort to investigate the quality of response to imatinib rechallenge in patients whose disease had progressed during treatment interruption after 1, 3, and 5 years of clinical response to imatinib.[12]

# Patients in Cohort	Inclusion Criteria	Study Groups	Stratification	Significance Demonstrated
N = 434	1. BRF14 criteria listed above. 2. Patients who received imatinib for 1, 3, or 5 y with nonprogressive disease followed by treatment interruption (n = 71)	Patients with secondary progression/ recurrence after treatment interruption (n = 51)	None	PFS correlated with time-to-treatment interruption Time to second progression correlated inversely with imatinib-free interval

In the study, of the 71 patients randomly assigned to treatment discontinuation, 54 of them had disease progression and 51 patients were rechallenged with imatinib. The median PFS correlated positively with time to treatment interruption, with PFS of 6.0, 7.1, and 10.8 months after treatment interruption at 1, 3, and 5 years. As expected, the quality of the first response to imatinib correlated positively with PFS off therapy, with the longest PFS in patients with CR at time of treatment discontinuation (10.5, 6.2, and 3.2 months in CR, PR and SD, respectively). When rechallenged, 96% of patients had treatment response. However, although objective response rates (ORR = CR + PR) at rechallenge were similar to objective response rates at initiation of imatinib therapy, the rate of clinical benefit (CR + PR + SD) did not meet initial response percentages. In addition, the time to second progression after rechallenge correlated inversely with the duration of the imatinib-free interval (or time to first progression), with a 2-year PFS of 30%, 62%, and 75% in patients who experienced relapse within 6 months, 6 to 12 months, and after 12 months, respectively.

The BFR14 study provides support for rechallenging with imatinib in patients with locally advanced or metastatic GIST with initial response to imatinib and disease progression after treatment interruption. These patients likely have persistent imatinib-sensitive disease. This interpretation is consistent with findings in patients whose disease progresses after adjuvant imatinib therapy, most of whom respond to the reintroduction of imatinib. However, it should be noted that those who relapse more quickly are less likely to have a prolonged benefit. It is unknown if the length of disease control on imatinib is altered by treatment interruption.

The role of imatinib rechallenge was further studied in a small, single-center double-blinded, placebo-controlled RCT.[13]

# Patients Randomized	Inclusion Criteria	Study Groups	Stratification	Significance Demonstrated	% Change Identified in Trial
N = 85	1. Histological-ly proven metastatic or unresect-able GISTs with pro-gression with at least imatinib and suniti-nib sequen-tially by RECIST v 1.0 2. Clinical benefit with first-line imatinib (CR, PR, SD) for at least 6 mo 3. ECOG per-formance status 0–3	Rechallenge with imatinib (n = 41) Rechallenge with placebo (n = 40)	None	PFS improved in rechallenge group	At median follow-up of 5.2 mo, median PFS 1.8 mo (95% CI, 1.7–3.6) with imatinib vs 0.9 (95% CI, 0.9–1.7) with placebo; P = .005

Abbreviation: ECOG, Eastern Cooperative Oncology Group.

Patients (n = 85) with metastatic or unresectable GIST with tumor progression by RECIST criteria after treatment with sequential imatinib and sunitinib, who derived clinical benefit on first-line imatinib therapy for at least 6 months, were randomly assigned to either rechallenge (n = 41) with imatinib, 400 mg daily, or placebo (n = 40). The primary endpoint was PFS, and crossover was allowed to the imatinib group. The study found significant improvement in PFS (HR, 0.46; 95% CI, 0.27–0.78; P = .005), although these improvements were small. At a median follow-up of 5.2 months, the median PFS of the imatinib rechallenge group was 1.8 months compared with 0.9 months in the placebo group. There was no difference in OS. This study showed 2 key points. First, patients with GIST whose disease has progressed on sunitinib are much more refractory to kinase therapy with imatinib. Second, progression of advanced disease is rapid off kinase-directed therapy, and kinase inhibition may allow for better palliation of symptoms and give patients the ability to transition to alternative therapies.

NOVEL TYROSINE KINASE INHIBITORS

Before 2010, sunitinib was the only available TKI that was studied in an RCT setting for the treatment of unresectable, imatinib-resistant GIST. An international study randomly assigned 312 patients with metastatic or unresectable GIST in a 2:1 fashion to either sunitinib (50mg daily for 4 weeks ,followed by 2 weeks of therapy) or placebo, which was the standard of care at the time.[14] In an intention-to-treat analysis, patients receiving sunitinib had a significantly longer time to tumor progression compared with placebo (27.3 wk; 95% CI, 16.0–32.1 vs 6.4 wk; 95% CI, 4.4–10). This finding established sunitinib as the standard care after disease progression on or intolerance to imatinib in the advanced GIST setting.

Regorafenib is a novel oral TKI that inhibits KIT and PDGFRA. The drug also targets RET, BRAF, FGFR, and VEGFR. Thus regorafenib, like sunitinib targets both the known oncogenic drivers of GIST and tumor angiogenesis. Regorafenib was approved by the US Food and Drug Administration for use in advanced colorectal cancer and GIST in 2013. The Gastrointestinal Stromal Tumours After Failure of Imatinib and Sunitinib (GRID) trial was a large, international, multicenter, double-blind, placebo-controlled phase III study in patients with histologically confirmed GIST with progression on or intolerance to imatinib and progression on sunitinib.[15]

# Patients Randomized	Inclusion Criteria	Study Groups	Stratification	Significance Demonstrated	% Change Identified in Trial
N = 199	1. Histologically confirmed metastatic of unresectable GIST with failure of previous imatinib (progression or intolerance) and sunitinib (progression only) 2. No history of VEGFR inhibitors other than sunitinib 3. ECOG performance status 0–1.	Regorafenib (n = 133) Placebo (n = 66)	1. Treatment line (failure of prior imatinib and sunitinib vs failure of prior imatinib, sunitinib, and other GIST therapies) 2. Geographic region (Asia vs rest of world).	Median PFS higher in regorafenib group compared with placebo	median PFS 4.8 mo (4.1–6.8) vs 0.9 mo (0.9–1.8) for placebo (HR, 0.27; 95% CI, 0.19–0.39); P<.0001

Abbreviation: ECOG, Eastern Cooperative Oncology Group.

Enrolled patients (n = 199) were randomly assigned in a 2:1 fashion to receive either regorafenib (n = 133) dosed at 160mg daily for 21 days, followed by 7 days of treatment or placebo (n = 66). The primary endpoint of the study was PFS. Treatment assignment was unmasked at the time of progression, and crossover from placebo to regorafenib was allowed. Median treatment duration was 22.9 weeks in the regorafenib arm compared with 7.0 weeks in the placebo arm; median PFS was 4.8 months for regorafenib compared with 0.9 months for placebo (HR, 0.27; 95%

CI, 0.19–0.39; *P*<.0001). As would be anticipated, patients receiving regorafenib experienced significantly higher rates of adverse events, with 60% experiencing grade 3 or higher, compared with 10% in the placebo group. Based on these results, regorafenib is commonly used in the third line in the treatment of metastatic, unresectable GIST. Interestingly, the benefit for treatment with regorafenib was seen in both exon 11 and exon 9 primary *KIT* mutations, unlike with sunitinib in which patients with exon 11 primary mutations were less likely to receive benefit.

Nilotinib, a selective TKI that inhibits the tyrosine kinase activity of KIT, PDGFRs, and ABL/BCR-ABL, is approved for the treatment of newly diagnosed and previously treated Philadelphia chromosome–positive chronic myeloid leukemia. Its efficacy has been studied in GIST in both the first-line and in refractory disease. An international, multicenter, open-label phase III RCT investigated nilotinib versus imatinib as first-line therapy for unresectable and metastatic GIST.[16]

# Patients Randomized	Inclusion Criteria	Study Groups	Stratification	Significance Demonstrated	% Change Identified in Trial
N = 647	Histologically confirmed metastatic or unresectable GIST with no previous systemic therapy or one recurrence within 6 mo of stopping adjuvant imatinib	Nilotinib (n = 324) Imatinib (n = 320)	1. Prior adjuvant imatinib therapy vs none.	2-y PFS higher in imatinib group than nilotinib group	2-y PFS 52.9% (95% CI, 50.9–66.5) vs 51.6% (95% CI, 43–0.59) HR, 1.47 (95% CI, 1.19–1.95)

In this study, patients (n = 647) with histologically confirmed unresectable or metastatic GIST with either no prior systemic therapy or recurrence more than 6 months after adjuvant imatinib were randomly selected to receive either nilotinib 400 mg twice dailty (n = 324) or imatinib 400 mg daily (n = 320). The primary endpoint was PFS. During a planned interim analysis for futility that included 397 patients with a median follow-up of 28 months, the 2-year PFS rate was higher in the imatinib group compared with the nilotinib group (59.2% vs 51.6%; HR, 1.47; 95% CI, 1.10–1.95). The study found similar rates of grade 3 to 4 toxicity between the 2 groups but a higher rate of total adverse events in the nilotinib group. This study was terminated early, and nilotinib is not recommended for broad use in first-line treatment of GIST. Of note, patients with exon 9 mutations had the option of receiving 400 mg of imatinib twice a day (double the standard dose) based on data suggesting improved PFS in patients with the higher dosage of imatinib. Subgroup analysis of patients with exon 9 mutations found improved PFS and OS in the imatinib group compared with imatinib, which was not observed with patients whose tumors contained a KIT exon 11 mutation. This finding suggests that nilotinib is a particularly poor therapeutic option for patients with GIST harboring the exon 9 mutation but may provide benefit for those with exon 11 mutations who may not be tolerant of imatinib.

Its efficacy was also studied in patients after progression or intolerance to imatinib and sunitinb.[17]

# Patients Randomized	Inclusion Criteria	Study Groups	Stratification	Significance Demonstrated	% Change Identified in Trial
N = 248	1. Histologically confirmed metastatic and/or unresectable GIST with either progression on imatinib and sunitinib therapy or intolerant to imatinib and/or sunitinib 2. No treatment with TKIs other than sunitinib or imatinib 3. WHO performance status of 0–2.	Nilotinib 400 mg BID (n = 165) Best supportive care ± imatinib or sunitinib (n = 83)	None	Median PFS not statistically significant between the 2 treatment arms In posthoc, subset analysis of patients truly receiving nilotinib in the third line, median OS greater in the nilotinib group	405 d vs 280 d, HR, 0.67; 95% CI, 0.48–0.95; P = .02

Abbreviation: WHO, World Health Organization.

In a phase III, open-label RCT, patients with histologically confirmed, unresectable or metastatic GIST with prior progression on imatinib and sunitinib or intolerance (n = 248) to either were randomly assigned to receive nilotinib (n = 165) or best supportive care (n = 83) with or without ongoing therapy with one of the TKIs, imatinib, or sunitinib, in a 2:1 fashion. The primary endpoint was PFS. Statistical analysis was completed in an intention-to-treat fashion. Most patients enrolled were resistant to therapy with imatinib and sunitinib, with only a small minority being intolerant (6.0% to imatinib, 13.7% to sunitinib). In this study, the difference in PFS was not statistically significant between the 2 treatment arms, with median PFS of 108 days on nilotinib versus 111 days in the control arm (HR, 0.90; 95% CI, 0.65–1.26, P = .56). However, the study authors completed a posthoc subset analysis of only patients (N = 197) who were truly receiving nilotinib or placebo in the third line. They found a significantly longer median OS in the nilotinib arm versus the control arm (405 days vs 280 days; HR, 0.67; 95% CI, 0.48–0.95, P = .02). Based on this posthoc analysis, nilotinib has been clinically used in the third-line in metastatic or unresectable GIST.

Yet another multitargeted TKI, masitinib, was studied in a small, phase II open-label multicenter RCT from France.[18] Masitinib targets KIT, PDGFR, and FGFR3.

# Patients Randomized	Inclusion Criteria	Study Groups	Stratification	Significance Demonstrated	% Change Identified in Trial
N = 44	1. Histological-ly confirmed GIST with KIT (CD117) detection with disease progression on imatinib- ≥400 mg/d 2. ECOG per-formance status 0–2. 3. No TKI ther-apy other than imatinib	Masitinib (n = 23) Sunitinib (n = 21)	1. *KIT* muta-tion (exon 11, vs exon 9, vs any other muta-tion or un-known mu-tation status)	Median OS higher in patients receiving masitinib	At median follow-up of 14 mo, median OS not reached, estimated at 1.2 mo (95% CI, 21.2-NR) vs 15.2 mo (95% CI, 9.4–21.7); $P = .016$

Abbreviation: ECOG, Eastern Cooperative Oncology Group; NR, not reached.

This study randomized patients (n = 44) with histoogically confirmed locally advanced inoperable or metastatic GIST with disease progression on imatinib, ≥400 mg daily, and no other TKI therapy, with treatment with masitinib (n = 23) or sunitinib (n = 21). The primary treatment efficacy endpoint was defined as PFS of greater than 3 months for masitinib; there was no comparison to sunitinib for this endpoint. With a median follow-up of 14 months, median PFS in the masitinib arm was 3.71 months, reaching its efficacy endpoint. Secondary endpoints were a comparison of OS and PFS between the 2 arms. The OS was significantly increased in the masitinib arm compared with the sunitinib arm (>21.2 months vs 15.2 months; HR, 0.27; 95% CI, 0.09–0.85; P = .016), which was sustained at a 26-month follow-up; it should be noted that patients on the masitinib arm were allowed to cross over to sunitinib, whereas the converse was not allowed. The statistical comparison of PFS between masitinib and sunitinib was not statistically different (3.7 vs 1.9 months; 95% CI, 1.8–4.4; HR, 1.1). Masitinib was found to have significantly fewer severe adverse events compared with sunitinib (52% vs 91%; P = .0008). The findings of this study are intriguing yet were based on a very small sample size, and the OS benefit may have been confounded by the addition of sunitinib as an additional active agent for the patients treated on this trial. Masitinib is a potentially promising alternative to sunitinib in second-line therapy, and a phase III clinical trial is currently underway to further assess its effectiveness (NCT01694277). A phase III clinical trial of masitinib compared with imatinib in first-line therapy for GIST is also currently underway (NCT00812240).

FUTURE DIRECTIONS

Since 2000, the treatment of GIST has significantly changed and led to better out-comes, especially for patients with advance disease. However, patients continue to progress on the available therapies, and it is not yet clear that adjuvant therapy is truly curing patients. The outcomes of adjuvant studies assessing longer imatinib therapy will be of interest especially with regard to cure rates; if there is not an improvement in long-term cures, the benefits will need to be balanced against the use of long-term chronic therapy and its associated with side effects.

Potential future directions to improve patient outcomes include investigating the role of immunotherapy in GIST; a phase I trial of dasatinib and ipilimumab has been completed (NCT01643278), and a trial of axitinib and pembrolizumab (NCT02636725) is including GIST patients. Studies assessing agents for subtypes of GIST are underway. A multicenter RCT is investigating the role of crenolanib, an inhibitor of class III receptor TKIs, FMS-like tyrosine kinase 3 and PDGFRA and PDGFRB, compared with placebo in patients with histologically confirmed advanced or metastatic GIST with a *PDGFRA* D842V mutation (NCT02847429). Preclinical and early phase I and II trials are also testing targeted combination therapies that may have the advantage of inhibiting several key biologic pathways thus limiting the emergence of resistance mechanisms.

REFERENCES

1. von Mehren M, Randall RL, Benjamin RS, et al. Featured updates to the NCCN guidelines. J Natl Compr Canc Netw 2014;12(4):473–83.
2. Coreless CL, Ballman KV, Antonescu CR, et al. Pathologic and molecular features correlate with long-term outcome after adjuvant therapy of resected primary GI stromal tumor: the ACOSOG Z9001 trial. J Clin Oncol 2014;32(15):1563–70.
3. Joensuu H, Eriksson M, Sundby Hall K, et al. One vs three years of adjuvant imatinib for operable gastrointestinal stromal tumor. JAMA 2012;307(12):1265–72.
4. Casali PG, Le Cesne A, Poveda Velasco A, et al. Time to definitive failure to the first tyrosine kinase inhibitor in localized GI stromal tumors treated with imatinib as an adjuvant: A European Organisation for Research and Treatment of Cancer Soft Tissue and Bone Sarcoma Group Intergroup Randomized Trial in Collaboration With the Australasian Gastro-Intestinal Trials Group, UNICANCER, French Sarcoma Group, Italian Sarcoma Group, and Spanish Group for Research on Sarcomas. J Clin Oncol 2015;33(36):4276–83.
5. Demetri GD, von Mehren M, Blanke CD, et al. Efficacy and safety of imatinib mesylate in advanced gastrointestinal stromal tumors. N Engl J Med 2002;347(7):472–80.
6. Blanke CD, Rankin C, Demetri GD, et al. Phase III randomized intergroup trial assessing imatinib mesylate at two dose levels in patients with unresectable or metastatic gist. J Clin Oncol 2008;626–32.
7. Verweij J, Casali PG, Zalcberg J, et al. Progression-free survival in gastrointestinal stromal tumours with high-dose imatinib: randomised trial. Lancet 2004;364(9440):1127–34.
8. Zalcberg JR, Verweij J, Casali PG, et al. Outcome of patients with advanced gastro-intestinal stromal tumours crossing over to a daily imatinib dose of 800 mg after progression on 400 mg. Eur J Cancer 2005;41(12):1751–7.
9. Blay JY, Le Cesne A, Ray-Coquard I, et al. Prospective Multicentric randomized phase III study of Imatinib in patients wiht advanced gastrointestinal stromal tumors comparing interruption versus continuation of treatment beyond 1 year: the French Sarcoma Group. J Clin Oncol 2007;1107–13.
10. Le Cesne A, Ray-Coquard I, Bui BN, et al. Discontinuation of Imatinib in patients with advanced gastrointestinalstromal tumours after 3 years of treatment: an open-label multicentre randomised phase 3 trial. Lancet Oncol 2010;11(10):942–9.

11. Ray-Coquard I, Bin Bui N, Adenis A, et al. Risk of relapse with imatinib (IM) discontinuation at 5 years in advanced GIST patients: results of the prospective BRF14 randomised phase III study comparing interruption versus continuation of IM at 5 years of treatment: a French Sarcoma Group Study. J Clin Oncol 2010;28:15s.

12. Patrikidou A, Chabaud S, Ray-Coquard I, et al. Influence of Imatinib interruption and rechallenge on the residual disease in patients with advanced GIST: results of the BFR14 prospective French Sarcoma Group randomised, phase III trial. Ann Oncol 2013;24(4):1087–98.

13. Kang YK, Ryu MH, Yoo C, et al. Resumption of Imatinib to control metastatic or unresected gastrointestinal stromal tumors after failure of imatinib and sunitinib (RIGHT): a randomized, placebo-controlled, phase 3 trial. Lancet Oncol 2013; 14(12):1175–82.

14. Demetri GD, van Oosterom AT, Garrett CR, et al. Efficacy and safety of sunitinib in patients with advanced gastrointestinal stromal tumor after failure of imatinib: a randomized controlled trial. Lancet 2006;368(9544):1329–38.

15. Demetri GD, Reichardt P, Kang YK, et al. Efficacy and safety of Regorafenib for advanced gastrointestional stromal tumours after failure of imatinib and sunitinib (GRID): an international, multicentre, randomised placebo-controlled phase III trial. Lancet Oncol 2013;381(9863):295–302.

16. Blay JY, Shen L, Kang YK, et al. Nilotinib versus Imatinib as first-line therapy for patients with unresectable or metastatic gastrointestinal stromal tumors (ENESTg1): a randomised phase 3 trial. Lancet Oncol 2015;16(5):550–60.

17. Reichardt P, Blay JY, Gelderblom H, et al. Phase III study of nilotinib versus best supportive care with or without a TKI in patients with gastrointestinal stromal tumors resistant to or intolerant of imatinib and sunitinib. Ann Oncol 2012;23(7): 1680–7.

18. Adenis A, Blay JY, Bui-Nguyen B, et al. Masitinib in advanced gastrointestinal stromal tumor (GIST) after failure of imatinib: a randomized controlled open-label trial. Ann Oncol 2014;25(9):1762–9.

An Update on Randomized Clinical Trials in Melanoma

Giorgos Karakousis, MD[a], Charlotte Ariyan, MD, PhD[b],*

KEYWORDS

- Melanoma • Management • Randomized controlled trials

KEY POINTS

- The results of trials have continued to demonstrate that more aggressive management of the regional lymph node basin is not associated with survival benefit.
- With the historical poor outcomes of chemotherapy in the treatment of melanoma, studies have focused on immunotherapy.
- The field of treatment of metastatic disease has been revolutionized by the advent of targeted therapies and checkpoint blockade, and for the first time, survival in Stage IV melanoma has improved.

INTRODUCTION

Despite many advances in the treatment of melanoma, it still continues to be a disease that affects many people. Fortunately, there have been a multitude of randomized trials that have refined the treatment of this prevalent disease. From 1975 to 2000, there were 154 prospective randomized trials on the treatment of local, regional, and metastatic melanoma. From 2001 to now, additional randomized trials have focused on the role of surgery, adjuvants to surgery, and treatment of metastatic disease. The results of the practice-changing trials are summarized in this review.

PRIMARY MELANOMA

Clinical trials on excision margins have failed to demonstrate a difference in survival with more aggressive surgery, and yet local recurrence is associated with a poor overall survival.[1] Therefore, investigation into the appropriate margin has continued. Two recent trials addressed the impact of excision margins of the primary lesion on outcome in patients with melanoma. A large European multicentric Phase III study

The authors have nothing to disclose.
[a] Department of Surgery, Hospital of the University of Pennsylvania, 3400 Spruce St # 4, Philadelphia, PA 19104, USA; [b] Department of Surgery, Memorial Sloan Kettering Cancer Center, 1275 York Avenue, New York, NY 10065, USA
* Corresponding author.
E-mail address: ariyanc@mskcc.org

Surg Oncol Clin N Am 26 (2017) 559–586
http://dx.doi.org/10.1016/j.soc.2017.05.002
1055-3207/17/© 2017 Elsevier Inc. All rights reserved.

surgonc.theclinics.com

from 9 European centers investigated the difference between 2-cm and 5-cm excision margins for melanomas less than 2.1 mm thick.[2] No significant difference was found in the number of recurrences, recurrence-free survival, or overall survival between the 2 excision margin groups. Another trial from the United Kingdom studied patients with melanomas 2 mm or greater in thickness randomized to either 1-cm or 3-cm margins.[3] This trial did not demonstrate a significant difference in overall survival or melanoma-specific survival but did establish an increase in locoregional recurrence in the 1-cm margin group as compared with the 3-cm margin group (hazard ratio [HR] 1.26; $P = .05$). Patients in this trial did not have staging with sentinel lymph node biopsy, so it is not clear if the increased locoregional recurrence is a result of unbalanced groups. Taken collectively, the results of all the randomized trials on excision margins suggest that reasonable practice is still 1-cm margin for lesions less than 1 mm in thickness, and 2-cm margins for thicker lesions. Whether 1-cm margins may yield outcomes equivalent to 2-cm margins for lesions of 1 to 2 mm remains to be addressed specifically by the MelmarT trial. This trial randomizes to 1-cm versus 2-cm margins and is currently accruing patients (https://clinicaltrials.gov/ct2/show/NCT02385214).

REGIONAL METASTATIC DISEASE

The results of trials have continued to demonstrate that more aggressive management of the regional lymph node basin is not associated with survival benefit. As shown in **Tables 1** and **2**, elective lymph node dissection (ELND) did not improve survival in patients with melanoma. Only the long-term follow-up of the Intergroup trial suggested a survival benefit in patients with nonulcerated limb melanomas with thickness 1 to 2 mm.[4] The sentinel lymph node (SLN) biopsy technique supplanted the need for further investigations into the merits of ELND and is the standard approach to evaluate clinically negative lymphatic basins. The Melanoma Selective Lymphadenectomy Trial (MSLT)-1 trial randomized patients with intermediate-thickness melanomas to either wide local excision (WLE) with nodal observation, or WLE in combination with SLN biopsy. Those patients with metastatic disease detected in the sentinel node underwent immediate completion lymph node dissection, whereas the patients in the observation arm underwent a therapeutic lymphadenectomy for clinically evident nodal disease. The study confirmed the prognostic value of the sentinel node status for patients with intermediate-thickness melanomas. MSLT-1 did not demonstrate any difference in melanoma-specific survival between the 2 groups, which was the primary endpoint of the trial. In a subset analysis of all patients with nodal metastases, however, there

Table 1
Surgical margin randomized trials before 2002

Trial	Thickness Melanoma	Margin	Comments
World Health Organization[39]	<2 mm	1 cm vs 3 cm	1-cm margin safe for melanoma <1 mm, increased local recurrence with 1-cm excision in melanoma >1 mm
Intergroup[4]	1–4 mm	2 cm vs 4 cm	2-cm margin safe for intermediate-thickness melanoma
Swedish[40]	0.8–2 mm	2 cm vs 5 cm	2-cm margin safe
European phase III[2]	<2.1 mm	2 cm vs 5 cm	2-cm safe
United Kingdom[3]	>2 mm	1 cm vs 3 cm	Increased locoregional recurrence rate with 1-cm excision, no sentinel lymph node biopsy performed

Table 2
Results of randomized ELND trials before 2002

Study	n	Site	Thickness, mm	F/U, y	OS: WLE	OS: WLE + ELND	P
Sim et al,[41] 1978	173	Excluded midline trunk, head and neck	Any	NR	85	85	NS
Veronesi et al,[42] 1982	553	Extremity	Any	8.2	72	74	NS
Balch et al,[43] 1996 (intergroup)	740	All	1–4	7.4	82	86	.25
Intergroup f/u[4]				10	73	77	.12
Cascinelli et al,[7] 1998	240	Trunk	>1.5	11	51	62	.09

Abbreviations: ELND, elective lymph node dissection; F/U, follow-up; NR, not reported; NS, not significant; OS, overall survival; WLE, wide local excision.

was a statistically significant improved 5-year survival rate in those patients who underwent SLN biopsy and immediate lymphadenectomy versus those who underwent delayed lymphadenectomy on clinically evident disease (72.3% vs 52.4%).[5]

The therapeutic value of completion lymph node (CLND) dissection for patients with a positive SLN biopsy is currently under investigation in the worldwide MSLT-II trial. This trial randomizes patients to CLND or observation with nodal ultrasound. In the meantime, a smaller replicate trial was performed in Germany, the DeCog trial. This trial did not demonstrate any evidence of difference in distant metastasis-free survival between groups.[6]

The role of prophylactic regional hyperthermic isolated limb perfusion (ILP) for patients with high-risk melanomas was examined in a cooperative-group trial that randomized 832 patients to ILP with melphalan.[7] No significant difference in survival was reported at the conclusion of the trial. Since 2001, the results of one additional randomized trial have been performed using ILP in the treatment of locally advanced melanoma (ACOSOG trial Z0020).[8] This trial randomized patients with locally advanced melanoma to standard hyperthermic limb perfusion with either melphalan alone or melphalan in combination with tumor necrosis factor (TNF). The trial was stopped early because of an increase in grade 4 toxicities, including amputations, in the combined treatment arm. The survival data, with short follow-up, was not different between the 2 groups. TNF is currently not approved for use in the United States; however, continued use at high-volume European centers has demonstrated efficacy and safety of this drug.[9]

ADJUVANT TREATMENT OF HIGH-RISK MELANOMA

With the historically poor outcomes of chemotherapy in the treatment of melanoma, studies have focused on immunotherapy. Adjuvant immunotherapies aim to activate the host immune through vaccines, interferons, and other immune modulators, such as Bacillus Calmette-Guerin (BCG) and checkpoint blockade.

Interferon (IFN) is a protein that is produced by the immune system in response to viral infection and foreign proteins. Exogenous administration of this compound, therefore, is in an effort to stimulate the immune system to recognize melanoma antigens. The results of adjuvant IFN treatment, on the whole, fail to demonstrate a survival benefit, but do demonstrate a modest improvement in recurrence-free survival. Investigations have therefore continued to attempt to identify if there is a subset of patients and a dosing regimen that will improve outcomes. IFN-alpha-2b was approved by the Food and Drug Administration as adjuvant treatment for high-risk patients with deep primary melanomas or regional lymph node metastatic disease after the Eastern Cooperative Oncology Group (ECOG) trial E1684.[10] This trial compared high-dose IFN-alpha-2b with observation, and found a significant improvement in disease-free and overall survival. The follow-up study compared observation, low-dose IFN-alpha-2b, and high-dose IFN-alpha-2b and found improved relapse-free survival but no overall survival difference.[11]

The continued inconsistency in results of IFN trials is demonstrated by 2 studies without significant results: the AIM HIGH Study and European Organisation for Research and Treatment of Cancer (EORTC) 18952. The AIM HIGH Study randomized patients to long-term low-dose IFN or observation after resection of stage IIB or III melanoma.[12] In this trial, there was an initial benefit in recurrence-free survival that disappeared after 3 years of follow-up and was not significant. Fifteen percent of patients in the IFN group withdrew from the study and toxicities were modest. These results were similar to those of the EORTC 18952 trial, which randomized patients after resection with stage IIb or III melanoma to 13 months or 25 months of intermediate-dose IFN or observation.[13] Recent results from the EORTC 18991,[14] which randomized patients with stage III melanoma after resection to pegylated IFN or observation also demonstrated additional promise for this immunotherapy. The trial demonstrated a small (6% at 4 years) improvement in recurrence-free survival with the pegylated interferon, which is potentially best noted in the subgroup of patients with N1 disease. It is possible that long-term follow-up of pegylated IFN will continue to show an improvement in patients with early stage III disease, and therefore it may have a more definitive role in the adjuvant setting than standard IFN, because it is also better tolerated.

IFN has also been combined with other immunologic and chemotherapeutic agents. Garbe and colleagues[15] randomized patients with stage III disease following surgery to adjuvant low-dose IFN with or without dacarbazine (DTIC) or to observation. Overall survival was significantly higher by multivariate analysis in patients with adjuvant low-dose IFN compared with surgery alone, but with the addition of dacarbazine, this survival benefit was lost. In another trial, high-dose IFN was compared with the ganglioside vaccine, GM2-KLH/QS-21, in patients with resected stage IIB and III melanomas.[16] The trial was halted on an interim analysis due to a significant recurrence-free survival and overall survival benefit in the high-dose IFN arm. In 2007, Mitchell and colleagues[17] reported on 604 patients who were randomized to 2 years of treatment with an allogeneic melanoma lysate and low-dose IFN or high-dose IFN. Overall and recurrence-free survival were the same between the 2 arms, providing another trial without any clear benefit to vaccine use in the adjuvant setting. Other immunotherapy trials have examined BCG in the adjuvant setting. Early trials reported improvements in disease-free survival with BCG use. To test this hypothesis, Agarwala and colleagues[18] randomized 734 patients with stage I-III melanoma into 4 groups that were assembled into 22 cohorts: (1) BCG versus BCG plus DTIC and (2) BCG versus observation. There was no benefit to BCG or BCG plus DTIC with any patients in the stage I-III categories of patients with melanoma.

The Canvaxin vaccine consisted of allogeneic melanoma cells with high antigen expression. Much excitement was generated when phase II studies showed an improvement in survival when used as an adjuvant in stage III patients.[19]

Unfortunately, a multicenter randomized phase III trial failed to confirm these results, and this therapy is no longer used.[20]

A recent adjuvant phase III trial (EORTC 18071) randomized patients with stage III disease, with 1 mm of tumor burden in the sentinel lymph node, to high-dose anti-CLA4 immunotherapy (ipilimumab at 10 mg/kg) versus placebo. The study demonstrated an improvement in recurrence-free survival, its primary endpoint, for the adjuvant ipilimumab group compared with control (40.8% vs 30.3% at 5 years, $P<.001$). Moreover, there was an improvement in overall survival observed at 5 years favoring the adjuvant immunotherapy group (65.4% vs 54.4%, $P = .001$). Notably, grade 3 or 4 immune-related adverse events occurred in 41.6% of patients in the adjuvant ipilimumab group, with 1.1% of patients in the treatment group having immune-related deaths.[21]

TREATMENT OF METASTATIC MELANOMA

The field of treatment of metastatic disease has been revolutionized by the advent of targeted therapies and checkpoint blockade, and for the first time, survival in stage IV melanoma has improved. Immunotherapy with CTLA-4 or PD1 blockade has demonstrated survival benefits in multiple trials. Furthermore, blockade of the MAP kinase pathway in patients with a BRAF mutation have also resulted in survival benefit. Unfortunately, targeted therapy inhibition leads to resistance and now most patients receive combination BRAF/MEK inhibition. This section reviews the historical trials leading up to and including the practice of changing trials of targeted inhibition and immunotherapy.

The Dartmouth regimen (cisplatin, carmustine, DTIC, and tamoxifen) and its components were the most commonly studied regimen in several large prospective randomized controlled trials (RCTs). Activity was demonstrated in the 1992 study by Cocconi and colleagues[22] that showed improved response rates and median survival with DTIC plus tamoxifen compared with DTIC alone. Chapman and colleagues[23] then performed a study that showed no difference between the Dartmouth regimen and DTIC with regard to tumor response, toxicity, or survival. At that time, DTIC alone was thus felt to be the optimal treatment. Temozolomide also has been used to treat patients with metastatic melanoma, and DTIC was compared with temozolomide in a study by the Royal Marsden Hospital.[24] Patients treated with temozolomide demonstrated equivalent progression-free survival (PFS), response rates, toxicity, and survival. Temozolomide also was studied in combination with cisplatin, with no benefit found in the combined regimen.[25]

Investigators have combined treatments with biologic agents and chemotherapies in an effort to maximize activity against melanoma. Unfortunately, most of these studies have not improved survival. As reviewed in the prior chapter, studies comparing interleukin (IL)-2/IFN-alpha and chemotherapy with IL-2/IFN-alpha alone or IL-2 with IL-2/IFN-alpha showed no difference in overall survival.[26,27] This review includes a bio-chemotherapy trial that is similar to other trials, such as EORTC 18951, in structure and outcomes, in that it compared cisplatin, vinblastine, and DTIC with cisplatin, vinblastine, dacarbazine, IL-2, and IFN-alpha and found no significant alteration in overall survival or durable responses.[28] There were higher response rates and a longer median PFS rate with the biochemotherapy, but there were significant toxicities associated with these regimens. The conclusion from these trials is that biochemotherapy with IL-2 and IFN-alpha are not recommended for treating metastatic melanoma.

Immunotherapy with CTLA-4 blockade was the first to demonstrate a survival benefit, although modest, of 10% in heavily pretreated patients with metastatic melanoma.[29] The durability of response with actual survivors alive at 10 years gave tremendous hope to the field.[30] Blockade of PD1 was also then shown to be effective, with a response rate of 30%.[31] The combination of CTLA-4 and PD1 blockade is now under investigation with initial response rates reported of more than 50%.[32]

Furthermore, knowledge about the genomic drivers of melanoma have expanded. BRAFV600E mutation is found in approximately 50% of cutaneous melanomas, and blockade of the MAP kinase pathway in patients with a BRAF mutation have also resulted in survival benefit.[33] Many of these patients develop resistance with single-agent blockade and now most patients receive combination BRAF/MEK inhibition.[34,35] Imatinib mesylate also has been used in a phase II trial with 21 patients who had melanoma cells that expressed c-kit.[36] At 400 mg twice a day, imatinib had little clinical efficacy, although it did have individual responders, suggesting a possible role for imatinib in patients with specific kit mutations.

LEVEL IA EVIDENCE IN MELANOMA
Surgical Trials

Khayat D, Rixe O, Martin G, et al. French Group of Research on Malignant Melanoma. Surgical margins in cutaneous melanoma (2 cm versus 5 cm for lesions measuring less than 2.1-mm thick). Cancer 2003;97(8):1941–6.

Hypothesis
A smaller excision margin (2-cm) of the primary tumor for patients with melanomas less than 2.1 mm in thickness may yield similar outcomes with regard to disease recurrence and survival as a wider (5-cm) excision margin.

No. Patients Randomized	Study Groups	Stratification	Significance Demonstrated	% Change Identified in Trial
337	2-cm margins n = 161 5-cm margins n = 165	Histology	None equivalent	None

Published abstract

Background This study addressed the question of whether limited surgery for primary malignant melanoma with a 2-cm margin is as good as a 5-cm margin. An update of a 16-year follow-up is provided.

Methods Nine European centers, over a period of 5 years, prospectively randomized 337 patients with melanoma measuring less than 2.1 mm in thickness to undergo a local excision with either a 2-cm or a 5-cm margin. Three hundred twenty-six patients were eligible for statistical analysis. Excluded from the trial were patients older than 70 years; those with melanomas from the toe, nail, or finger; and those with acral-lentiginous melanoma. A separate randomization was performed to independently test an adjuvant treatment with a nonspecific immunostimulant, isoprinosine, compared with observation. The median follow-up time was 192 months (16 years) for the estimation of survival and disease recurrences.

Results There were 22 tumor recurrences in the 2-cm arm and 33 in the 5-cm arm. The median time to disease recurrence was 43 months and 37.6 months, respectively. The 10-year disease-free survival rates were 85% for the group with a 2-cm margin and 83% for the group with a 5-cm margin. There was no difference in the 10-year overall survival rates (87% vs 86%). Isoprinosine did not demonstrate any activity in this setting.

Conclusions The authors concluded that for melanoma less than 2.1-mm thick, a margin of excision of 2 cm is sufficient. A larger margin of 5 cm does not appear to have any impact on either the rate or the time to disease recurrence or on survival.

Editor's summary and comments
This multicenter European trial investigated the role of surgical margins for melanoma lesions less than 2.1 mm in thickness by randomizing patients to either 2-cm or 5-cm excisional margins in patients (those older than 70 years and with acral lentiginous lesions were excluded). There was no difference in local tumor recurrence rates, disease-free survival or overall survival with a median follow-up of 16 years between the 2 excision margin groups. This study reinforces the results of the Swedish Melanoma Study group (2-cm vs 5-cm margin groups for 0.8 to 2-mm thickness lesions) and the prior WHO trial discussed above. As a secondary randomization, patients in each excisional margin arm were assigned to receive isoprinosine, shown to have immunostimulation properties toward natural killer cells against melanoma in vitro, or to observation. There was no difference seen in median overall survival or disease-free survival between the groups receiving adjuvant immunotherapy and those followed with observation alone using any subgroup analysis of tumor characteristics or surgery extent, although the numbers in each final randomized group were fairly small (76–89 patients).

Thomas JM, Newton-Bishop J, A'Hern R, et al. United Kingdom Melanoma Study Group; British Association of Plastic Surgeons; Scottish Cancer Therapy Network. Excision margins in high-risk malignant melanoma. N Engl J Med 2004;350(8):757–66.

Hypothesis
Narrow (1-cm) excision margins for high risk melanoma lesions (>2 mm) may be insufficient as compared with wider (3-cm) margins.

No. Patients Randomized	Study Groups	Stratification	Significance Demonstrated	% Change Identified in Trial
453	1-cm margin (n = 453)	Histology	Increase in loco-regional recurrence (LR) with 1-cm margin	HR 1.26 for LR in 1-cm vs 3-cm margin group (P = .05)
	3-cm margin (n = 447)			

Published abstract
Background Controversy exists concerning the necessary margin of excision for cutaneous melanoma 2 mm or greater in thickness.

Methods We conducted a randomized clinical trial comparing 1-cm and 3-cm margins.

Results Of the 900 patients who were enrolled, 453 were randomly assigned to undergo surgery with a 1-cm margin of excision and 447 with a 3-cm margin of excision; the median follow-up was 60 months. A 1-cm margin of excision was associated with a significantly increased risk of locoregional recurrence. There were 168 locoregional recurrences (as first events) in the group with 1-cm margins of excision, as compared with 142 in the group with 3-cm margins (hazard ratio, 1.26; 95% confidence interval, 1.00–1.59; P = .05). There were 128 deaths attributable to melanoma in the group with 1-cm margins, as compared with 105 in the group with 3-cm margins (hazard ratio, 1.24; 95% confidence interval, 0.96–1.61; P = .1); overall survival was similar in the two groups (hazard ratio for death, 1.07; 95% confidence interval, 0.85–1.36; P = .6).

Conclusions A 1-cm margin of excision for melanoma with a poor prognosis (as defined by a tumor thickness of at least 2 mm) is associated with a significantly greater risk of regional recurrence than is a 3-cm margin, but with a similar overall survival rate.

Editor's summary and comments
This well-designed randomized trial addresses the important question as to whether 1-cm margins are adequate for higher risk melanoma lesions greater than 2 mm in thickness. Interestingly, the comparison arm to the 1-cm margin is a 3-cm margin and not 2-cm, which is the standard margin size routinely performed for intermediate-thickness lesions (adapted largely from the results of the Intergroup trial). The study design does directly complement the design of the WHO trial though, which compared 1-cm to 3-cm margins for lesions less than 2 mm. The investigators found a decrease in the incidence of loco-regional recurrence (which included local, in transit or regional nodal recurrences) favoring the 3-cm margin group. This did not however translate into a statistically different disease-free survival or overall survival though between the 2 randomized arms, although there was a trend toward increased disease-specific mortality associated with the narrow margin (HR 1.24, P = .1), a trend that continued in long-term follow-up.[37] It should be noted that patients in the study did not undergo SLN biopsy, and it remains unclear how the use of this technique, which is routinely performed in this patient population, would have impacted the results.

Morton DL, Thompson JF, Cochran AJ, et al, MSLT Group. Sentinel-node biopsy or nodal observation in melanoma. N Engl J Med 2006;355(13):1307–17, and 10-year follow-up N Engl J Med 2014;377:7.

Hypothesis
Patients with intermediate-thickness melanomas undergoing SLN biopsy for staging with immediate lymphadenectomy for SLN metastases would have an improved survival as compared with patients with simple excision of their primary lesion and therapeutic lymphadenectomy on detection of clinically evident regional nodal disease.

No. Patients Randomized	Study Groups	Stratification	Significance Demonstrated	% Change Identified in Trial
1347	Nodal observation with therapeutic lymphadenectomy for clinically evident disease (n = 500) SLN biopsy and immediate lymphadenectomy for SLN metastases (n = 769)	Tumor thickness Tumor site	None	None[a] Melanoma-specific survival at 10 y 78.3% vs 81.4 (P = .18)

[a] See editor's comments.

Published abstract
Background We evaluated the contribution of sentinel-node biopsy to outcomes in patients with newly diagnosed melanoma.

Methods Patients with a primary cutaneous melanoma were randomly assigned to wide excision and postoperative observation of regional lymph nodes with lymphadenectomy if nodal relapse occurred, or to wide excision and sentinel-node biopsy with immediate lymphadenectomy if nodal micrometastases were detected on biopsy.

Results Among 1269 patients with an intermediate-thickness primary melanoma, the mean ($\pm$SE) estimated 5-year disease-free survival rate for the population was 78.3% $\pm$ 1.6% in the biopsy group and 73.1% $\pm$ 2.1% in the observation group (hazard ratio for recurrence[corrected], 0.74; 95% confidence interval [CI], 0.59–0.93; $P = .009$). Five-year melanoma-specific survival rates were similar in the 2 groups (87.1% $\pm$ 1.3% and 86.6% $\pm$ 1.6%, respectively). In the biopsy group, the presence of metastases in the sentinel node was the most important prognostic factor; the 5-year survival rate was 72.3% $\pm$ 4.6% among patients with tumor-positive sentinel nodes and 90.2% $\pm$ 1.3% among those with tumor-negative sentinel nodes (hazard ratio for death, 2.48; 95% CI, 1.54–3.98; $P<.001$). The incidence of sentinel-node micrometastases was 16.0% (122 of 764 patients), and the rate of nodal relapse in the observation group was 15.6% (78 of 500 patients). The corresponding mean number of tumor-involved nodes was 1.4 in the biopsy group and 3.3 in the observation group ($P<.001$), indicating disease progression during observation. Among patients with nodal metastases, the 5-year survival rate was higher among those who underwent immediate lymphadenectomy than among those in whom lymphadenectomy was delayed (72.3% $\pm$ 4.6% vs 52.4% $\pm$ 5.9%; hazard ratio for death, 0.51; 95% CI, 0.32–0.81; $P = .004$). This held up in the 10-year follow-up of patients with a 62.1% survival for the SLN biopsy group compared with 45.5% in the nodal recurrence group ($P = .006$).

Conclusions The staging of intermediate-thickness (1.2–3.5 mm) primary melanomas according to the results of sentinel-node biopsy provides important prognostic information and identifies patients with nodal metastases whose survival can be prolonged by immediate lymphadenectomy.

Editor's summary and comments
This trial randomizes patients with intermediate-thickness melanomas to either SLN biopsy and immediate lymphadenectomy for those patients with metastatic disease in the SLNs versus observation and therapeutic lymphadenectomy for patients who develop clinically evident nodal disease. Several important conclusions can be drawn from this well-designed study requiring tremendous international efforts for its implementation. First, the study confirms the prognostic role of SLN status in patients with intermediate-thickness melanomas. On Cox multivariate analysis, SLN status conferred an HR (positive vs negative) of 3.04 ($P<.001$) for disease recurrence and 2.48 for melanoma-specific mortality ($P<.001$). Second, the incidence of SLN positivity and clinically evident disease in the observation group were almost identical (16% vs 15.6% respectively), suggesting the patients randomized in the 2 groups shared similar characteristics and that the natural progression of SLN positivity would be the development of clinically evident nodal disease. Finally, although the study showed no difference in melanoma-specific survival between the 2 randomized arms (primary endpoint), in a subset analysis focusing on patients with

nodal metastases, those patients with positive SLN biopsy who underwent immediate lymphadenectomy demonstrated an improved melanoma-specific survival when compared with patients in the observation group with clinically evident nodal disease who underwent a therapeutic lymphadenectomy. This observation strongly held up in the 10-year survival analysis as well.[5] Although the staging information of an SLN biopsy remain well accepted, the survival of subset analysis has been the subject of ongoing controversy regarding the possible therapeutic value of an SLN biopsy.

Leiter U, Stadler R, Mauch C, et al, German Dermatologic Cooperative Oncology Group (DeCOG). Complete lymph node dissection versus no dissection in patients with sentinel lymph node biopsy positive melanoma (DeCOG-SLT): a multicenter, randomized, phase 3 trial. Lancet Oncol 2016;17(6):757–67.

No. Patients Randomized	Study Groups	Stratification	Outcome	% Change Identified in Trial
483	Completion lymph node dissection vs nodal observation with ultrasound	1:1	Distant metastasis-free survival	None, at 3 y DMM 74.9% vs 77%

Hypothesis
Completion lymph node dissection is equivalent to nodal observation in patients with melanoma.

Published abstract
Background Complete lymph node dissection is recommended in patients with positive sentinel lymph node biopsy results. To date, the effect of complete lymph node dissection on prognosis is controversial. In the DeCOG-SLT trial, we assessed whether complete lymph node dissection resulted in increased survival compared with observation.

Methods In this multicenter, randomized, phase 3 trial, we enrolled patients with cutaneous melanoma of the torso, arms, or legs from 41 German skin cancer centers. Patients with positive sentinel lymph node biopsy results were eligible. Patients were randomly assigned (1:1) to undergo complete lymph node dissection or observation with permuted blocks of variable size and stratified by primary tumor thickness, ulceration of primary tumor, and intended adjuvant interferon therapy. Treatment assignment was not masked. The primary endpoint was distant metastasis-free survival and analyzed by intention to treat. All patients in the intention-to-treat population of the complete lymph node dissection group were included in the safety analysis. This trial is registered with ClinicalTrials.gov, number NCT02434107. Follow-up is ongoing, but the trial no longer recruiting patients.

Findings Between Jan 1, 2006, and Dec 1, 2014, 5547 patients were screened with sentinel lymph node biopsy and 1269 (23%) patients were positive for micrometastasis. Of these, 483 (39%) agreed to randomization into the clinical trial; due to difficulties enrolling and a low event rate the trial closed early on Dec 1, 2014. A total of 241 patients were randomly assigned to the observation group and 242 to the complete lymph node dissection group. Ten patients did not meet the inclusion criteria, so 233 patients were analyzed in the observation group and 240 patients were analyzed in the complete lymph node dissection group, as the intention-to-treat population. A total of 311 (66%) patients (158 in the observation group and 153 in the dissection group) had sentinel lymph node metastases of 1 mm or less. Median follow-up was 35 months (interquartile range 20–54). Distant metastasis-free survival at 3 years was 77.0% (90% CI 71.9–82.1; 55 events) in the observation group and 74.9% (69.5–80.3; 54 events) in the complete lymph node dissection group. In the complete lymph node dissection group, grade 3 and 4 events occurred in 15 patients (6%) and 19 patients (8%) patients, respectively. Adverse events included lymph edema (grade 3 in 7 patients, grade 4 in 13 patients), lymph fistula (grade 3 in 1 patient, grade 4 in 2 patients), seroma (grade 3 in 3 patients, no grade 4), infection (grade 3 in 3 patients, no grade 4), and delayed wound healing (grade 3 in 1 patient, grade 4 in 4 patients); no serious adverse events were reported.

Interpretation Although we did not achieve the required number of events, leading to the trial being underpowered, our results showed no difference in survival in patients treated with complete lymph node dissection compared with observation only. Consequently, complete lymph node dissection should not be recommended in patients with melanoma with lymph node micrometastases of at least a diameter of 1 mm or smaller.

Editor's note
This trial (DeCOG-SLT) accrued patients from 41 skin centers in Germany comparing completion lymph node dissection versus observation in patients with micrometastasis in the regional nodes identified by SLN biopsy. There is no difference in distant metastasis-free survival at 3 years between the 2 groups. In the completion lymphadenectomy group, grade 3 and 4 complications occurred in 14% of patients. Notable limitations of this study included relatively short follow-up (35 months) and exclusion of patients with head and neck primaries. Moreover, due to the difficulty in trial accrual, the study was felt to be underpowered. Interestingly, patients were more likely to withdraw from the trial if randomized to the surgery arm as compared with the observation arm (36 patients in surgery arm vs 3 in observation arm). Results from 2 additional investigations are eagerly awaited, the MSLT2 randomized trial and the EORTC 1208 (Minitub) prospective registry study, to help direct the optimal surgical management of patients with melanoma micrometastases identified in the sentinel lymph nodes.

Adjuvant Treatment

Prospective Randomized Trial of Interferon Alfa-2b and Interleukin-2 as Adjuvant Treatment for Resected Intermediate- and High-Risk Primary Melanoma Without Clinically Detectable Node Metastasis.

Hauschild A, Weichenthal M, Balda BR, et al. Prospective randomized trial of interferon alfa-2b and interleukin-2 as adjuvant treatment for resected intermediate- and high-risk primary melanoma without clinically detectable node metastasis. J Clin Oncol 2003;21:2883–8.

Hypothesis
The addition of low-dose IL-2 to adjuvant low-dose IFN-alpha-2b will improve survival.

No. Patients Randomized	Study Groups	Stratification	Significance Demonstrated	% Change Identified in Trial
225	Surgery, low-dose IFN-alpha, low-dose IL-2 Surgery, observation		None	None

Published abstract
Background Low-dose IFN-alfa has been shown to have limited effects in the adjuvant treatment of patients with intermediate- and high-risk primary melanoma. We hypothesized that a combination regimen with low-dose interleukin-2 (IL-2) may improve survival prospects in these patients.

Patients and methods After wide excision of primary melanoma without clinically detectable lymph node metastasis (pT3 to 4, cN0, M0), 225 patients from 10 participating centers were randomly assigned to receive either subcutaneous low-dose IFN-alpha-2b (3 million international units [MU]/m2/d, days 1–7, week 1; 3 times weekly, weeks 3–6, repeated all 6 weeks) plus IL-2 (9 MU/m2/d, days 1–4, week 2 of each cycle) for 48 weeks, or observation alone. The primary end point was prolongation of a relapse-free interval.

Results Of the 225 enrolled patients, 223 were found to be eligible. Median follow-up time was 79 months. All evaluated prognostic factors were well balanced between the 2 arms of the study. Relapses were noticed in 36 of 113 patients treated with IFN-alpha-2b plus IL-2 and in 34 of 110 patients with observation alone. Five-year disease-free survival of those who had routine surgery supplemented by IFN-alpha-2b and IL-2 treatment was 70.1% (95% confidence interval [CI], 61.3% to 78.9%), compared with 69.9% in those receiving surgery and observation alone (95% CI, 60.7% to 79.1%) in the intention-to-treat analysis. Evaluation of the overall survival did not show any difference between treated and untreated melanoma patients ($P = .93$).

Conclusion Adjuvant treatment of intermediate- and high-risk melanoma patients with low-dose IFN-alpha-2b and IL-2 is safe and well tolerated by most patients, but it does not improve disease-free or overall survival.

Editor's summary and comments
Prior studies showed that low-dose IFN-alpha improved relapse-free survival, but not overall survival in patients with resectable melanoma. This trial randomized patients to receive adjuvant low-dose IFN and IL-2 or observation. At a median follow-up of 79 months, 5-year disease-free survival was 70% in the treatment arm and 69.9% in the observation arm. Although the therapy was well tolerated, with 104 patients receiving more than 90% of the intended therapy, there was no benefit in the adjuvant setting.

  Sondak VK, Liu PY, Tuthill RJ, et al. Adjuvant immunotherapy of resected, intermediate-thickness, node-negative melanoma with an allogeneic tumor vaccine: overall results of a randomized trial of the Southwest Oncology Group. *J Clin Oncol* 2002;20:2058–66.

Hypothesis
Adjuvant allogeneic melanoma vaccine will improve recurrence-free survival in patients with node-negative intermediate-thickness melanoma.

No. Patients Randomized	Study Groups	Stratification	Significance Demonstrated	% Change Identified in Trial
689	Surgery plus allogeneic melanoma vaccine for 2 y Surgery alone	Sex Thickness Nodal stage	None	None

Published abstract
Background Patients with clinically negative nodes constitute over 85% of new melanoma cases. There is no adjuvant therapy for intermediate-thickness, node-negative melanoma patients.

Patients and methods The Southwest Oncology Group conducted a randomized phase III trial of an allogeneic melanoma vaccine for 2 years versus observation in patients with intermediate-thickness (1.5–4.0 mm or Clark's level IV if thickness unknown), clinically or pathologically node-negative melanoma (T3N0M0).

Results Six hundred eighty-nine patients were accrued over 4.5 years; 89 patients (13%) were ineligible. Surgical node staging was performed in 24%, the remainder were clinical N0. Thirteen eligible patients refused assigned treatment: 7 on the observation arm and 6 on the vaccine arm. Most vaccine patients experienced mild to moderate local toxicity, but 26 (9%) experienced grade 3 toxicity. After a median follow-up of 5.6 years, there were 107 events (tumor recurrences or deaths) among the 300 eligible patients randomized to vaccine compared with 114 among the 300 eligible patients randomized to observation (hazard ratio, 0.92; Cox-adjusted $P2 \_ 0.51$). There was no difference in vaccine efficacy among patients with tumors less than 3 mm or greater than 3 mm.

Conclusion This represents one of the largest randomized, controlled trials of adjuvant vaccine therapy in human cancer reported to date. Compliance with randomization was excellent, with only 2% refusing assigned therapy. There is no evidence of improved disease-free survival among patients randomized to receive vaccine, although the power to detect a small but clinically significant difference was low. Future investigations of adjuvant vaccine approaches for patients with intermediate-thickness melanoma should involve larger numbers of patients and ideally should include sentinel node biopsy staging.

Editor's summary and comments
There is a prior phase III study that showed an allogeneic melanoma cell lysate had a slightly improved response rate and survival (although not significant) when compared with a group treated with the Dartmouth regimen. There was, however, no control arm of surgery alone, so this trial was developed to answer the question of the benefit of an allogeneic melanoma cell lysate used in the adjuvant setting compared with the control arm of surgery alone. The vaccine constituted 15 melanoma-associated antigens. The primary outcome of the trial, disease-free survival, showed no difference between the 2 groups. Secondary analyses of groups with different thicknesses also showed no difference.

   Garbe C, Radny P, Linse R, et al. Adjuvant low-dose interferon {alpha}2a with or without dacarbazine compared with surgery alone: a prospective-randomized phase III DeCOG trial in melanoma patients with regional lymph node metastasis. Ann Oncol 2008;19:1195–201.

Hypothesis
IFN-alpha-2a with or without dacarbazine improves disease-free survival and overall survival in patients after nodal dissection with positive lymph nodes.

No. Patients Randomized	Study Groups	Stratification	Significance Demonstrated	% Change Identified in Trial
444	Adjuvant IFN-alpha-2a (n = 146)	None	Disease-free survival	59% (IFN) vs 45% (combination) vs 42% (observation) (P = .0045 IFN vs observation, P = .76 for combination vs observation)
	Adjuvant IFN-alpha-2a plus DTIC (n = 148) Observation (n = 147)		Overall survival	IFN alone HR .609 (P = .005)

Published abstract

Background More than half of patients with melanoma that has spread to regional lymph nodes develop recurrent disease within the first 3 years after surgery. The aim of the study was to improve disease-free survival (DFS) and overall survival (OS) with interferon (IFN) alpha2a with or without dacarbazine (DTIC) compared with observation alone.

Patients and methods A total of 444 patients from 42 centers of the German Dermatologic Cooperative Oncology Group who had received a complete lymph node dissection for pathologically proven regional node involvement were randomized to receive either 3 MU s.c. of IFN-alpha-2a three times a week for 2 years (Arm A) or combined treatment with same doses of IFN-alpha-2a plus DTIC 850 mg/m(2) every 4 to 8 weeks for 2 years (Arm B) or to observation alone (Arm C). Treatment was discontinued at first sign of relapse.

Results A total of 441 patients were eligible for intention-to-treat analysis. Kaplan-Meier 4-year OS rate of those who had received IFN-alpha-2a was 59%. For those with surgery alone, survival was 42% (A vs C, P = .0045). No improvement of survival was found for the combined treatment Arm B with 45% survival rate (B vs C, P = .76). Similarly, DFS rates showed significant benefit for Arm A, and not for Arm B. Multivariate Cox model confirmed that Arm A has an impact on OS (P = .005) but not Arm B (P = .34).

Conclusions 3 MU interferon alpha 2a given s.c. three times a week for 2 years significantly improved OS and DFS in patients with melanoma that had spread to the regional lymph nodes. Interestingly, the addition of DTIC reversed the beneficial effect of adjuvant interferon alpha 2a therapy.

Editor's summary and comments
Given the high mortality rates of patients with metastatic melanoma, the goal of this trial was to attempt to improve on disease-free survival and overall survival in patients with positive lymph nodes by using a combination of low-dose IFN-alpha-2a, DTIC, and observation. The study was well powered, with 441 total patients, and designed to detect a significant difference of 15% in the 4-year survival rate. The overall survival of patients in the IFN-alpha-2a group was significantly higher than the surgery-alone group (59% vs 42%, P = .0045). It was interesting to see there was a lower overall survival in the combination group, with an overall survival rate of 45%. These trends were similar, with multivariate analysis with an HR of 0.609 for the IFN-alone group (P = .005) and 0.854 for the combination group (P = .343). These findings are relevant for 2 reasons: (1) low-dose IFN-alpha in this study showed an increase in disease-specific and overall survival after 2 years of treatment, and (2) the addition of DTIC

to low-dose IFN negated the benefit of low-dose IFN. The 5-year overall survival in Hancock and colleagues'[12] low-dose IFN group was 44% for all patients, which is lower than the 59% overall survival at 4 years in this year, raising questions about the patient populations in both studies.

Hancock BW, Wheatley K, Harris S, et al. Adjuvant interferon in high-risk melanoma: the AIM HIGH Study—United Kingdom Coordinating Committee on Cancer Research randomized study of adjuvant low-dose extended-duration interferon Alfa-2a in high-risk resected malignant melanoma. J Clin Oncol 2004;22:53–61.

Hypothesis
Low-dose extended adjuvant IFN-alpha-2a improves recurrence-free survival and overall survival in patients with resected high-risk melanomas.

No. Patients Randomized	Study Groups	Stratification	Significance Demonstrated	% Change Identified in Trial
674	IFN-alpha (n = 338) Observation (n = 336)	None	None	None

Published abstract

Purpose To evaluate low-dose extended-duration IFN-alpha-2a as adjuvant therapy in patients with thick (>4 mm) primary cutaneous melanoma and/or locoregional metastases.

Patients and methods In this randomized controlled trial involving 674 patients, the effect of IFN-alpha-2a (3 megaunits three times per week for 2 years or until recurrence) on overall survival (OS) and recurrence-free survival (RFS) was compared with that of no further treatment in radically resected stage IIB and stage III cutaneous malignant melanoma.

Results The OS and RFS rates at 5 years were 44% (SE, 2.6) and 32% (SE, 2.1), respectively. There was no significant difference in OS or RFS between the IFN-treated and control arms (odds ratio [OR], 0.94; 95% CI, 0.75–1.18; $P = .6$; and OR, 0.91; 95% CI, 0.75–1.10; $P = .3$; respectively). Male sex ($P = .003$) and regional lymph node involvement ($P = .0009$), but not age ($P = .7$), were statistically significant adverse features for OS. Subgroup analysis by disease stage, age, and sex did not show any clear differences between IFN-treated and control groups in either OS or RFS. IFN-related toxicities were modest: grade 3 (and in only one case, grade 4) fatigue or mood disturbance was seen in 7% and 4%, respectively, of patients. However, there were 50 withdrawals (15%) from IFN treatment due to toxicity.

Conclusion The results from this study, taken in isolation, do not indicate that extended-duration low-dose IFN is significantly better than observation alone in the initial treatment of completely resected high-risk malignant melanoma.

Editor's summary and comments
This study was initiated in response to several phase I and phase II trials that showed some improvement in recurrence-free survival in patients with metastatic melanoma who were treated with IFN-alpha. The original target accrual was 1000 patients to achieve a 90% chance of detecting a 10% absolute difference in recurrence-free survival and overall survival, but accrual was halted after 674 patients due to the belief

that additional patients would not change the preliminary analysis. Patients were randomized to low-dose IFN-alpha for 2 years or until disease recurrence after resection of high-risk melanomas (≥4 mm and/or locoregional metastases). Similar to prior RCTs that examined adjuvant IFN, there was an initial benefit in recurrence-free survival that disappeared after 3 years of follow-up and was not significant. In addition, 15% of patients in the IFN group withdrew from the study and toxicities were modest. Given there was no effect on overall survival demonstrated with low-dose IFN, there is no clear benefit to using it as treatment for patients with high-risk melanoma in the adjuvant setting.

Eggermont AM, Suciu S, Santinami M, et al, EORTC Melanoma Group. Adjuvant therapy with pegylated interferon alfa-2b versus observation alone in resected stage III melanoma: final results of EORTC 18991, a randomised phase III trial. Lancet 2008;372:117–26.

Hypothesis
Pegylated IFN-alpha-2b is well tolerated and will improve recurrence-free survival in patients after resection of stage III melanoma.

No. Patients Randomized	Study Groups	Stratification	Significance Demonstrated	% Change Identified in Trial
1256	Observation (n = 629)	Microscopic vs macroscopic nodal involvement	Recurrence-free survival	45.6% vs 38.9% at 4 y (HR .82, $P = .01$)
	Pegylated IFN-alpha-2b (n = 627)	Number of positive nodes		
		Ulceration Tumor thickness		

Published abstract
Background Any benefit of adjuvant IFN-alpha-2b for melanoma could depend on dose and duration of treatment. Our aim was to determine whether pegylated IFN-alpha-2b can facilitate prolonged exposure while maintaining tolerability.

Methods 1256 patients with resected stage III melanoma were randomly assigned to observation (n = 629) or pegylated IFN-alpha-2b (n = 627) 6 μg/kg per week for 8 weeks (induction) then 3 μg/kg per week (maintenance) for an intended duration of 5 years. Randomization was stratified for microscopic (N1) versus macroscopic (N2) nodal involvement, number of positive nodes, ulceration and tumor thickness, sex, and center. Randomization was done with a minimization technique. The primary endpoint was recurrence-free survival. Analyses were done by intention to treat. This study is registered with ClinicalTrials.gov, number NCT00006249.

Results All randomized patients were included in the primary efficacy analysis. 608 patients in the interferon group and 613 patients in the observation group were included in safety analyses. The median length of treatment with pegylated IFN-alpha-2b was 12 (IQR 3.8–33.4) months. At 3.8 (3.2–4.2) years median follow-up, 328 recurrence events had occurred in the IFN group compared with 368 in the observation group (HR 0.82, 95% CI 0.71–0.96; $P = .01$); the 4-year rate of recurrence-free survival was 45.6% (SE 2.2) in the IFN group and 38.9% (2.2) in the observation group. There was no difference in overall survival between the groups. Grade 3 adverse events occurred in 246 (40%)

patients in the IFN group and 60 (10%) in the observation group; grade 4 adverse events occurred in 32 (5%) patients in the IFN group and 14 (2%) in the observation group. In the IFN group, the most common grade 3 or 4 adverse events were fatigue (97 patients, 16%), hepatotoxicity (66, 11%), and depression (39, 6%). Treatment with pegylated IFN-alpha-2b was discontinued because of toxicity in 191 (31%) patients.

Conclusions Adjuvant pegylated IFN-alpha-2b for stage III melanoma has a significant, sustained effect on recurrence-free survival.

Editor's summary and comments
In this trial, patients were randomized to observation or adjuvant pegylated IFN-alpha-2b after resection of stage III melanoma. This is the first randomized trial to examine the utility of pegylated IFN in the adjuvant setting. The theoretic advantage to using pegylated IFN is that it is better tolerated, allows for a longer treatment period, and maintains maximum exposure of IFN. The study reported a significant difference in recurrence-free survival at 4 years, with 45.6% of the IFN group compared with 38.9% of the observation group free of recurrence. There was no difference in overall survival between the 2 groups. When the groups were broken down into subgroups, the greatest effect of IFN treatment was in the group with earlier stage III disease, specifically microscopic nodal disease or only 1 positive node. There was, however, no statistically significant difference in overall survival in these groups. The only subgroup with a difference in overall survival was in the 96 patients treated with pegylated IFN who had an ulcerated lesion, in which the overall survival was 65% compared with 45.4% (HR .61, $P = .03$). There was a large difference between the toxicities found in the 2 groups, as in the IFN group, 40% of patients had grade 3 toxicities, compared with 10% of patients in the observation arm. Although the greatest benefit was in patients with limited N1 disease, this was at 4-year follow-up, which is too short of a period for patients with positive nodal disease. This regimen may be an alternative to patients who are offered high-dose adjuvant IFN, but its utility is not fully proven yet, and again there was no difference in overall survival outside of small subgroup analyses.

Mitchell MS, Abrams J, Thompson JA, et al. Randomized trial of an allogeneic melanoma lysate vaccine with low-dose interferon alfa-2b compared with high-dose interferon alfa-2b for resected stage III cutaneous melanoma. J Clin Oncol 2007;25:2078–85.

Hypothesis
Adjuvant allogeneic melanoma lysate vaccine and low-dose IFN-alpha-2b will improve overall survival compared with high-dose IFN-alpha-2b.

No. Patients Randomized	Study Groups	Stratification	Significance Demonstrated	% Change Identified in Trial
604	Allogeneic lysates and low-dose IFN- alpha-2b (n = 300) High-dose IFN-alpha-2b (n = 300)	Sex Number of nodes	None	None

Published abstract
Background To compare the overall survival (OS) of patients with resected stage III melanoma administered active specific immunotherapy and low-dose IFN-alpha-2b (IFN-a-2b) with the OS achieved using high-dose IFN-a-2b.

Patients and methods An Ad Hoc Melanoma Working Group of 25 investigators treated 604 patients from April 1997 to January 2003. Patients were stratified by sex and number of nodes and were randomly assigned to receive either 2 years of treatment with active specific immunotherapy with allogeneic melanoma lysates and low-dose IFN-a-2b (arm 1) or high-dose IFN-a-2b alone for 1 year (arm 2). Active specific immunotherapy was injected subcutaneously (SC) weekly for 4 weeks, at week 8, and bimonthly thereafter. IFN-a-2b SC was begun on week 4 and continued thrice weekly at 5 MU/m2 for 2 years. IFN-a-2b in arm 2 was administered according to the Eastern Cooperative Oncology Group 1684 study regimen.

Results Median follow-up time was 32 months for all patients and 42 months for surviving patients. Median OS time exceeds 84 months in arm 1 and is 83 months in arm 2 ($P = .56$). Five-year OS rate is 61% in arm 1% and 57% in arm 2. Estimated 5-year relapse-free survival (RFS) rate is 50% in arm 1% and 48% in arm 2, with median RFS times of 58 and 50 months, respectively. The incidence of serious adverse events as a result of treatment was the same in both arms, but more severe neuropsychiatric toxicity was seen in arm 2.

Conclusion OS and RFS achieved by active specific immunotherapy and low-dose IFN-a-2b were indistinguishable from those achieved by high-dose IFN-a-2b. Long RFS and OS times were observed in both treatment arms.

Editor's summary and comments
This trial examined the difference in recurrence-free survival and overall survival in patients with stage III melanoma. The study was powered to detect a 1-year difference in recurrence-free survival with 90% statistical power. At a median follow-up of 32 months, overall survival and relapse-free survival were similar between the 2 groups. There were also similar toxicities between the 2 treatment regimens. The survival times in both arms of this trial were longer than historical controls (eg, ECOG 1684), as approximately 70% of patients in this study were alive at 36 to 42 months. This study, however, probably is a more accurate representative of modern survival rates, as many patients had microscopically positive nodal disease due to the sentinel node procedure. One difficulty in analyzing the results of this trial is that there was no control arm without IFN. In addition, the study was not powered to show equivalence between the 2 groups, so it is not clear that the results of this study can be used to argue for low-dose IFN and allogeneic melanoma lysate.

No. Patients Randomized	Study Groups	Stratification	Significance Demonstrated	% Change Identified in Trial
951	Ipilimumab vs placebo		Recurrence free survival (RFS), overall survival (OS)	40 vs 30% RFS, 65% vs 54 OS

Background On the basis of data from a phase 2 trial that compared the checkpoint inhibitor ipilimumab at doses of 0.3 mg, 3 mg, and 10 mg per kilogram of body weight in patients with advanced melanoma, this phase 3 trial evaluated ipilimumab at a dose of 10 mg per kilogram in patients who had undergone complete resection of stage III melanoma.

Methods After patients had undergone complete resection of stage III cutaneous melanoma, we randomly assigned them to receive ipilimumab at a dose of 10 mg per kilogram (475 patients) or placebo (476) every 3 weeks for 4 doses, then every 3 months for up to 3 years or until disease recurrence or an unacceptable level of toxic effects occurred. Recurrence-free survival was the primary end point. Secondary end points included overall survival, distant metastasis-free survival, and safety.

Results At a median follow-up of 5.3 years, the 5-year rate of recurrence-free survival was 40.8% in the ipilimumab group, as compared with 30.3% in the placebo group (hazard ratio for recurrence or death, 0.76; 95% confidence interval [CI], 0.64–0.89; $P<.001$). The rate of overall survival at 5 years was 65.4% in the ipilimumab group, as compared with 54.4% in the placebo group (hazard ratio for death, 0.72; 95.1% CI, 0.58–0.88; $P = .001$). The rate of distant metastasis-free survival at 5 years was 48.3% in the ipilimumab group, as compared with 38.9% in the placebo group (hazard ratio for death or distant metastasis, 0.76; 95.8% CI, 0.64–0.92; $P = .002$). Adverse events of grade 3 or 4 occurred in 54.1% of the patients in the ipilimumab group and in 26.2% of those in the placebo group. Immune-related adverse events of grade 3 or 4 occurred in 41.6% of the patients in the ipilimumab group and in 2.7% of those in the placebo group. In the ipilimumab group, 5 patients (1.1%) died owing to immune-related adverse events.

Conclusions As adjuvant therapy for high-risk stage III melanoma, ipilimumab at a dose of 10 mg per kilogram resulted in significantly higher rates of recurrence-free survival, overall survival, and distant metastasis-free survival than placebo. There were more immune-related adverse events with ipilimumab than with placebo.

Editors notes
This landmark trial demonstrates that adjuvant ipilimumab improves survival in stage III melanoma. However, there was significant toxicity with the treatment, including death. For this reason, the use of adjuvant ipilimumab requires a careful discussion with patients, and perhaps reserved for the patients at highest risk. Because ipilimumab is effective in stage IV disease, patients who recur may be salvaged by effective systemic treatment, and therefore avoiding the toxicity in patients who did not need it.

Systemic Treatments (Metastatic Disease)

Atkins MB, Hsu J, Lee S, et al, Eastern Cooperative Oncology Group. Phase III trial comparing concurrent biochemotherapy with cisplatin, vinblastine, dacarbazine, interleukin-2, and interferon alfa-2b with cisplatin, vinblastine, and dacarbazine alone in patients with metastatic malignant melanoma (E3695): a trial coordinated by the Eastern Cooperative Oncology Group. J Clin Oncol 2008;26:5748–54.

Hypothesis
Biochemotherapy with IL-2 and IFN-alpha-2b added to a regimen of cisplatin, vinblastine, and DTIC will improve survival.

No. Patients Randomized	Study Groups	Stratification	Significance Demonstrated	% Change Identified in Trial
415	Cisplatin, vinblastine, and DTIC (n = 195)	None	Median progression-free survival	4.8 mo vs 2.9 mo (P = .015)
	Cisplatin, vinblastine, DTIC, IL-2, IFN-alpha-2b (n = 200)		Rate of grade 3 or worse toxicities	95% vs 73% (P = .001)

Published abstract
Background Phase II trials with biochemotherapy (BCT) have shown encouraging response rates in metastatic melanoma, and meta-analyses and one phase III trial have suggested a survival benefit. In an effort to determine the relative efficacy of BCT compared with chemotherapy alone, a phase III trial was performed within the United States Intergroup.

Patients and methods Patients were randomly assigned to receive cisplatin, vinblastine, and dacarbazine (CVD) either alone or concurrent with interleukin-2 and IFN-alpha-2b (BCT). Treatment cycles were repeated at 21-day intervals for a maximum of 4 cycles. Tumor response was assessed after cycles 2 and 4, then every 3 months.

Results Four hundred fifteen patients were enrolled, and 395 patients (CVD, n = 195; BCT, n = 200) were deemed eligible and assessable. The 2 study arms were well balanced for stratification factors and other prognostic factors. Response rate was 19.5% for BCT and 13.8% for CVD (P = .140). Median progression-free survival was significantly longer for BCT than for CVD (4.8 v 2.9 months; (P = .015), although this did not translate into an advantage in either median overall survival (9.0 v 8.7 months) or the percentage of patients alive at 1 year (41% v 36.9%). More patients experienced grade 3 or worse toxic events with BCT than CVD (95% v 73%; P = .001).

Conclusion Although BCT produced slightly higher response rates and longer median progression-free survival than CVD alone, this was not associated with either improved overall survival or durable responses. Considering the extra toxicity and complexity, this concurrent BCT regimen cannot be recommended for patients with metastatic melanoma.

Editor's summary and comments
This phase III trial was initiated in response to phase II trials that showed encouraging response rates with biochemotherapy in patients with metastatic melanoma. The only significant finding in this trial was a longer median time to progression (4.8 months compared with 2.9 months, P = .015). This did not, however, translate into any difference in overall survival or percentage of patients alive at 1 year. Given that 95% of the patients in the biochemotherapy group experienced a toxicity that was grade 3 or higher, the conclusion of this trial is that biochemotherapy is not indicated for treatment of patients with metastatic melanoma. Clearly these treatments need further optimization to balance the quality of life with treatment in patients with metastatic melanoma.

   Chapman PB, Hauschild A, Robert C, et al, BRIM-3 Study Group. *Improved survival with vemurafenib in melanoma with BRAF V600E mutation. N Eng J Med 2011;264:2507.*

Hypothesis
BRAF inhibition in patients with BRAF V600 E mutation will improve survival.

No. Patients Randomized	Study Groups	Stratification	Significance Demonstrated	% Change Identified in Trial
675	Vemurafenib vs DTIC	None	Progression free survival, overall survival	6.9 vs 1.6 mo, (HR 0.38, 95% CI 0.32–0.46), overall survival 12.5 vs 9.5 mo

Published abstract
Background Phase 1 and 2 clinical trials of the BRAF kinase inhibitor vemurafenib (PLX4032) have shown response rates of more than 50% in patients with metastatic melanoma with the BRAF V600 E mutation.

Methods We conducted a phase 3 randomized clinical trial comparing vemurafenib with dacarbazine in 675 patients with previously untreated, metastatic melanoma with the BRAF V600 E mutation. Patients were randomly assigned to receive either vemurafenib (960 mg orally twice daily) or dacarbazine (1000 mg per square meter of body-surface area intravenously every 3 weeks). Coprimary end points were rates of overall and progression-free survival. Secondary end points included the response rate, response duration, and safety. A final analysis was planned after 196 deaths and an interim analysis after 98 deaths.

Results At 6 months, overall survival was 84% (95% confidence interval [CI], 78–89) in the vemurafenib group and 64% (95% CI, 56–73) in the dacarbazine group. In the interim analysis for overall survival and final analysis for progression-free survival, vemurafenib was associated with a relative reduction of 63% in the risk of death and of 74% in the risk of either death or disease progression, as compared with dacarbazine ($P<.001$ for both comparisons). After review of the interim analysis by an independent data and safety monitoring board, crossover from dacarbazine to vemurafenib was recommended. Response rates were 48% for vemurafenib and 5% for dacarbazine. Common adverse events associated with vemurafenib were arthralgia, rash, fatigue, alopecia, keratoacanthoma or squamous-cell carcinoma, photosensitivity, nausea, and diarrhea; 38% of patients required dose modification because of toxic effects.

Conclusions Vemurafenib produced improved rates of overall and progression-free survival in patients with previously untreated melanoma with the BRAF V600 E mutation.

Editor's comments
This was the first article to demonstrate in an RCT that targeted therapy in melanoma could improve survival. Although the response rate is high, most patients progress with a median progression-free survival (PFS) of 6.9 months. Since this paper, additional studies have proven the efficacy of BRAF inhibition with dabrafenib, or MEK inhibition with trametinib.

> *Long GV, Storyakovskiy D, Gogas H, et al. Dabrafenib and trametinib versus dabrafenib and placebo for Val600BRAF-mutant melanoma: a multicenter, double-blind, phase 3 randomised controlled trial. Lancet 2015;386(9992):444–51.*

Hypothesis
Combined RAF/MEK inhibition will improve survival in melanoma with BRAF mutation.

No. Patients Randomized	Study Groups	Stratification	Significance Demonstrated	% Change Identified in Trial
423	Dabrafenib + trametinib vs Dabrafenib + placebo	All V600E or K mutation, no prior treatment	PFS, overall survival	11 vs 8 mo, (HR 0.67, 95% CI 0.53–0.84), overall survival 25.1 vs 18.7 mo

Background Previously, a study of ours showed that the combination of dabrafenib and trametinib improves progression-free survival compared with dabrafenib and placebo in patients with BRAF Val600Lys/Glu mutation-positive metastatic melanoma. The study was continued to assess the secondary endpoint of overall survival, which we report in this article.

Methods We did this double-blind phase 3 study at 113 sites in 14 countries. We enrolled previously untreated patients with BRAF Val600Glu or Val600Lys mutation-positive unresectable stage IIIC or stage IV melanoma. Participants were computer-randomized (1:1) to receive a combination of dabrafenib (150 mg orally twice daily) and trametinib (2 mg orally once daily), or dabrafenib and placebo. The primary endpoint was progression-free survival and overall survival was a secondary endpoint. This study is registered with ClinicalTrials.gov, number NCT01584648.

Findings Between May 4, 2012, and Nov 30, 2012, we screened 947 patients for eligibility, of whom 423 were randomly assigned to receive dabrafenib and trametinib (n = 211) or dabrafenib only (n = 212). The final data cutoff was Jan 12, 2015, at which time 222 patients had died. Median overall survival was 25.1 months (95% CI 19.2–not reached) in the dabrafenib and trametinib group versus 18.7 months (15.2–23.7) in the dabrafenib only group (hazard ratio [HR] 0.71, 95% CI 0.55–0.92; P = .0107). Overall survival was 74% at 1 year and 51% at 2 years in the dabrafenib and trametinib group versus 68% and 42%, respectively, in the dabrafenib-only group. Based on 301 events, median progression-free survival was 11.0 months (95% CI 8.0–13.9) in the dabrafenib and trametinib group and 8.8 months (5.9–9.3) in the dabrafenib-only group (HR 0.67, 95% CI 0.53–0.84; P = .0004; unadjusted for multiple testing). Treatment-related adverse events occurred in 181 (87%) of 209 patients in the dabrafenib and trametinib group and 189 (90%) of 211 patients in the dabrafenib-only group; the most common was pyrexia (108 patients, 52%) in the dabrafenib and trametinib group, and hyperkeratosis (70 patients, 33%) in the dabrafenib-only group. Grade 3 or 4 adverse events occurred in 67 (32%) patients in the dabrafenib and trametinib group and 66 (31%) patients in the dabrafenib only group.

Interpretation The improvement in overall survival establishes the combination of dabrafenib and trametinib as the standard targeted treatment for BRAF Val600 mutation-positive melanoma. Studies assessing dabrafenib and trametinib in combination with immunotherapies are ongoing.

Editor's comments
Single-agent BRAF inhibition is associated with reactivation of the MAP kinase pathway, and also accumulation of multiple squamous cell cancers secondary to paradoxic activation of wild-type cells. This article demonstrates the efficacy of dual-agent MAP kinase inhibition with BRAF and MEK inhibitors, with improvement in PFS and overall survival. The results of this trial have been repeated with dabrafenib + trametinib demonstrating improved survival over vemurafenib alone, and vemurafenib + cobimetinib demonstrating improved survival over vemurafenib alone. In addition, the incidence of squamous cell cancer and keratoacanthomas was significantly decreased with the combination agents. Therefore, single-agent therapy has been largely supplanted by combination BRAF/MEK inhibition in patients who can tolerate it.

Hodi FS, O'Day SJ, McDermott DF, et al. Improved survival with ipilimumab in patients with metastatic melanoma. N Engl J Med 2010;363:711.

Hypothesis
Checkpoint blockade will improve survival over vaccination.

No. Patients Randomized	Study Groups	Stratification	Significance Demonstrated	% Change Identified in Trial
676	Ipilimumab + gp100 vaccine vs Ipilimumab vs gp100 vaccine		Overall survival	Overall survival 10 vs 6.4 mo (HR 0.68)

Background An improvement in overall survival among patients with metastatic melanoma has been an elusive goal. In this phase 3 study, ipilimumab—which blocks cytotoxic T-lymphocyte-associated antigen 4 to potentiate an antitumor T-cell response—administered with or without a glycoprotein 100 (gp100) peptide vaccine was compared with gp100 alone in patients with previously treated metastatic melanoma.

Methods A total of 676 HLA-A*0201–positive patients with unresectable stage III or IV melanoma, whose disease had progressed while they were receiving therapy for metastatic disease, were randomly assigned, in a 3:1:1 ratio, to receive ipilimumab plus gp100 (403 patients), ipilimumab alone (137), or gp100 alone (136). Ipilimumab, at a dose of 3 mg per kilogram of body weight, was administered with or without gp100 every 3 weeks for up to 4 treatments (induction). Eligible patients could receive reinduction therapy. The primary end point was overall survival.

Results The median overall survival was 10.0 months among patients receiving ipilimumab plus gp100, as compared with 6.4 months among patients receiving gp100 alone (hazard ratio for death, 0.68; $P<.001$). The median overall survival with ipilimumab alone was 10.1 months (hazard ratio for death in the comparison with gp100 alone, 0.66; $P = .003$). No difference in overall survival was detected between the ipilimumab groups (hazard ratio with ipilimumab plus gp100, 1.04; $P = .76$). Grade 3 or 4 immune-related adverse events occurred in 10% to 15% of patients treated with ipilimumab and in 3% treated with gp100 alone. There were 14 deaths related to the study drugs (2.1%), and 7 were associated with immune-related adverse events.

Conclusions Ipilimumab, with or without a gp100 peptide vaccine, as compared with gp100 alone, improved overall survival in patients with previously treated metastatic melanoma. Adverse events can be severe, long-lasting, or both, but most are reversible with appropriate treatment.

Editor's note
This is the first RCT to demonstrate efficacy of immunotherapy with checkpoint blockade. There was no benefit of the gp100 vaccine to ipilimumab. Subsequent trials demonstrated improved survival of ipilimumab over DTIC as well.[38] Although the response rate is low, the responses are durable.

Robert C, Schachter J, Long GV, et al. Pembrolizumab versus ipilimumab in advanced melanoma. N Engl J Med 2015;372:2521.

Hypothesis
PD-1 blockade will improve survival over CTLA-4 blockade.

No. Patients Randomized	Study Groups	Stratification	Significance Demonstrated	% Change Identified in Trial
834	Pembrolizumab 10 mg every 2 wk, pembrolizumab 10 mg/kg every 3 wk, ipilimumab 3 mg/kg every 3 wk for 4 doses		PFS and overall survival	PFS 39 and 38 vs 19% at 12 mo, overall survival 2-y survival 55, 55 vs 43% (HR 0.68)

Background The immune checkpoint inhibitor ipilimumab is the standard-of-care treatment for patients with advanced melanoma. Pembrolizumab inhibits the programmed cell death 1 (PD-1) immune checkpoint and has antitumor activity in patients with advanced melanoma.

Methods In this randomized, controlled, phase 3 study, we assigned 834 patients with advanced melanoma in a 1:1:1 ratio to receive pembrolizumab (at a dose of 10 mg per kilogram of body weight) every 2 weeks or every 3 weeks or 4 doses of ipilimumab (at 3 mg per kilogram) every 3 weeks. Primary end points were progression-free and overall survival.

Results The estimated 6-month progression-free survival rates were 47.3% for pembrolizumab every 2 weeks, 46.4% for pembrolizumab every 3 weeks, and 26.5% for ipilimumab (hazard ratio for disease progression, 0.58; $P<.001$ for both pembrolizumab regimens vs ipilimumab; 95% confidence intervals [CIs], 0.46–0.72 and 0.47–0.72, respectively). Estimated 12-month survival rates were 74.1%, 68.4%, and 58.2%, respectively (hazard ratio for death for pembrolizumab every 2 weeks, 0.63; 95% CI, 0.47–0.83; $P = .0005$; hazard ratio for pembrolizumab every 3 weeks, 0.69; 95% CI, 0.52–0.90; $P = .0036$). The response rate was improved with pembrolizumab administered every 2 weeks (33.7%) and every 3 weeks (32.9%), as compared with ipilimumab (11.9%) ($P<.001$ for both comparisons). Responses were ongoing in 89.4%, 96.7%, and 87.9% of patients, respectively, after a median follow-up of 7.9 months. Efficacy was similar in the 2 pembrolizumab groups. Rates of treatment-related adverse events of grade 3 to 5 severity were lower in the pembrolizumab groups (13.3% and 10.1%) than in the ipilimumab group (19.9%).

Conclusions The anti-PD-1 antibody pembrolizumab prolonged progression-free survival and overall survival and had less high-grade toxicity than did ipilimumab in patients with advanced melanoma.

Editor's note
PD-1 was the second checkpoint inhibitor to demonstrate efficacy in the treatment of metastatic melanoma and be approved for use. It is notable for a higher response rate, and a lower toxicity profile than CTLA-4 blockade.

Larkin J, Chiarion-Sileni V, Gonzalez R, et al. Combined nivolumab and ipilimumab or monotherapy in untreated melanoma. N Engl J Med 2015;373:23.

Hypothesis
Combination CTLA-4 and PD-1 blockade improved survival in patients with melanoma.

No. Patients Randomized	Study Groups	Stratification	Significance Demonstrated	% Change Identified in Trial
945	Nivolumab + ipilimumab Versus nivolumab vs ipilimumab		PFS and overall survival	PFS 39 and 38 vs 19% at 12 mo, overall survival 2-y survival 55, 55 vs 43% (HR 0.68)

Background Nivolumab (a programmed death 1 [PD-1] checkpoint inhibitor) and ipilimumab (a cytotoxic T-lymphocyte-associated antigen 4 [CTLA-4] checkpoint inhibitor) have been shown to have complementary activity in metastatic melanoma. In this randomized, double-blind, phase 3 study, nivolumab alone or nivolumab plus ipilimumab was compared with ipilimumab alone in patients with metastatic melanoma.

Methods We assigned, in a 1:1:1 ratio, 945 previously untreated patients with unresectable stage III or IV melanoma to nivolumab alone, nivolumab plus ipilimumab, or ipilimumab alone. Progression-free survival and overall survival were coprimary end points. Results regarding progression-free survival are presented here.

Results The median progression-free survival was 11.5 months (95% confidence interval [CI], 8.9–16.7) with nivolumab plus ipilimumab, as compared with 2.9 months (95% CI, 2.8–3.4) with ipilimumab (hazard ratio for death or disease progression, 0.42; 99.5% CI, 0.31–0.57; $P<.001$), and 6.9 months (95% CI, 4.3–9.5) with nivolumab (hazard ratio for the comparison with ipilimumab, 0.57; 99.5% CI, 0.43–0.76; $P<.001$). In patients with tumors positive for the PD-1 ligand (PD-L1), the median progression-free survival was 14.0 months in the nivolumab-plus-ipilimumab group and in the nivolumab group, but in patients with PD-L1-negative tumors, progression-free survival was longer with the combination therapy than with nivolumab alone (11.2 months [95% CI, 8.0 to not reached] vs 5.3 months [95% CI, 2.8–7.1]). Treatment-related adverse events of grade 3 or 4 occurred in 16.3% of the patients in the nivolumab group, 55.0% of those in the nivolumab-plus-ipilimumab group, and 27.3% of those in the ipilimumab group.

Conclusions Among previously untreated patients with metastatic melanoma, nivolumab alone or combined with ipilimumab resulted in significantly longer progression-free survival than ipilimumab alone. In patients with PD-L1-negative tumors, the combination of PD-1 and CTLA-4 blockade was more effective than either agent alone.

Editor's note
This trial was based on earlier reports of markedly improved response rates in combination immunotherapy. The increased response rate with combination ipilimumab/nivolumab are associated with increased side effects. Data have suggested that high PD-L1 expression can identify those patients who do not need to have combination treatment, but these data need to be confirmed.

REFERENCES

1. Dong XD, Tyler D, Johnson JL, et al. Analysis of prognosis and disease progression after local recurrence of melanoma. Cancer 2000;88:1063–71.

2. Khayat D, Rixe O, Martin G, et al, French Group of Research on Malignant Melanoma. Surgical margins in cutaneous melanoma (2 cm versus 5 cm for lesions measuring less than 2.1-mm thick). Cancer 2003;97:1941–6.

3. Thomas JM, Newton-Bishop J, A'Hern R, et al, United Kingdom Melanoma Study Group, British Association of Plastic Surgeons, Scottish Cancer Therapy Network. Excision margins in high-risk malignant melanoma. N Engl J Med 2004;350: 757–66.

4. Balch CM, Soong S, Ross MI, et al. Long-term results of a multi-institutional randomized trial comparing prognostic factors and surgical results for intermediate thickness melanomas (1.0 to 4.0 mm). Intergroup Melanoma Surgical Trial. Ann Surg Oncol 2000;7:87–97.

5. Morton DL, Thompson JF, Cochran AJ, et al. Final trial report of sentinel-node biopsy versus nodal observation in melanoma. N Engl J Med 2014;370:599–609.

6. Leiter U, Stadler R, Mauch C, et al, German Dermatologic Cooperative Oncology Group (DeCOG). Complete lymph node dissection versus no dissection in patients with sentinel lymph node biopsy positive melanoma (DeCOG-SLT): a multicentre, randomised, phase 3 trial. Lancet Oncol 2016;17:757–67.

7. Cascinelli N, Morabito A, Santinami M, et al. Immediate or delayed dissection of regional nodes in patients with melanoma of the trunk: a randomised trial. WHO Melanoma Programme. Lancet 1998;351:793–6.

8. Cornett WR, McCall LM, Petersen RP, et al, American College of Surgeons Oncology Group Trial Z0020. Randomized multicenter trial of hyperthermic isolated limb perfusion with melphalan alone compared with melphalan plus tumor necrosis factor: American College of Surgeons Oncology Group Trial Z0020. J Clin Oncol 2006;24:4196–201.

9. Deroose JP, Eggermont AM, van Geel AN, et al. 20 years experience of TNF-based isolated limb perfusion for in-transit melanoma metastases: TNF dose matters. Ann Surg Oncol 2012;19:627–35.

10. Kirkwood JM, Strawderman MH, Ernstoff MS, et al. Interferon alfa-2b adjuvant therapy of high-risk resected cutaneous melanoma: the Eastern Cooperative Oncology Group Trial EST 1684. J Clin Oncol 1996;14:7–17.

11. Kirkwood JM, Ibrahim JG, Sondak VK, et al. High- and low-dose interferon alfa-2b in high-risk melanoma: first analysis of intergroup trial E1690/S9111/C9190. J Clin Oncol 2000;18:2444–58.

12. Hancock BW, Wheatley K, Harris S, et al. Adjuvant interferon in high-risk melanoma: the AIM HIGH Study–United Kingdom Coordinating Committee on Cancer Research randomized study of adjuvant low-dose extended-duration interferon Alfa-2a in high-risk resected malignant melanoma. J Clin Oncol 2004;22:53–61.

13. Eggermont AM, Suciu S, MacKie R, et al. Post-surgery adjuvant therapy with intermediate doses of interferon alfa 2b versus observation in patients with stage IIb/III melanoma (EORTC 18952): randomised controlled trial. Lancet 2005;366: 1189–96.

14. Eggermont AM, Suciu S, Santinami M, et al. Adjuvant therapy with pegylated interferon alfa-2b versus observation alone in resected stage III melanoma: final results of EORTC 18991, a randomised phase III trial. Lancet 2008;372:117–26.

15. Garbe C, Radny P, Linse R, et al. Adjuvant low-dose interferon {alpha}2a with or without dacarbazine compared with surgery alone: a prospective-randomized phase III DeCOG trial in melanoma patients with regional lymph node metastasis. Ann Oncol 2008;19:1195–201.

16. Kirkwood JM, Ibrahim JG, Sosman JA, et al. High-dose interferon alfa-2b significantly prolongs relapse-free and overall survival compared with the GM2-KLH/QS-21 vaccine in patients with resected stage IIB-III melanoma: results of intergroup trial E1694/S9512/C509801. J Clin Oncol 2001;19:2370–80.

17. Mitchell MS, Abrams J, Thompson JA, et al. Randomized trial of an allogeneic melanoma lysate vaccine with low-dose interferon Alfa-2b compared with high-dose interferon Alfa-2b for Resected stage III cutaneous melanoma. J Clin Oncol 2007;25:2078–85.

18. Agarwala SS, Neuberg D, Park Y, et al. Mature results of a phase III randomized trial of bacillus Calmette-Guerin (BCG) versus observation and BCG plus dacarbazine versus BCG in the adjuvant therapy of American Joint Committee on Cancer Stage I-III melanoma (E1673): a trial of the Eastern Oncology Group. Cancer 2004;100:1692–8.

19. Morton DL, Hsueh EC, Essner R, et al. Prolonged survival of patients receiving active immunotherapy with Canvaxin therapeutic polyvalent vaccine after complete resection of melanoma metastatic to regional lymph nodes. Ann Surg 2002;236:438–48 [discussion 448–9].

20. Shu S, Cochran AJ, Huang RR, et al. Immune responses in the draining lymph nodes against cancer: implications for immunotherapy. Cancer Metastasis Rev 2006;25:233–42.

21. Eggermont AM, Chiarion-Sileni V, Grob JJ, et al. Prolonged survival in stage III melanoma with ipilimumab adjuvant therapy. N Engl J Med 2016;375:1845–55.

22. Cocconi G, Bella M, Calabresi F, et al. Treatment of metastatic malignant melanoma with dacarbazine plus tamoxifen. N Engl J Med 1992;327:516–23.

23. Chapman PB, Einhorn LH, Meyers ML, et al. Phase III multicenter randomized trial of the Dartmouth regimen versus dacarbazine in patients with metastatic melanoma. J Clin Oncol 1999;17:2745–51.

24. Middleton MR, Grob JJ, Aaronson N, et al. Randomized phase III study of temozolomide versus dacarbazine in the treatment of patients with advanced metastatic malignant melanoma. J Clin Oncol 2000;18:158–66.

25. Bafaloukos D, Tsoutsos D, Kalofonos H, et al. Temozolomide and cisplatin versus temozolomide in patients with advanced melanoma: a randomized phase II study of the Hellenic Cooperative Oncology Group. Ann Oncol 2005;16:950–7.

26. Keilholz U, Goey SH, Punt CJ, et al. Interferon alfa-2a and interleukin-2 with or without cisplatin in metastatic melanoma: a randomized trial of the European Organization for Research and Treatment of Cancer Melanoma Cooperative Group. J Clin Oncol 1997;15:2579–88.

27. Sparano JA, Fisher RI, Sunderland M, et al. Randomized phase III trial of treatment with high-dose interleukin-2 either alone or in combination with interferon alfa-2a in patients with advanced melanoma. J Clin Oncol 1993;11:1969–77.

28. Atkins MB, Hsu J, Lee S, et al. Phase III trial comparing concurrent biochemotherapy with cisplatin, vinblastine, dacarbazine, interleukin-2, and interferon alfa-2b with cisplatin, vinblastine, and dacarbazine alone in patients with metastatic malignant melanoma (E3695): a trial coordinated by the Eastern Cooperative Oncology Group. J Clin Oncol 2008;26:5748–54.

29. Hodi FS, O'Day SJ, McDermott DF, et al. Improved survival with ipilimumab in patients with metastatic melanoma. N Engl J Med 2010;363:711–23.

30. Prieto PA, Yang JC, Sherry RM, et al. CTLA-4 blockade with ipilimumab: long-term follow-up of 177 patients with metastatic melanoma. Clin Cancer Res 2012;18:2039–47.

31. Topalian SL, Hodi FS, Brahmer JR, et al. Safety, activity, and immune correlates of anti-PD-1 antibody in cancer. N Engl J Med 2012;366:2443–54.

32. Wolchok JD, Kluger H, Callahan MK, et al. Nivolumab plus ipilimumab in advanced melanoma. N Engl J Med 2013;369:122–33.

33. Flaherty KT, Puzanov I, Kim KB, et al. Inhibition of mutated, activated BRAF in metastatic melanoma. N Engl J Med 2010;363:809–19.
34. Ribas A, Gonzalez R, Pavlick A, et al. Combination of vemurafenib and cobimetinib in patients with advanced BRAF(V600)-mutated melanoma: a phase 1b study. Lancet Oncol 2014;15:954–65.
35. Long GV, Stroyakovskiy D, Gogas H, et al. Dabrafenib and trametinib versus dabrafenib and placebo for Val600 BRAF-mutant melanoma: a multicentre, double-blind, phase 3 randomised controlled trial. Lancet 2015;386:444–51.
36. Kim KB, Eton O, Davis DW, et al. Phase II trial of imatinib mesylate in patients with metastatic melanoma. Br J Cancer 2008;99:734–40.
37. Hayes AJ, Maynard L, Coombes G, et al, UK Melanoma Study Group, British Association of Plastic, Reconstructive and Aesthetic Surgeons, Scottish Cancer Therapy Network. Wide versus narrow excision margins for high-risk, primary cutaneous melanomas: long-term follow-up of survival in a randomised trial. Lancet Oncol 2016;17:184–92.
38. Robert C, Thomas L, Bondarenko I, et al. Ipilimumab plus dacarbazine for previously untreated metastatic melanoma. N Engl J Med 2011;364:2517–26.
39. Veronesi U, Cascinelli N. Narrow excision (1-cm margin). A safe procedure for thin cutaneous melanoma. Arch Surg 1991;126:438–41.
40. Ringborg U, Andersson R, Eldh J, et al. Resection margins of 2 versus 5 cm for cutaneous malignant melanoma with a tumor thickness of 0.8 to 2.0 mm: randomized study by the Swedish Melanoma Study Group. Cancer 1996;77:1809–14.
41. Sim FH, Taylor WF, Ivins JC, et al. A prospective randomized study of the efficacy of routine elective lymphadenectomy in management of malignant melanoma. Preliminary results. Cancer 1978;41:948–56.
42. Veronesi U, Adamus J, Bandiera DC, et al. Delayed regional lymph node dissection in stage I melanoma of the skin of the lower extremities. Cancer 1982;49:2420–30.
43. Balch CM, Soong SJ, Bartolucci AA, et al. Efficacy of an elective regional lymph node dissection of 1 to 4 mm thick melanomas for patients 60 years of age and younger. Ann Surg 1996;224:255–63 [discussion: 263–6].

An Update on Randomized Clinical Trials in Breast Cancer

 CrossMark

Kayla Barnard, MD, V. Suzanne Klimberg, MD, PhD*

KEYWORDS

- Breast cancer • Randomized clinical trials (RCT) • Axillary staging
- Lymphadenectomy • Sentinel lymph node (SLN) • Breast conservation therapy (BCT)

KEY POINTS

- Numerous clinical trials reveal new innovations and therapies that continually change the treatment and prevention of breast cancer.
- Earlier trials have changed the standard of care from radical mastectomy to breast conservation therapy and individualized treatment based on tumor-specific biology.
- As research continues and long-term follow-up results become available, updated reviews on randomized clinics trials become exceedingly important in discerning the most effective and oncologically safe therapies to provide optimal outcomes.

INTRODUCTION

In 2016, more than 250,000 women were predicted to be diagnosed with breast cancer. Representing 14.6% of all new cancer cases in the United States, breast cancer is the most common cancer among women. Numerous clinical trials reveal new innovations and therapies that continually change the treatment and prevention of breast cancer. Earlier trials have changed the standard of care from radical mastectomy to breast conservation therapy (BCT) and individualized treatment based on tumor-specific biology. The landmark randomized clinical trials (RCT) in breast cancer were published in the 2002 and 2010 editions of this publication. As research continues and long-term follow-up results become available, updated reviews on RCTs become exceedingly important in discerning the most effective and oncologically safe therapies to provide optimal outcomes. Many of the published RCTs in the last 7 years have focused on decreasing the overtreatment of breast cancer.

Disclosure: The authors have nothing to disclose.
Winthrop P. Rockefeller Cancer Institute, Little Rock, AR, USA
* Corresponding author.
E-mail address: klimberg1954@gmail.com

Surg Oncol Clin N Am 26 (2017) 587–620
http://dx.doi.org/10.1016/j.soc.2017.05.013
1055-3207/17/Published by Elsevier Inc.

LEVEL IA EVIDENCE: PROSPECTIVE RANDOMIZED SURGICAL TRIALS AND META-ANALYSES IN BREAST CANCER

Litiere S, Werutsky G, Fentiman IS, et al. Breast conserving therapy versus mastectomy for stage I-II breast cancer: 20 year follow-up of the EORTC 10801 phase 3 randomized trial. Lancet Oncol 2012;13(4):412–19.[1]

Hypothesis

BCT is an oncologically safe treatment of breast cancer.

Published Abstract

Background
The European Organisation for Research and Treatment of Cancer (EORTC) 10801 trial compared BCT with modified radical mastectomy (MRM) in patients with tumors 5 cm or smaller and axillary node-negative or node-positive disease. Compared with BCT, MRM resulted in better local control, but did not affect overall survival (OS) or time to distant metastases. This study reports 20-year follow-up results.

Methods
The EORTC 10801 trial was open for accrual between 1980 and 1986 in 8 centers in the United Kingdom, the Netherlands, Belgium, and South Africa. The trial randomized 448 patients to BCT and 420 to MRM. Randomization was done centrally, stratifying patients by institute, carcinoma stage (I or II), and menopausal status. BCT comprised lumpectomy and complete axillary clearance, followed by breast radiotherapy and a tumor-bed boost. The primary end point was time to distant metastasis. This analysis was done on all eligible patients, as they were randomized.

Findings
After a median follow-up of 22.1 years (interquartile range [IQR], 18.5–23.8), 175 patients (42%) had distant metastases in the MRM group versus 207 (46%) in the BCT group. Furthermore, 506 patients (58%) died (232 [55%] in the MRM group and 274 [61%] in the BCT group). No significant difference was observed between BCT and MRM for time to distant metastases (hazard ratio [HR], 1.13; 95% confidence interval [CI], 0.92–1.38; $P = .23$) or for time to death (HR, 1.11; 95% CI, 0.94–1.33; $P = .23$). Cumulative incidence of distant metastases at 20 years was 42.6% (95% CI, 37.8–47.5) in the MRM group and 46.9% (42.2–51.6) in the BCT group. Twenty-year OS was estimated to be 44.5% (95% CI, 39.3–49.5) in the MRM group and 39.1% (34.4–43.9) in the BCT group. There was no difference between the groups in time to distant metastases or OS by age (time to distant metastases: <50 years 1.09 [95% CI, 0.79–1.51] vs ≥50 years 1.16 [0.90–1.50]; OS <50 years 1.17 [0.86–1.59] vs ≥50 years 1.10 [0.89–1.37]).

Interpretation
BCT, including radiotherapy, offered as standard care to patients with early breast cancer seems to be justified, because long-term follow-up in this trial showed similar survival to that after mastectomy.

Editorial comments RCTs have established the safety of BCT compared with mastectomy. The National Surgical Adjuvant Breast and Bowel Project (NSABP) B-06 trial compared patients with tumors less than 4 cm undergoing partial mastectomy and axillary node dissection or MRM. At 20 years, there was no difference in OS or disease-free survival (DFS). However, local recurrence was increased in the BCT group compared with the MRM group. Furthermore, results showed ipsilateral breast tumor recurrence (IBTR) to be higher in the group that underwent partial mastectomy versus partial mastectomy followed by whole-breast radiation.[2] Likewise, the Milan trial compared radical mastectomy with partial mastectomy followed by radiation in women with invasive breast cancer less than 2 cm. The long-term results have reflected those of NSABP B-06 with a significant difference in local recurrence: 8.8% for BCT versus 2.3% for radical mastectomy.[3] Survival outcomes were not significantly different between the two groups. At the time of EORTC 10801 enrollment, patients with breast tumors less than 5 cm were randomized to BCT or MRM. Results have been consistent with the previous similar trials showing an increase in local recurrence, but no significant difference in OS or time to distant metastasis. Death rates were also increased with tumor size greater than 2 cm and lymph node metastasis across both treatment groups, showing the safety of BCT in patients with larger tumors and/or axillary metastasis.[4] Also of consideration is the 48% rate of positive margins in the BCT group when comparing EORTC 10801 with the previously mentioned trials. Local recurrence rates were higher in the EORTC study, supporting that resection to negative margins is essential.[5,6]

LEVEL IA EVIDENCE: PROSPECTIVE RANDOMIZED TRIALS AND META-ANALYSES ON EVALUATION AND MANAGEMENT OF THE AXILLA IN BREAST CANCER

Krag DN, Anderson SJ, Julian TB, et al. Sentinel-lymph-node resection compared with conventional axillary-lymph-node dissection in clinically node-negative patients with breast cancer: overall survival findings from the NSABP B-32 randomized phase 3 trial. Lancet Oncol 2010;11:927–33.[7]

Hypothesis

Sentinel lymph node (SLN) dissection is equal to axillary lymph node dissection.

Published Abstract

Background
SLN surgery was designed to minimize the side effects of lymph node surgery but still offer outcomes equivalent to axillary lymph node dissection (ALND). The aims of NSABP trial B-32 were to establish whether SLN resection in patients with breast cancer achieves the same survival and regional control as ALND, but with fewer side effects.

Methods
NSABP B-32 was a randomized controlled phase 3 trial done at 80 centers in Canada and the United States between May 1, 1999, and February 29, 2004. Women with invasive breast cancer were randomly assigned to either SLN resection plus ALND (group 1) or to SLN resection alone with ALND only if the SLNs were positive (group 2). Random assignment was done at the NSABP Biostatistical Center (Pittsburgh, PA) with a biased-coin minimization approach in an allocation ratio of 1:1. Stratification variables were age at entry ($\leq$49 years, $\geq$50 years), clinical tumor size ($\leq$2.0 cm, 2.1–4.0 cm, $\geq$4.1 cm), and surgical plan (lumpectomy, mastectomy). SLN resection was done with a blue dye and radioactive tracer. Outcome analyses were done in patients who were assessed as having pathologically negative sentinel nodes and for whom follow-up data were available. The primary end point was OS. Analyses were done on an intention-to-treat basis. All deaths, irrespective of cause, were included. The mean time on study for the SLN-negative patients with follow-up information was 95.6 months (range, 70.1–126.7). This study is registered with ClinicalTrials. gov, number NCT00003830.

Findings

A total of 5611 women were randomly assigned to the treatment groups, and 3989 had pathologically negative SLN. Three-hundred and nine deaths were reported in the 3986 SLN-negative patients with follow-up information: 140 of 1975 patients in group 1 and 169 of 2011 in group 2. Log-rank comparison of OS in groups 1 and 2 yielded an unadjusted HR of 1.20 (95% CI, 0.96–1.50; $P = .12$). Eight-year Kaplan-Meier estimates for OS were 91.8% (95% CI, 90.4–93.3) in group 1 and 90.3% (95% CI, 88.8–91.8) in group 2. Treatment comparisons for DFS yielded an unadjusted HR of 1.05 (95% CI, 0.90–1.22; $P = .54$). Eight-year Kaplan-Meier estimates for DFS were 82.4% (95% CI, 80.5–84.4) in group 1 and 81.5% (95% CI, 79.6–83.4) in group 2. There were 8 regional-node recurrences as first events in group 1 and 14 in group 2 ($P = .22$). Patients are continuing follow-up for longer-term assessment of survival and regional control. The most common adverse events were allergic reactions, mostly related to the administration of the blue dye.

Interpretation

OS, DFS, and regional control were statistically equivalent between groups. When the SLN is negative, SLN surgery alone with no further ALND is an appropriate, safe, and effective therapy for patients with breast cancer with clinically negative lymph nodes.

Editorial comments The results of this large, well-run, and well-supervised trial in terms of the appropriateness, safety, and effectiveness of SLN biopsy (SLNB) in patients with favorable node-negative disease showed equivalence in terms of DFS, OS, and locoregional recurrence but significantly lower risk of lymphedema.

Giuliano AE, Ballman K, McCall L, et al. Locoregional recurrence after sentinel lymph node dissection with or without axillary dissection in patients with sentinel lymph node metastases: long-term follow-up from the American College of Surgeons Oncology Group (Alliance) ACOSOG Z0011 Randomized Trial. Ann Surg 2016;264(3):413–20.[8]

Hypothesis

ALND does not decrease local regional recurrence in SLN-positive patients receiving BCT with 2 or fewer SLNs.

Published Abstract

Background and objective

The early results of the American College of Surgeons Oncology Group (ACOSOG) Z0011 trial showed no difference in locoregional recurrence for patients with positive SLNs randomized either to ALND or SLN dissection (SLND) alone. This study now reports long-term locoregional recurrence results.

Methods

ACOSOG Z0011 prospectively examined OS of patients with SLN metastases undergoing BCT randomized to undergo ALND after SLND or no further axillary specific treatment. Locoregional recurrence was prospectively evaluated and compared between the groups.

Results

Four-hundred and forty-six patients were randomized to SLND alone and 445 to SLND and ALND. Both groups were similar with respect to age, Bloom-Richardson score, estrogen receptor (ER) status, adjuvant systemic therapy, histology, and tumor size. Patients randomized to ALND had a median of 17 axillary nodes removed compared with a median of only 2 SLNs removed with SLND alone (P<.001). ALND, as expected, also removed more positive lymph nodes (P<.001). At a median follow-up of 9.25 years, there was no statistically significant difference in local recurrence-free survival (P = .13). The cumulative incidence of nodal recurrences at 10 years was 0.5% in the ALND arm and 1.5% in the SLND alone arm (P = .28). Ten-year cumulative locoregional recurrence was 6.2% with ALND and 5.3% with SLND alone (P = .36).

Conclusions
Despite the potential for residual axillary disease after SLND, SLND without ALND offers excellent regional control for selected patients with early metastatic breast cancer treated with BCT and adjuvant systemic therapy.

Editorial comments This trial was heavily criticized for lack of enrollment, low power, crossover between arms, nonstandardization of radiation therapy, and short follow-up in a very favorable group of patients. This 10-year follow-up shows no difference in survival between ALND or SLND in patients with breast cancer undergoing BCT. However, the original report of this study showed no statistically significant difference in lymphedema between these two randomized arms, perhaps because of x-ray therapy (XRT) to the axilla. This report gives no further insight to that issue.

Galimberti V, Cole BF, Zurrida S, et al. Axillary dissection versus no axillary dissection in patients with sentinel lymph-node micrometastases (IBCSG 23–01): a phase 3 randomised controlled trial. Lancet Oncol 2013;14:297–305.[9]

Hypothesis
Axillary dissection is overtreatment of patients with SLN micrometastases.

Published Abstract

Background
For patients with breast cancer and metastases in the sentinel nodes, axillary dissection has been standard treatment. However, for patients with limited sentinel node involvement, axillary dissection might be overtreatment. The IBCSG (International Breast Cancer Study Group) trial 23-01 was designed to determine whether no axillary dissection was noninferior to axillary dissection in patients with 1 or more micrometastatic ($\leq$2 mm) sentinel nodes and tumors of a maximum 5 cm.

Methods
In this multicenter, randomized, noninferiority, phase 3 trial, patients were eligible if they had clinically nonpalpable axillary lymph nodes and a primary tumor of 5 cm or less and who, after sentinel node biopsy, had 1 or more micrometastatic ($\leq$2 mm) SLNs with no extracapsular extension. Patients were randomly assigned (in a 1:1 ratio) to either undergo axillary dissection or not to undergo axillary dissection. Randomization was stratified by center and menopausal status. Treatment assignment was not masked. The primary end point was DFS. Noninferiority was defined as an HR of less than 1.25 for no axillary dissection versus axillary dissection. The analysis was by intention to treat. Per protocol, disease and survival information continue to be collected yearly. This trial is registered with ClinicalTrials.gov, NCT00072293.

Findings
Between April 1, 2001, and February 28, 2010, 465 patients were randomly assigned to axillary dissection and 469 to no axillary dissection. After the exclusion of 3 patients, 464 patients were in the axillary dissection group and 467 patients were in the no

axillary dissection group. After a median follow-up of 5.0 (IQR, 3.6–7.3) years, we recorded 69 DFS events in the axillary dissection group and 55 events in the no axillary dissection group. Breast cancer–related events were recorded in 48 patients in the axillary dissection group and 47 in the no axillary dissection group (10 local recurrences in the axillary dissection group and 8 in the no axillary dissection group; 3 and 9 contralateral breast cancers; 1 and 5 [corrected] regional recurrences; and 34 and 25 distant relapses). Other non–breast cancer events were recorded in 21 patients in the axillary dissection group and 8 in the no axillary dissection group (20 and 6 second nonbreast malignancies; and 1 and 2 deaths not caused by a cancer event). Five-year DFS was 87.8% (95% CI, 84.4–91.2) in the group without axillary dissection and 84.4% (95% CI, 80.7–88.1) in the group with axillary dissection (log-rank $P = .16$; HR for no axillary dissection vs axillary dissection was 0.78, 95% CI, 0.55–1.11; noninferiority $P = .0042$). Patients with reported long-term surgical events (grade 3–4) included 1 sensory neuropathy (grade 3), 3 lymphedema (2 grade 3 and 1 grade 4), and 3 motor neuropathy (grade 3), all in the group that underwent axillary dissection, and 1 grade 3 motor neuropathy in the group without axillary dissection. One serious adverse event was reported: a postoperative infection in the axilla in the group with axillary dissection.

Interpretation
Axillary dissection could be avoided in patients with early breast cancer and limited sentinel node involvement, thus eliminating complications of axillary surgery with no adverse effect on survival.

Editorial comments Similar to Z-0011, IBCSG 23091 supports the finding that ALND can safely be omitted in selected patients who are clinically node negative. In contrast with Z-0011, in this study all SLN metastases were less than 2 mm, 28% of patients receiving BCT received intraoperative partial breast irradiation (PBI), and 9% of the patients had a mastectomy, connoting the possibility of extended indications to PBI and mastectomy patients with micrometastasis. In this study, 13% of patients with micrometastatic SLNs had additional involved lymph nodes on ALND. The present National Comprehensive Cancer Network (NCCN) guidelines recommend considering using tumor molecular markers (Oncotype DX, Genomic Health Redwood City, CA) for determination of systemic treatment when micrometastatic disease only is present. Whether ALND is needed to determine which patients have truly N1 disease and would benefit from more aggressive systemic treatment is unknown from this study. The results of the ALND compared with SLNB showed no effect of the rate of administration of chemotherapy. Overall, sequelae from ALND were worse than those from SLNB.

Donker M, van Tienhoven G, Straver ME, et al. Radiotherapy or surgery of the axilla after a positive sentinel node in breast cancer (EORTC 10981–22023 AMAROS): a randomized, multicenter, open-label phase 3 non-inferiority trial. Lancet Oncol 2014;15(12):1303–10.[10]

Hypothesis
Axillary radiation provides equal control compared with axillary node dissection in patients with nodal metastases.

Published Abstract

Background
If treatment of the axilla is indicated in patients with breast cancer who have a positive sentinel node, ALND is the present standard. Although ALND provides excellent regional control, it is associated with harmful side effects. The study aimed to assess

whether axillary radiotherapy provides comparable regional control with fewer side effects.

Methods

Patients with T1 to T2 primary breast cancer and no palpable lymphadenopathy were enrolled in the randomized, multicenter, open-label, phase 3 noninferiority EORTC 10981-22023 after mapping of the axilla: radiotherapy or surgery(AMAROS) trial. Patients were randomly assigned (1:1) by a computer-generated allocation schedule to receive either ALND or axillary radiotherapy in case of a positive sentinel node, stratified by institution. The primary end point was noninferiority of 5-year axillary recurrence, considered to be not more than 4% for the axillary radiotherapy group compared with an expected 2% in the ALND group. Analyses were by intention to treat and per protocol. The AMAROS trial is registered with ClinicalTrials.gov, number NCT00014612.

Findings

Between February 19, 2001, and April 29, 2010, 4823 patients were enrolled at 34 centers from 9 European countries, of whom 4806 were eligible for randomization. The study randomly assigned 2402 patients to receive ALND and 2404 to receive axillary radiotherapy. Of the 1425 patients with a positive sentinel node, 744 had been randomly assigned to ALND and 681 to axillary radiotherapy; these patients constituted the intention-to-treat population. Median follow-up was 6.1 years (IQR, 4.1–8.0) for the patients with positive SLNs. In the ALND group, 220 (33%) of 672 patients who underwent ALND had additional positive nodes. Axillary recurrence occurred in 4 of 744 patients in the ALND group and 7 of 681 in the axillary radiotherapy group. Five-year axillary recurrence was 0.43% (95% CI, 0.00–0.92) after ALND versus 1.19% (95% CI, 0.31–2.08) after axillary radiotherapy. The planned noninferiority test was underpowered because of the low number of events. The 1-sided 95% CI for the underpowered noninferiority test on the HR was 0.00 to 5.27, with a noninferiority margin of 2. Lymphedema in the ipsilateral arm was noted significantly more often after ALND than after axillary radiotherapy at 1 year, 3 years, and 5 years.

Interpretation

ALND and axillary radiotherapy after a positive sentinel node provide excellent and comparable axillary control for patients with T1 to T2 primary breast cancer and no palpable lymphadenopathy. Axillary radiotherapy results in significantly less morbidity.

Editorial comments The AMAROS trial, although underpowered for a noninferiority test, showed equivalent survival as well as axillary recurrence compared with axillary XRT in SLN-positive patients. Lymphedema by arm circumference at 5 years was significant higher for ALND (13%) versus XRT (6%), although this was not true of shoulder function or quality of life. "10%" at the beginning of a sentence? of the randomized patients did not have an ALND and nearly 10% of XRT patients crossed over to the ALND group; two-thirds of these had additional positive nodes. In addition, 6% of patients in the ALND group and 2% of patients in the XRT group receive both ALND and XRT. Regardless of the problems with the trial and in light of the results of the preceding trials ACOSOG Z0011 and IBCSG 23-01, most of these patients could have been treated with no further axillary treatment. Most patient (77%) had only 1 positive lymph node and 40% only micrometastatic disease or isolated tumor cells. As such, caution should be exercised in applying these data to patients with more aggressive disease in order to avoid additional toxicity and cost to patient care. Nevertheless, knowledge of full ALND contents did not seem to affect administration of chemotherapy. In addition, the AMAROS trial excluded patients treated with neoadjuvant chemotherapy and thus the results are awaited of Alliance 11202 (NCT01901094), which randomizes patients receiving neoadjuvant chemotherapy and who are SLN positive to ALND or axillary XRT.

Boughey JC, Suman VJ, Mittendorf EA, et al. Sentinel lymph node surgery after neoadjuvant chemotherapy in patients with node-positive breast cancer: The ACOSOG Z1071 (Alliance) clinical trial. JAMA 2013;310:1455–61.[11]

Hypothesis

Using dual mapping (blue dye and radioactivity) to excise the SLNs in patients having undergone neoadjuvant chemotherapy, the false-negative rate (FNR) would be acceptably low (<10%).

Published Abstract

Importance
SLN surgery provides reliable nodal staging information with less morbidity than ALND for patients with clinically node-negative (cN0) breast cancer. The application of SLN surgery for staging the axilla following chemotherapy for women who initially had node-positive cN1 breast cancer is unclear because of high false-negative results reported in previous studies.

Objective
To determine the FNR for SLN surgery following chemotherapy in women initially presenting with biopsy-proven cN1 breast cancer.

Design, setting, and patients
The ACOSOG Z1071 trial enrolled women from 136 institutions from July 2009 to June 2011 who had clinical T0 through T4, N1 through N2, and M0 breast cancer and were receiving neoadjuvant chemotherapy. Following chemotherapy, patients underwent both SLN surgery and ALND. SLN surgery using both blue dye (isosulfan blue or methylene blue), and a radiolabeled colloid mapping agent was encouraged.

Main outcomes and measures
The primary end point was the FNR of SLN surgery after chemotherapy in women who presented with cN1 disease. The Study evaluated the likelihood that the FNR in patients with 2 or more SLNs examined was greater than 10%, which is the rate expected for women undergoing SLN surgery who present with cN0 disease.

Results
Seven-hundred and fifty-six women were enrolled in the study. Of 663 evaluable patients with cN1 disease, 649 underwent chemotherapy followed by both SLN surgery and ALND. An SLN could not be identified in 46 patients (7.1%). Only 1 SLN was excised in 78 patients (12.0%). Of the remaining 525 patients with 2 or more SLNs removed, no cancer was identified in the axillary lymph nodes of 215 patients, yielding a pathologic complete nodal response of 41.0% (95% CI, 36.7%–45.3%). In 39 patients, cancer was not identified in the SLNs but was found in lymph nodes obtained with ALND, resulting in an FNR of 12.6% (90% bayesian credible interval, 9.85%–16.05%).

Conclusions and relevance
Among women with cN1 breast cancer receiving neoadjuvant chemotherapy who had 2 or more SLNs examined, the FNR was not found to be 10% or less. Given this FNR threshold, changes in approach and patient selection that result in greater sensitivity would be necessary to support the use of SLN surgery as an alternative to ALND.

Editorial comments In ACOSOG Z1071 the FNR for SLNB in patients with cN1 breast cancer receiving neoadjuvant chemotherapy(CTX) was unacceptably high. Patient factors, tumor factors, pathologic nodal response to chemotherapy, and site of tracer injection did not affect SLN FNR. However, further analysis of this study showed that the FNR could be reduced by using dual tracer (10.8% vs 20.3%) and examination of at least 3 nodes (9.1% vs 21.1%). In a subsequent analyses, obtaining the clip with the SLN reduced the FNR to 6.8%.[12,13]

Kuehn T, Bauerfeind I, Fehm T, et al. Sentinel-lymph-node biopsy in patients with breast cancer before and after neoadjuvant chemotherapy (SENTINA): A prospective, multicenter cohort study. Lancet Oncol 2013;14:609–18.[14]

Hypothesis

SLN biopsy can be performed reliably after neoadjuvant chemotherapy.

Published Abstract

Background

The optimum timing of SLNB for patients with breast cancer treated with neoadjuvant chemotherapy is uncertain. The SENTINA (SENTinel NeoAdjuvant) study was designed to evaluate a specific algorithm for timing of a standardized SLNB procedure in patients who undergo neoadjuvant chemotherapy.

Methods

SENTINA is a 4-arm, prospective, multicenter cohort study undertaken at 103 institutions in Germany and Austria. Women with breast cancer who were scheduled for neoadjuvant chemotherapy were enrolled into the study. Patients with clinically node-negative disease (cN0) underwent SLNB before neoadjuvant chemotherapy (arm A). If the sentinel node was positive (pN1), a second SLNB procedure was done after neoadjuvant chemotherapy (arm B). Women with clinically node-positive disease (cN+) received neoadjuvant chemotherapy. Those who converted to clinically node-negative disease after chemotherapy (ycN0; arm C) were treated with SLNB and axillary dissection. Only patients whose clinical nodal status remained positive (ycN1) underwent axillary dissection without SLNB (arm D). The primary end point was accuracy (FNR) of SLNB after neoadjuvant chemotherapy for patients who converted from cN1 to ycN0 disease during neoadjuvant chemotherapy (arm C). Secondary end points included comparison of the detection rate of SLNB before and after neoadjuvant chemotherapy, and also the FNR and detection rate of SLNB after removal of the SLN. Analyses were done according to treatment received (per protocol).

Findings

Of 1737 patients who received treatment, 1022 women underwent SLNB before neoadjuvant chemotherapy (arms A and B), with a detection rate of 99.1% (95% CI, 98.3–99.6; 1013 of 1022 patients). In patients who converted after neoadjuvant chemotherapy from cN+ to ycN0 (arm C), the detection rate was 80.1% (95% CI, 76.6–83.2; 474 of 592 patients) and FNR was 14.2% (95% CI, 9.9–19.4; 32 of 226 patients). The FNR was 24.3% (17 of 70 patients) for women who had 1 node removed and 18.5% (10 of 54 patients) for those who had 2 sentinel nodes removed (arm C). In patients who had a second SLNB procedure after neoadjuvant chemotherapy (arm B), the detection rate was 60.8% (95% CI, 55.6–65.9; 219 of 360 patients) and the FNR was 51.6% (95% CI, 38.7–64.2; 33 of 64 patients).

Interpretation

SLNB is a reliable diagnostic method before neoadjuvant chemotherapy. After systemic treatment or early SLNB, the procedure has a lower detection rate and a higher FNR compared with SLNB done before neoadjuvant chemotherapy. These limitations should be considered if biopsy is planned after neoadjuvant chemotherapy.

Editorial comments In this trial, two-thirds of the SLNBs were done using a single tracer. SLN before chemotherapy had a 99% localization rate whether with single or dual tracer. A second SLN after a positive initial SLN had a poor localization rate (80.1%) regardless of the use of lymphoscintigraphy as well as a poor FNR (51.6%). Conversion of a clinically positive node to a clinically negative node (arm C) had an FNR of 16.0% with radiocolloid alone and 8.6% with dual tracer. Overall, FNR reduced with the increased number of SLNs removed. Clips placed in clinically N1 lymph nodes and the impact on FNR were not analyzed. Localization in all groups favored periareolar injection rather than peritumoral or subcutaneous injection. In a subsequent analysis of the ultrasonography data obtained prospectively on the study, Schwentner and colleagues[15] showed that clinical evaluation after neoadjuvant chemotherapy was very poor whether by palpation or ultrasonography. In those patients initially presenting with cN1, the accuracy of nodal evaluation after neoadjuvant chemotherapy by palpation had a sensitivity of 8.3%, specificity of 94.8%, and a negative predictive value (NPV) of 46.6%. Ultrasonography alone revealed a sensitivity of 23.9%, specificity of 91.7%, and an NPV of 50.3%. Palpation and ultrasonography together resulted in a sensitivity of 24.4%, specificity of 91.4%, and an NPV of 50.3%. Placement of clips in cN1(by ultrasonography) patients followed by chemotherapy and then SLNB clearly gives patients the best chance for the least morbid procedure because as many as 40% of these patients convert to node-negative status. An SLNB ahead of time if positive predetermines these patients for an ALND or XRT because the accuracy of a second SLN is so poor.

LEVEL IA EVIDENCE: PROSPECTIVE RANDOMIZED TRIALS AND META-ANALYSES ON RADIATION IN BREAST CANCER

Wapnir IL, Dignam JJ, Fisher B, et al. Long-term outcomes of invasive ipsilateral breast tumor recurrences after lumpectomy in NSABP B-17 and B-24 randomized clinical trials for DCIS. J Natl Cancer Inst. 2011;103(6):478–88.[16]

Hypothesis

In NSABP studies on ductal carcinoma in situ (DCIS), IBTR would negatively affect survival.

Published Abstract

Background
IBTR is the most common failure event after lumpectomy for DCIS. This study evaluated invasive IBTR (I-IBTR) and its influence on survival among participants in 2 NSABP randomized trials for DCIS.

Methods
In the NSABP B-17 trial (accrual period: October 1, 1985, to December 31, 1990), patients with localized DCIS were randomly assigned to the lumpectomy only (LO; n = 403) group or to the lumpectomy followed by radiotherapy (LRT; n = 410) group. In the NSABP B-24 double-blinded, placebo-controlled trial (accrual period: May 9, 1991, to April 13, 1994), all accrued patients were randomly assigned to LRT

plus placebo (n = 900) or LRT plus tamoxifen (TAM; n = 899). End points included I-IBTR, DCIS-IBTR, contralateral breast cancers, overall and breast cancer–specific survival, and survival after I-IBTR. Median follow-up was 207 months for the B-17 trial (N = 813 patients) and 163 months for the B-24 trial (N = 1799 patients).

Results

Of 490 IBTR events, 263 (53.7%) were invasive. Radiation reduced I-IBTR by 52% in the LRT group compared with LO (B-17, HR of risk of I-IBTR = 0.48; 95% CI, 0.33–0.69; P<.001). LRT plus TAM reduced I-IBTR by 32% compared with LRT plus placebo (B-24, HR of risk of I-IBTR = 0.68, 95% CI, 0.49–0.95, P = .025). The 15-year cumulative incidence of I-IBTR was 19.4% for LO, 8.9% for LRT (B-17), 10.0% for LRT plus placebo (B-24), and 8.5% for LRT plus TAM. The 15-year cumulative incidence of all contralateral breast cancers was 10.3% for LO, 10.2% for LRT (B-17), 10.8% for LRT plus placebo (B-24), and 7.3% for LRT plus TAM. I-IBTR was associated with increased mortality risk (HR of death = 1.75; 95% CI, 1.45–2.96; P<.001), whereas recurrence of DCIS was not. Twenty-two of 39 deaths after I-IBTR were attributed to breast cancer. Among all patients (with or without I-IBTR), the 15-year cumulative incidence of breast cancer death was 3.1% for LO, 4.7% for LRT (B-17), 2.7% for LRT plus placebo (B-24), and 2.3% for LRT plus TAM.

Conclusions

Although I-IBTR increased the risk for breast cancer–related death, radiation therapy and tamoxifen reduced I-IBTR, and long-term prognosis remained excellent after breast-conserving surgery for DCIS.

Editorial comments As expected, a recurrence of DCIS does not affect survival. An invasive recurrence would be expected to affect survival, and the relative risk is 1.75. Long-term prognosis with lumpectomy alone versus lumpectomy plus tamoxifen plus XRT is less than 5% and virtually the same regardless of treatment. However, the psychosocial impact of any recurrence should not be underestimated.

Hughes KS, Schnaper LA, Bellon JR, et al. Lumpectomy plus tamoxifen with or without irradiation in women age 70 years or older with early breast cancer: long-term follow-up of CALGB 9343. J Clin Oncol 2013; 31 (19):2382–87.[17]

Hypothesis

Adjuvant radiation does not provide meaningful benefit in a specific subgroup with favorable tumor biology.

Published Abstract

Purpose

To determine whether there is a benefit to adjuvant radiation therapy after breast-conserving surgery and tamoxifen in women aged 70 years and older with early-stage breast cancer.

Methods

Between July 1994 and February 1999, 636 women (aged ≥ 70 years) who had clinical stage I (T1N0M0 according to TNM [tumor, node, metastasis] classification) ER (ER)–positive breast carcinoma treated by lumpectomy were randomly assigned to receive tamoxifen plus radiation therapy (TamRT; 317 women) or tamoxifen alone (Tam; 319 women). Primary end points were time to local or regional recurrence, frequency of mastectomy, breast cancer–specific survival, time to distant metastasis, and OS.

Results
Median follow-up for treated patients is now 12.6 years. At 10 years, 98% of patients receiving TamRT (95% CI, 96%–99%) compared with 90% of those receiving Tam (95% CI, 85%–93%) were free from local and regional recurrences. There were no significant differences in time to mastectomy, time to distant metastasis, breast cancer–specific survival, or OS between the two groups. Ten-year OS was 67% (95% CI, 62%–72%) and 66% (95% CI, 61%–71%) in the TamRT and Tam groups, respectively.

Conclusions
With long-term follow-up, the previously observed small improvement in locoregional recurrence with the addition of radiation therapy remains. However, this does not translate into an advantage in OS, distant DFS, or breast preservation. Depending on the value placed on local recurrence, Tam remains a reasonable option for women aged 70 years or older with ER-positive early-stage breast cancer.

Editorial comments This study of patients aged 70 years or older with early-stage favorable breast cancer originally published a 5-year follow-up that showed no significant difference in locoregional recurrence rate, which was highly touted. Because recurrence steadily increases over time, especially with favorable tumors, the most recent publication shows an 8% locoregional recurrence-free advantage with XRT and tamoxifen versus tamoxifen alone. Again, the psychosocial impact of any recurrence should not be underestimated but this study does give room for patient choice and for less morbid alternatives, such as intracavitary hyperthermia.

Early Breast Cancer Trialists' Collaborative Group (EBCTCG), Darby S, McGale P, Correa C, et al. Effect of radiotherapy after breast-conserving surgery on 10-year recurrence and 15-year breast cancer death: meta-analysis of individual patient data for 10,801 women in 17 randomised trials. Lancet 2011;378(9804):1707–16.[18]

Hypothesis
The benefit of radiation may vary by tumor and patient characteristics.

Published Abstract

Background
After breast-conserving surgery, radiotherapy reduces recurrence and breast cancer death, but it may do so more for some groups of women than for others. This study describes the absolute magnitude of these reductions according to various prognostic and other patient characteristics, and relates the absolute reduction in 15-year risk of breast cancer death to the absolute reduction in 10-year recurrence risk.

Methods
The study undertook a meta-analysis of individual patient data for 10,801 women in 17 randomized trials of radiotherapy versus no radiotherapy after breast-conserving surgery, 8337 of whom had pathologically confirmed node-negative (pN0) or node-positive (pN+) disease.

Findings
Overall, radiotherapy reduced the 10-year risk of any (ie, locoregional or distant) first recurrence from 35.0% to 19.3% (absolute reduction, 15.7%; 95% CI, 13.7–17.7; 2-sided significance level [2P]<.00001) and reduced the 15-year risk of breast cancer death from 25.2% to 21.4% (absolute reduction, 3.8%; 95% CI, 1.6–6.0; 2P = .00005). In women with pN0 disease (n = 7287), radiotherapy reduced these risks from

31.0% to 15.6% (absolute recurrence reduction 15.4%, 13.2–17.6, 2P<.00001) and from 20.5% to 17.2% (absolute mortality reduction, 3.3%; 0.8–5.8; 2P = .005), respectively. In these women with pN0 disease, the absolute recurrence reduction varied according to age, grade, ER status, tamoxifen use, and extent of surgery, and these characteristics were used to predict large (≥20%), intermediate (10%–19%), or lower (<10%) absolute reductions in the 10-year recurrence risk. Absolute reductions in 15-year risk of breast cancer death in these 3 prediction categories were 7.8% (95% CI, 3.1–12.5), 1.1% (95% CI, −2.0 to 4.2), and 0.1% (95% CI, −7.5 to 7.7) respectively (trend in absolute mortality reduction, 2P = .03). In the few women with pN+ disease (n=1050), radiotherapy reduced the 10-year recurrence risk from 63.7% to 42.5% (absolute reduction, 21.2%; 95% CI, 14.5–27.9; 2P<.00001) and the 15-year risk of breast cancer death from 51.3% to 42.8% (absolute reduction, 8.5%; 95% CI, 1.8–15.2; 2P = .01). Overall, about 1 breast cancer death was avoided by year 15 for every 4 recurrences avoided by year 10, and the mortality reduction did not differ significantly from this overall relationship in any of the 3 prediction categories for pN0 disease or for pN+ disease.

Interpretation
After breast-conserving surgery, radiotherapy to the conserved breast halves the rate at which the disease recurs and reduces the breast cancer death rate by about a sixth. These proportional benefits vary little between different groups of women. By contrast, the absolute benefits from radiotherapy vary substantially according to the characteristics of the patient and they can be predicted at the time when treatment decisions need to be made.

Editorial comments In this meta-analysis of cooperative trials in more than 10,000 patients treated with BCT with or without XRT the investigators show a 16% decrease (19% vs 35%) in the risk of breast cancer recurrence and a 4% decrease in the risk of death with adjuvant XRT. The study shows a 50% proportional reduction in 10-year recurrence, greater than that of systemic therapy, which highlights the importance of local control. The reduction of recurrence depends on biological subtype, with the benefit of XRT twice as great for ER-positive disease as for ER-negative disease. The benefit for XRT is greater in earlier-stage favorable disease (ER positive, node negative) than later because the likelihood of systemic spread is less and local control is more important. This finding is supported by this meta-analysis showing that, for every 4 local recurrences avoided by 10 years, approximately 1 breast cancer–related death is avoided by 15 years.

Early Breast Cancer Trialists' Collaborative Group (EBCTCG), McGale P, Taylor C, Correa C, et al. Effect of radiotherapy after mastectomy and axillary surgery on 10-year recurrence and 20-year breast cancer mortality: meta-analysis of individual patient data for 8135 women in 22 randomised trials. Lancet 2014;383(9935):2127–35.[19]

Hypothesis
Postmastectomy radiation decreases recurrence and mortality in patients with 1 to 3 positive nodes.

Published Abstract

Background
Postmastectomy radiotherapy was shown in previous meta-analyses to reduce the risks of both recurrence and breast cancer mortality in all women with node-positive disease considered together. However, the benefit in women with

only 1 to 3 positive lymph nodes is uncertain. This study aimed to assess the effect of radiotherapy in these women after mastectomy and axillary dissection.

Methods
The study involved a meta-analysis of individual data for 8135 women randomly assigned to treatment groups during 1964 to 1986 in 22 trials of radiotherapy to the chest wall and regional lymph nodes after mastectomy and axillary surgery versus the same surgery but no radiotherapy. Follow-up lasted 10 years for recurrence and to January 1, 2009, for mortality. Analyses were stratified by trial, individual follow-up year, age at entry, and pathologic nodal status.

Findings
A total of 3786 women had axillary dissection to at least level II and had 0, 1 to 3, or 4 or more positive nodes. All were in trials in which radiotherapy included the chest wall, supraclavicular or axillary fossa (or both), and internal mammary chain. For 700 women with axillary dissection and no positive nodes, radiotherapy had no significant effect on locoregional recurrence ($2P > .1$), overall recurrence (rate ratio [RR], irradiated vs not, 1.06; 95% CI, 0.76–1.48; $2P > .1$), or breast cancer mortality (RR, 1.18; 95% CI, 0.89–1.55; $2P > .1$). For 1314 women with axillary dissection and 1 to 3 positive nodes, radiotherapy reduced locoregional recurrence ($2P < .00001$), overall recurrence (RR, 0.68; 95% CI, 0.57–0.82; $2P = .00006$), and breast cancer mortality (RR, 0.80; 95% CI, 0.67–0.95; $2P = .01$). Of these 1314 women, 1133 were in trials in which systemic therapy (cyclophosphamide, methotrexate, fluorouracil, or tamoxifen) was given in both trial groups and, for them, radiotherapy again reduced locoregional recurrence ($2P < .00001$), overall recurrence (RR, 0.67; 95% CI, 0.55–0.82; $2P = .00009$), and breast cancer mortality (RR, 0.78; 95% CI, 0.64–0.94; $2P = .01$). For 1772 women with axillary dissection and 4 or more positive nodes, radiotherapy reduced locoregional recurrence ($2P < .00001$), overall recurrence (RR, 0.79; 95% CI, 0.69–0.90; $2P = .0003$), and breast cancer mortality (RR, 0.87; 95% CI, 0.77–0.99; $2P = .04$).

Interpretation
After mastectomy and axillary dissection, radiotherapy reduced both recurrence and breast cancer mortality in the women with 1 to 3 positive lymph nodes in these trials even when systemic therapy was given. For women, who in many countries are at lower risk of recurrence, absolute gains might currently be smaller but proportional gains might be larger because of more effective radiotherapy.

Editorial comments Postmastectomy XRT improved locoregional DFS, overall DFS, and breast cancer–specific survival, independent of systemic therapy, in patents with any metastases to the axillary nodes. Local control depends on the multimodality therapy chosen, its extent (nodal sampling vs axillary node dissection), and its effectiveness as well as the extent and aggressiveness of the disease. In this meta-analysis of postmastectomy XRT, 1 breast cancer death is avoided for every 15 recurrences avoided at 10 years.

Whelan TJ, Olivotto IA, Parulekar WR et al. Regional nodal irradiation in early-stage breast cancer. N Engl J Med 2015 23;373(4):307–16.[20]

Hypothesis

In patients with node-positive breast cancer undergoing BCT and systemic therapy, the addition of regional nodal irradiation (RNI) would improve locoregional recurrence and survival.

Published Abstract

Background
Most women with breast cancer who undergo breast-conserving surgery receive whole-breast irradiation. This study examined whether the addition of RNI to whole-breast irradiation improved outcomes.

Methods
The study randomly assigned women with node-positive or high-risk node-negative breast cancer who were treated with breast-conserving surgery and adjuvant systemic therapy to undergo either whole-breast irradiation plus RNI (including internal mammary, supraclavicular, and axillary lymph nodes; nodal-irradiation group) or whole-breast irradiation alone (control group). The primary outcome was OS. Secondary outcomes were DFS, isolated locoregional DFS, and distant DFS.

Results
Between March 2000 and February 2007, a total of 1832 women were assigned to the nodal-irradiation group or the control group (916 women in each group). The median follow-up was 9.5 years. At the 10-year follow-up, there was no significant between-group difference in survival, with a rate of 82.8% in the nodal-irradiation group and 81.8% in the control group (HR, 0.91; 95% CI, 0.72–1.13; $P = .38$). The rates of DFS were 82.0% in the nodal-irradiation group and 77.0% in the control group (HR, 0.76; 95% CI, 0.61–0.94; $P = .01$). Patients in the nodal-irradiation group had higher rates of grade 2 or greater acute pneumonitis (1.2% vs 0.2%; $P = .01$) and lymphedema (8.4% vs 4.5%; $P = .001$).

Conclusions
Among women with node-positive or high-risk node-negative breast cancer, the addition of RNI to whole-breast irradiation did not improve OS but reduced the rate of breast cancer recurrence. (Funded by the Canadian Cancer Society Research Institute and others; MA.20 ClinicalTrials.gov number, NCT00005957.)

Editorial comments The MA.20 study failed to show a survival advantage and reported higher rates of lymphedema but lower rates of local regional recurrence. A similar RCT by Poortmans and colleagues[21] that studied adding RNI to whole breast or thoracic chest wall after surgery in more than 4000 patients did not a benefit in OS but did show a 2.1% benefit in breast cancer–related mortality. The number needed to treat to avoid on death from breast cancer was 39. Because RNI has a small risk of cardiac toxicity, careful selection of the patients who would benefit the most is advised.

Karlsson P, Cole BF, Price KN, et al. *Timing of radiation therapy and chemotherapy after breast-conserving surgery for node-positive breast cancer: long-term results from International Breast Cancer Study Group trials VI and VII.* IJRO 2016;2016:273–79.[22]

Hypothesis

That a delay in XRT until after systemic therapy is finished does not affect local control or survival.

Published Abstract

Purpose
To update the previous report from 2 RCTs, now with a median follow-up of 16 years, to analyze the effect of radiation therapy timing on local failure and DFS.

Patients and methods

From July 1986 to April 1993, International Breast Cancer Study Group trial VI randomly assigned 1475 premenopausal/perimenopausal women with node-positive breast cancer to receive 3 or 6 cycles of initial chemotherapy. International Breast Cancer Study Group trial VII randomly assigned 1212 postmenopausal women with node-positive breast cancer to receive tamoxifen for 5 years, or tamoxifen for 5 years with 3 early cycles of initial chemotherapy. For patients who received breast-conserving surgery (BCS), radiation therapy (RT) was delayed until initial chemotherapy was completed; 4 or 7 months after BCS for trial VI and 2 or 4 months for trial VII. The study compared RT timing groups among 433 patients on trial VI and 285 patients on trial VII who received BCS plus RT. End points were local failure, regional/distant failure, and DFS.

Results

Among premenopausal/perimenopausal patients there were no significant differences in disease-related outcomes. The 15-year DFS was 48.2% in the group allocated 3 months of initial chemotherapy and 44.9% in the group allocated 6 months of initial chemotherapy (HR, 1.12; 95% CI, 0.87–1.45). Among postmenopausal patients, the 15-year DFS was 46.1% in the no-initial-chemotherapy group and 43.3% in the group allocated 3 months of initial chemotherapy (HR, 1.11; 95% CI, 0.82–1.51). Corresponding HRs for local failures were 0.94 (95% CI, 0.61–1.46) in trial VI and 1.51 (95% CI, 0.77–2.97) in trial VII. For regional/distant failures, the respective HRs were 1.15 (95% CI, 0.80–1.63) and 1.08 (95% CI, 0.69–1.68).

Conclusions

This study confirms that, after more than 15 years of follow-up, it is reasonable to delay RT until after the completion of standard chemotherapy.

Editorial comments This long-term follow-up for patients randomized to CTX regimens that consequently delayed XRT until the CTX was finished (2, 4, and 7 months) confirms that delaying XRT until after CTX does not affect local failure, DFS, or OS.

Vaidya JS, Wenz F, Bulsara M. Risk-adapted targeted intraoperative radiotherapy versus whole-breast radiotherapy for breast cancer: 5-year results for local control and overall survival from the TARGIT–A randomised trial. Lancet 2014;383(9917):603–13.[23]

Hypothesis

Because most local recurrences in conserved breasts appear in the original tumor bed, intraoperative XRT of the tumor bed should be equivalent in local control to whole-breast XRT.

Published Abstract

Background

The TARGIT-A trial compared risk-adapted radiotherapy using single-dose targeted intraoperative radiotherapy (TARGIT) versus fractionated external beam radiotherapy (EBRT) for breast cancer. The study reported 5-year results for local recurrence and the first analysis of OS.

Methods

TARGIT-A was a randomized, noninferiority trial. Women aged 45 years and older with invasive ductal carcinoma were enrolled and randomly assigned in a 1:1 ratio to receive TARGIT or whole-breast EBRT, with blocks stratified by center and by timing of delivery of targeted intraoperative radiotherapy: randomization occurred either before lumpectomy (prepathology stratum, TARGIT concurrent with lumpectomy) or after lumpectomy (postpathology stratum, TARGIT given subsequently by reopening the wound). Patients in the TARGIT group received supplemental EBRT (excluding a boost) if unforeseen adverse features were detected on final pathology, thus radiotherapy was risk adapted. The primary outcome was absolute difference in local recurrence in the conserved breast, with a prespecified noninferiority margin of 2.5% at 5 years; prespecified analyses included outcomes as per timing of randomization in relation to lumpectomy. Secondary outcomes included complications and mortality. This study is registered with ClinicalTrials.gov, number NCT00983684.

Findings

Patients were enrolled at 33 centers in 11 countries, between March 24, 2000, and June 25, 2012. The study randomized 1721 patients to TARGIT and 1730 to EBRT. Supplemental EBRT after TARGIT was necessary in 15.2% (239 of 1571) of patients who received TARGIT (21.6% prepathology, 3.6% postpathology). There was a median follow-up of 2 years and 5 months (IQR 12–52 months) in 3451 patients, 2020 of 4 years, and 1222 of 5 years. The 5-year risk for local recurrence in the conserved breast was 3.3% (95% CI, 2.1–5.1) for TARGIT versus 1.3% (0.7–2.5) for EBRT (P = .042). TARGIT concurrent with lumpectomy (prepathology, n = 2298) had much the same results as EBRT: 2.1% (1.1–4.2) versus 1.1% (0.5–2.5; P = .31). With delayed TARGIT (postpathology, n = 1153) the between-group difference was larger than 2.5% (TARGIT, 5.4% [3.0–9.7] vs EBRT, 1.7% [0.6–4.9]; P = .069). Overall, breast cancer mortality was much the same between groups (2.6% [1.5–4.3] for TARGIT vs 1.9% [1.1–3.2] for EBRT; P = .56) but there were significantly fewer non–breast cancer deaths with TARGIT (1.4% [0.8–2.5] vs 3.5% [2.3–5.2]; P = .0086), which was attributable to fewer deaths from cardiovascular causes and other cancers. Overall mortality was 3.9% (2.7–5.8) for TARGIT versus 5.3% (3.9–7.3) for EBRT (P = .099). Wound-related complications were much the same between groups but grade 3 or 4 skin complications were significantly reduced with TARGIT (4 of 1720 vs 13 of 1731; P = .029).

Interpretation

TARGIT concurrent with lumpectomy within a risk-adapted approach should be considered as an option for eligible patients with breast cancer carefully selected as per the TARGIT-A trial protocol, as an alternative to postoperative EBRT.

Editorial comments In this updated publication of the TARGIT-A trial with a median follow-up of 29 months, the external beam arm recurrences have approximately doubled to 11 and, with the TARGIT-A arm, quadrupled to 23 from the prior report. This finding indicates that recurrences in this favorable group of patients have not yet reached the plateau of recurrences. Although these results are encouraging, widespread application should await long-term follow-up. The percentage differences are small and the benefits of using a single procedure are manifold.

Veronesi U, Orecchia R, Maisonneuve P et al. Intraoperative radiotherapy versus external radiotherapy for early breast cancer (ELIOT): a randomised controlled equivalence trial. Lancet Oncol 2013;14:1269–77.[24]

Hypothesis

Intraoperative XRT is equivalent to whole-breast XRT to provide local control.

Published Abstract

Background

Intraoperative radiotherapy with electrons allows the substitution of conventional postoperative whole-breast irradiation with 1 session of radiotherapy with the same equivalent dose during surgery. However, its ability to control for recurrence of local disease required confirmation in a randomized controlled trial.

Methods

This study was done at the European Institute of Oncology (Milan, Italy). Women aged 48 to 75 years with early breast cancer, a maximum tumor diameter of up to 2.5 cm, and suitable for BCS were randomly assigned in a 1:1 ratio (using a random permuted block design, stratified for clinical tumor size [<1.0 cm vs 1.0–1.4 cm vs ≥1.5 cm]) to receive either whole-breast external radiotherapy or intraoperative radiotherapy with electrons. Study coordinators, clinicians, and patients were aware of the assignment. Patients in the intraoperative radiotherapy group received 1 dose of 21 Gy to the tumor bed during surgery. Those in the external radiotherapy group received 50 Gy in 25 fractions of 2 Gy, followed by a boost of 10 Gy in 5 fractions. This study was an equivalence trial; the prespecified equivalence margin was local recurrence of 7.5% in the intraoperative radiotherapy group. The primary end point was occurrence of IBTR; OS was a secondary outcome. The main analysis was by intention to treat. This trial is registered with ClinicalTrials.gov, number NCT01849133.

Findings

The study randomized 1305 patients (654 to external radiotherapy and 651 to intraoperative radiotherapy) between November 20, 2000, and December 27, 2007. After a medium follow-up of 5.8 years (IQR, 4.1–7.7), 35 patients in the intraoperative radiotherapy group and 4 patients in the external radiotherapy group had had an IBTR ($P<.0001$). The 5-year event rate for IBRT was 4.4% (95% CI, 2.7–6.1) in the intraoperative radiotherapy group and 0.4% (0.0–1.0) in the external radiotherapy group (HR 9.3; 95% CI, 3.3–26.3). During the same period, 34 women allocated to intraoperative radiotherapy and 31 to external radiotherapy died ($P = .59$). Five-year OS was 96.8% (95% CI, 95.3–98.3) in the intraoperative radiotherapy group and 96.9% (95.5–98.3) in the external radiotherapy group. In patients with data available (n = 464 for intraoperative radiotherapy; n = 412 for external radiotherapy) there were significantly fewer skin side effects in women in the intraoperative radiotherapy group than in those in the external radiotherapy group ($P = .0002$).

Interpretation

Although the rate of IBTR in the intraoperative radiotherapy group was within the prespecified equivalence margin, the rate was significantly greater than with external radiotherapy, and OS did not differ between groups. Improved selection of patients could reduce the rate of IBTR with intraoperative radiotherapy with electrons.

Editorial comments ELIOT versus external beam radiation had a 10-fold higher local recurrence rate over a median follow-up of 5.8 years, although both arms were low (4.4% vs 0.4%, respectively). However, in a group of low-risk women the 5-year IBTR was 1.5% but 11.3% for those patient with high-risk factors. Regardless, OS was the same. In an era when only ~80% of women with BCT complete their XRT dose, single-dose intraoperative completion provides a lot of advantages for busy and/or noncompliant patients. In addition, patients who live distant to XRT treatment facilities or in rural areas can still undergo BCT. The main drawback with ELIOT is the cost of the equipment and the costly coordination and extra time spent in the operating theater.

LEVEL IA EVIDENCE: PROSPECTIVE RANDOMIZED CHEMOTHERAPY TRIALS AND META-ANALYSES IN BREAST CANCER

Slamon D, Eirmann W, Robert N, et al. Adjuvant trastuzumab in HER2-positive breast cancer. N Engl J Med 2011;365(14):1273–83.[25]

Hypothesis

Use of a new nonanthracycline regimen with trastuzumab would have equivalent or improved survival with less toxicity.

Published Abstract

Background

Trastuzumab improves survival in the adjuvant treatment of Human epidermal growth factor receptor (HER)-positive breast cancer, although combined therapy with anthracycline-based regimens has been associated with cardiac toxicity. The study evaluated the efficacy and safety of a new nonanthracycline regimen with trastuzumab.

Methods

The study randomly assigned 3222 women with human epidermal growth factor receptor 2 (HER2)–positive early-stage breast cancer to receive doxorubicin and cyclophosphamide followed by docetaxel every 3 weeks (AC-T), the same regimen plus 52 weeks of trastuzumab (AC-T plus trastuzumab), or docetaxel and carboplatin plus 52 weeks of trastuzumab (TCH). The primary study end point was DFS. Secondary end points were OS and safety.

Results

At a median follow-up of 65 months, 656 events triggered this protocol-specified analysis. The estimated DFS rates at 5 years were 75% among patients receiving AC-T, 84% among those receiving AC-T plus trastuzumab, and 81% among those receiving TCH. Estimated rates of OS were 87%, 92%, and 91%, respectively. No significant differences in efficacy (DFS or OS) were found between the 2 trastuzumab regimens, whereas both were superior to AC-T. The rates of congestive heart failure and cardiac dysfunction were significantly higher in the group receiving AC-T plus trastuzumab than in the TCH group (*P*<.001). Eight cases of acute leukemia were reported: 7 in the groups receiving the anthracycline-based regimens and 1 in the TCH group after receiving an anthracycline outside the study.

Conclusions

The addition of 1 year of adjuvant trastuzumab significantly improved DFS and OS among women with HER2-positive breast cancer. The risk/benefit ratio favored the nonanthracycline TCH regimen rather than AC-T plus trastuzumab, given its similar efficacy, fewer acute toxic effects, and lower risks of cardiotoxicity and leukemia.

Editorial comments

This article by Slamon and colleagues[25] from the Breast Cancer International Research Group is the fifth prospective RCT with trastuzumab, all of which showed a substantial increase in DFS and OS with 52-week therapy in patients overexpressing HER2. The critical question here is whether anthracyclines are necessary for the treatment of HER-2–positive breast cancer in order to avoid the cardiotoxicity of anthracyclines. The third group was randomized to a nonanthracycline regimen (docetaxel and carboplatin with trastuzumab every 3 weeks for 6 cycles) followed by a year of trastu-zumab. The non–anthracycline-containing regimen showed equivalency to the standard regimen in terms of DFS and OS but showed fewer cardiac and leukemia complications. Further prospective studies are determining just how positive (1+ or 2+) the HER2 oncogene has to be to benefit from trastuzumab. Combined analysis of NSABP B-31 and the North Central Cancer Treatment Group trials showed a relative reduction in DFS and death rate of 48% and 39% respectively.[26] The next RCTs study combinations of HER tyrosine kinase inhibitors.

Robidoux A, Tang G, Rastogi P, et al. Lapatinib as a component of neoadjuvant therapy for HER2-positive operable breast cancer (NSABP protocol B-41): an open-label, randomized phase 3 trial. Lancet Oncol 2013;14(12):1183–92.

Hypothesis

Dual blockade of the HER2 oncogene with lapatinib added to trastuzumab would increase therapeutic response.

Published Abstract

Background
The authors studied the effect on tumor response to neoadjuvant therapy for the substitution of lapatinib for trastuzumab in combination with weekly paclitaxel after doxorubicin plus cyclophosphamide treatment, and of the addition of lapatinib and trastuzumab combined after doxorubicin plus cyclophosphamide treatment in patients with HER2-positive operable breast cancer to determine whether there would be a benefit of dual HER2 blockade in these patients.

Methods
For this open-label, randomized phase 3 trial the study recruited women aged 18 years or older with an ECOG performance status of 0 or 1 with operable HER2-positive breast cancer. Each received 4 cycles of standard doxorubicin 60 mg/m^2 and cyclophosphamide 600 mg/m^2 intravenously on day 1 every 3 weeks followed by 4 cycles of weekly paclitaxel (80 mg/m^2) intravenously on days 1, 8, and 15, every 4 weeks. Concurrently with weekly paclitaxel, patients received either trastuzumab (4 mg/kg load, then 2 mg/kg intravenously) weekly until surgery, lapatinib (1250 mg orally) daily until surgery, or weekly trastuzumab plus lapatinib (750 mg orally) daily until surgery. After surgery, all patients received trastuzumab to complete 52 weeks of HER2-targeted therapy. Randomization (ratio 1:1:1) was done centrally with stratification by clinical tumor size, clinical nodal status, hormone-receptor status, and age. The primary end point was the pathologic complete response in the breast, and analysis was performed on an intention-to-treat population.

Findings
Patient accrual started on July 16, 2007, and was completed on June 30, 2011; 529 women were enrolled in the trial. The pathologic response determined in 519 patients. Breast pathologic complete response was noted in 93 (52.5%; 95% CI, 44.9–59.5) of 177 patients in the trastuzumab group, 91 (53.2%; 45.4–60.3) of 171 patients in the lapatinib group (*P* = .9852); and 106 (62.0%; 54.3–68.8) of 171 patients in the combination group (*P* = .095). The most common grade 3 and 4 toxic effects were neutropenia in 29 patients (16%) in the trastuzumab group (grade 4 in 5 patients [3%]), 28 patients (16%) in the lapatinib group (grade 4 in 8 patients [5%]), and 29 patients (17%) in the combination group (grade 4 in 9 patients [5%]) and grade 3 diarrhea in 4 patients (2%) in the trastuzumab group, 35 patients (20%) in the lapatinib group,

and 46 patients (27%) in the combination group (P<.0001). Symptomatic congestive heart failure, defined as New York Heart Association class III or IV events, occurred in 7 patients (4%) in the trastuzumab group, 7 (4%) in the lapatinib group, and 1 (<1%) in the combination group (P = .185).

Interpretation
Substitution of lapatinib for trastuzumab in combination with chemotherapy resulted in similar high percentages of pathologic complete response. Combined HER2-targeted therapy produced a numerically but insignificantly higher pathologic complete response percentage than single-agent HER2-directed therapy; these findings are consistent with results from other studies. Trials are being undertaken to further assess these findings in the adjuvant setting.

Editorial comments Lapatinib in combination with trastuzumab was not significantly better than single agent. Anti-HER2 agents under investigation include heat shock protein 90 inhibitors, small molecules that inhibit HER2 tyrosine kinase activity (eg lapatinib), monoclonal antibodies directed at other epitopes of the HER2 extracellular domain (eg, pertuzumab), and antibody-drug conjugates (eg, trastuzumab-DM1),[27] or in combination. These agents are covered in systematic reviews.[28,29]

Swain SM, Kim S-B, Cortés J, et al. Overall survival benefit with pertuzumab, trastuzumab, and docetaxel for HER2-positive metastatic breast cancer in CLEOPATRA, a randomised Phase 3 study. Lancet Oncol 2014;14(6):461–71.[30]

Hypothesis

Dual blockade of the HER2 oncogene with pertuzumab added to trastuzumab increases therapeutic response.

Background
Primary results from the randomized, double-blind, phase 3 study CLEOPATRA showed significantly improved median progression-free survival (PFS) with pertuzumab plus trastuzumab plus docetaxel versus placebo plus trastuzumab plus docetaxel in patients with HER2-positive first-line metastatic breast cancer (MBC). OS data at the primary analysis showed a strong trend in favor of the pertuzumab arm but did not reach statistical significance. This study reports confirmatory OS results after 1 additional year of follow-up.

Methods
Patients were randomly assigned to study treatment. OS and investigator-assessed PFS were analyzed using the Kaplan-Meier approach and log-rank tests stratified by geographic region and prior treatment status. This trial is registered with ClinicalTrials.gov, NCT00567190.

Findings
In the intent-to-treat population (808 patients), 267 deaths had occurred at data cutoff (placebo arm, 154 of 406 [37.9%]; pertuzumab arm, 113 of 402 [28.1%]). Treatment with pertuzumab plus trastuzumab plus docetaxel resulted in a 34% reduction in the risk of death during the course of the study (HR, 0.66; 95% CI, 0.52–0.84; P = .0008). Median OS was 37.6 months in the placebo arm and was not yet reached in the pertuzumab arm. A descriptive follow-up analysis of investigator-assessed PFS showed a median PFS of 12.4 and 18.7 months in the placebo versus pertuzumab arm (HR, 0.69; 95% CI, 0.58–0.81). No new safety concerns were identified with 1 additional year of follow-up. Adverse events were similar to those reported at the primary analysis with respect to incidence, severity, and specificity.

Interpretation

This OS analysis showed statistically significant and clinically meaningful survival benefit with pertuzumab plus trastuzumab plus docetaxel in patients with HER2-positive MBC. Updated analyses of investigator-assessed PFS and safety were consistent with the results from the primary analysis.

Editorial comments Adding pertuzumab to the combination of taxanes and trastuzumab significantly reduced risk of death by 34% with acceptable toxicity in metastatic patients. A combination of vinorelbine, pertuzumab, and trastuzumab offers an alternative for patients who cannot receive the standard anthracyclines for first-line treatment of HER2-positive locally advanced or metastatic disease.[31]

Rugo HS, Olopade OI, DeMichele A, et al. Adaptive randomization of veliparib-carboplatin treatment in breast cancer. N Engl J Med 2016;375(1):23–34.[32]

Hypothesis

Neoadjuvant chemotherapy containing poly(ADP-ribose) polymerase (PARP) inhibitors would provide improved pathologic complete response.

The genetic and clinical heterogeneity of breast cancer makes the identification of effective therapies challenging. The investigators designed I-SPY 2, a phase 2, multicenter, adaptively randomized trial to screen multiple experimental regimens in combination with standard neoadjuvant chemotherapy for breast cancer. The goal is to match experimental regimens with responding cancer subtypes. The study reports results for veliparib, a PARP inhibitor, combined with carboplatin.

Methods

In this ongoing trial, women are eligible for participation if they have stage II or III breast cancer with a tumor 2.5 cm or larger in diameter; cancers are categorized into 8 biomarker subtypes from their status with regard to human epidermal growth factor receptor 2 (HER2), hormone receptors, and a 70-gene assay. Patients undergo adaptive randomization within each biomarker subtype to receive regimens that have better performance than the standard therapy. Regimens are evaluated within 10 biomarker signatures (ie, prospectively defined combinations of biomarker subtypes). Veliparib-carboplatin plus standard therapy was considered for HER2-negative tumors and was therefore evaluated in 3 signatures. The primary end point is pathologic complete response. Tumor volume changes measured by MRI during treatment are used to predict whether a patient will have a pathologic complete response. Regimens move on from phase 2 if they have a high bayesian predictive probability of success in a subsequent phase 3 neoadjuvant trial within the biomarker signature in which they performed well.

Results

With regard to triple-negative breast cancer, veliparib-carboplatin had an 88% predicted probability of success in a phase 3 trial. A total of 72 patients were randomly assigned to receive veliparib-carboplatin, and 44 patients were concurrently assigned to receive control therapy; at the completion of chemotherapy, the estimated rates of pathologic complete response in the triple-negative population were 51% (95% bayesian probability interval [PI], 36%–66%) in the veliparib-carboplatin group versus 26% (95% PI, 9%–43%) in the control group. The toxicity of veliparib-carboplatin was greater than that of the control.

Conclusions

The process used in our trial showed that veliparib-carboplatin added to standard therapy resulted in higher rates of pathologic complete response than standard therapy alone specifically in triple-negative breast cancer. (Funded by the QuantumLeap Healthcare Collaborative and others; I-SPY 2 TRIAL ClinicalTrials.gov number, NCT01042379.)

Editorial comments PARP enzymes are essential for processing and repair of DNA breaks. BRCA-1/2 breast cancers, lacking this functionality, have been shown to be highly sensitive to PARP inhibitors. Therefore, the investigators thought that the response in triple-negative breast cancer would be similar. The I-SPY 2 is a phase 2, multicenter, adaptively randomized trial to screen multiple experimental regimens in combination with standard neoadjuvant chemotherapy for breast cancer in order to speed their adoption into practice. From the I-SPY2 came this small phase III trialed that showed that neoadjuvant treatment with the PARP inhibitor (veliparib) produced a greater pathologic complete response compared with treatment with carboplatin alone as well as greater toxicity.

Early Breast Cancer Trialists' Collaborative Group (EBCTCG), Peto R, Davies C, Godwin J et al. Comparisons between different polychemotherapy regimens for early breast cancer: meta-analyses of long-term outcome among 100,000 women in 123 randomised trials. Lancet 2012;379(9814):432–44.[33]

Hypothesis

Evaluation by a patient-level meta-analyses of available RCT could detect differences in efficacy between treatment regimens for breast cancer.

Published Abstract

Background
Moderate differences in efficacy between adjuvant chemotherapy regimens for breast cancer are plausible, and could affect treatment choices. This study sought any such differences.

Methods
The study undertook individual-patient-data meta-analyses of the randomized trials comparing any taxane plus anthracycline–based regimen versus the same, or more, nontaxane chemotherapy (n = 44,000); 1 anthracycline-based regimen versus another (n = 7000) or versus cyclophosphamide, methotrexate, and fluorouracil (CMF; n = 18,000); and polychemotherapy versus no chemotherapy (n = 32,000). The scheduled dosages of these 3 drugs and of the anthracyclines doxorubicin (A) and epirubicin (E) were used to define standard CMF, standard four cycles of doxorubicin + cyclophosphamide (4AC), and cyclophosphamide, doxorubicin, fluorouracil (CAF) and cyclophosphamide, epirubicin, fluorouracil (CEF). Log-rank breast cancer mortality ratios (RRs) are reported.

Findings
In trials adding 4 separate cycles of a taxane to a fixed anthracycline-based control regimen, extending treatment duration, breast cancer mortality was reduced (RR, 0.86; standard error [SE], 0.04; 2P = .0005). In trials with 4 such extra cycles of a taxane counterbalanced in controls by extra cycles of other cytotoxic drugs, roughly doubling nontaxane dosage, there was no significant difference (RR, 0.94; SE, 0.06; 2P = .33). Trials with CMF-treated controls showed that standard 4AC and standard CMF were

equivalent (RR, 0.98; SE, 0.05; 2P = .67), but that anthracycline-based regimens with substantially higher cumulative dosage than standard 4AC (eg, CAF or CEF) were superior to standard CMF (RR, 0.78; SE, 0.06; 2P = .0004). Trials versus no chemotherapy also suggested greater mortality reductions with CAF (RR, 0.64; SE, 0.09; 2P<.0001) than with standard 4AC (RR, 0.78; SE, 0.09; 2P = .01) or standard CMF (RR, 0.76; SE, 0.05; 2P<.0001). In all meta-analyses involving taxane-based or anthracycline-based regimens, proportional risk reductions were little affected by age, nodal status, tumor diameter or differentiation (moderate or poor; few were well differentiated), ER status, or tamoxifen use. Hence, largely independently of age (up to at least 70 years) or the tumor characteristics currently available for the patients selected to be in these trials, some taxane plus anthracycline–based or higher cumulative dosage anthracycline–based regimens (not requiring stem cells) reduced breast cancer mortality by, on average, about one-third. Ten-year overall mortality differences paralleled breast cancer mortality differences, despite taxane, anthracycline, and other toxicities.

Interpretation
Ten-year gains from a one-third breast cancer mortality reduction depend on absolute risks without chemotherapy (which, for ER-positive disease, are the risks remaining with appropriate endocrine therapy). Low absolute risk implies low absolute benefit, but information was lacking about tumor gene expression markers or quantitative immunohistochemistry that might help to predict risk, chemosensitivity, or both.

Editorial comments This study clearly shows that polychemotherapy with CMF or standard 4AC decreases breast cancer mortality and an even greater effect can be seen by increasing the cumulative dose of anthracycline, but with a concomitant increase in cardiac mortality. An unexpected and important finding is that the proportional reduction in breast cancer mortality with polychemotherapy was independent of receptor status (ER+ vs ER−) or age. A limitation of this meta-analysis is that the effect of molecular heterogeneity on the benefits and risks of chemotherapy cannot be assessed.

LEVEL IA EVIDENCE: PROSPECTIVE RANDOMIZED TRIALS (AND META-ANALYSES) ADDRESSING THE ROLE OF ENDOCRINE THERAPY IN BREAST CANCER PREVENTION AND TREATMENT

Davies C, Pan H, Godwin J, et al. Long-term effects of continuing adjuvant tamoxifen to 10 years versus stopping at 5 years after diagnosis of oestrogen receptor-positive breast cancer: ATLAS, a randomised trial. Lancet 2013;381(9869):805–16.[34]

Hypothesis
Extending tamoxifen therapy to 10 versus 5 years would reduce breast cancer mortality.

Published Abstract

Background
For women with ER-positive early breast cancer, treatment with tamoxifen for 5 years substantially reduces the breast cancer mortality throughout the first 15 years after diagnosis. The study aimed to assess the further effects of continuing tamoxifen to 10 years instead of stopping at 5 years.

Methods
In the worldwide Adjuvant Tamoxifen: Longer Against Shorter (ATLAS) trial, 12,894 women with early breast cancer who had completed 5 years of treatment

with tamoxifen were randomly allocated to continue tamoxifen to 10 years or stop at 5 years (open control). Allocation (1:1) was by central computer, using minimization. After entry (between 1996 and 2005), yearly follow-up forms recorded any recurrence, second cancer, hospital admission, or death. The study reported effects on breast cancer outcomes among the 6846 women with ER-positive disease, and side effects among all women (with positive, negative, or unknown ER status). Long-term follow-up still continues. This study is registered, number ISRCTN19652633.

Findings

Among women with ER-positive disease, allocation to continue tamoxifen reduced the risk of breast cancer recurrence (617 recurrences in 3428 women allocated to continue vs 711 in 3418 controls; $P = .002$), reduced breast cancer mortality (331 deaths vs 397 deaths; $P = .01$), and reduced overall mortality (639 deaths vs 722 deaths; $P = .01$). The reductions in adverse breast cancer outcomes seemed to be less extreme before than after year 10 (recurrence RR 0.90 [95% CI, 0.79–1.02] during years 5 to 9 and 0.75 [95% CI, 0.62–0.90] in later years; breast cancer mortality RR, 0.97 [95% CI, 0.79–1.18] during years 5 to 9 and 0.71 [95% CI, 0.58–0.88] in later years). The cumulative risk of recurrence during years 5 to 14 was 21.4% for women allocated to continue versus 25.1% for controls; breast cancer mortality during years 5 to 14 was 12.2% for women allocated to continue versus 15.0% for controls (absolute mortality reduction 2.8%). Treatment allocation seemed to have no effect on breast cancer outcome among 1248 women with ER-negative disease, and an intermediate effect among 4800 women with unknown ER status. Among all 12,894 women, mortality without recurrence from causes other than breast cancer was little affected (691 deaths without recurrence in 6454 women allocated to continue vs 679 deaths in 6440 controls; RR, 0.99 [0.89–1.10]; $P = .84$). For the incidence (hospitalization or death) rates of specific diseases, RRs were as follows: pulmonary embolus 1.87 (95% CI, 1.13–3.07; $P = .01$ [including 0.2% mortality in both treatment groups]), stroke 1.06 (0.83–1.36), ischemic heart disease 0.76 (0.60–0.95; $P = .02$), and endometrial cancer 1.74 (1.30–2.34; $P = .0002$). The cumulative risk of endometrial cancer during years 5 to 14 was 3.1% (mortality 0.4%) for women allocated to continue versus 1.6% (mortality 0.2%) for controls (absolute mortality increase 0.2%).

Interpretation

For women with ER-positive disease, continuing tamoxifen to 10 years rather than stopping at 5 years produces a further reduction in recurrence and mortality, particularly after year 10. These results, taken together with results from previous trials of 5 years of tamoxifen treatment versus none, suggest that 10 years of tamoxifen treatment can approximately halve breast cancer mortality during the second decade after diagnosis.

Editorial comments ER status is the only recorded factor importantly predictive of the proportional reductions with tamoxifen.[35] Extending treatment beyond 5 years in ER+ patients in the overview analysis significantly improved DFS but also significantly increased the risks of death caused by endometrial cancer and stoke, whereas there was a significant decrease in cardiac mortality.

Early Breast Cancer Trialists' Collaborative Group (EBCTCG), Dowsett M, Forbes JF, Bradley R, et al. Aromatase inhibitors versus tamoxifen in early breast cancer: patient-level meta-analysis of the randomised trials. Lancet 2015;386(10001):1341–52.[36]

Hypothesis

Aromatase inhibitors provide superior DFS compared with tamoxifen in estrogen-positive disease.

Published Abstract

Background
The optimal ways of using aromatase inhibitors or tamoxifen as endocrine treatment of early breast cancer remains uncertain.

Methods
The study undertook meta-analyses of individual data on 31,920 postmenopausal women with ER-positive early breast cancer in the randomized trials of 5 years of aromatase inhibitor versus 5 years of tamoxifen; of 5 years of aromatase inhibitor versus 2 to 3 years of tamoxifen then aromatase inhibitor to year 5; and of 2 to 3 years of tamoxifen then aromatase inhibitor to year 5 versus 5 years of tamoxifen. Primary outcomes were any recurrence of breast cancer, breast cancer mortality, death without recurrence, and all-cause mortality. Intention-to-treat log-rank analyses, stratified by age, nodal status, and trial, yielded aromatase inhibitor versus tamoxifen first-event RRs.

Findings
In the comparison of 5 years of aromatase inhibitor versus 5 years of tamoxifen, recurrence RRs favored aromatase inhibitors significantly during years 0 to 1 (RR, 0.64; 95% CI, 0.52–0.78) and 2 to 4 (RR, 0.80; 0.68–0.93), and nonsignificantly thereafter. Ten-year breast cancer mortality was lower with aromatase inhibitors than with tamoxifen (12.1% vs 14.2%; RR, 0.85, 0.75–0.96; $2P = .009$). In the comparison of 5 years of aromatase inhibitor versus 2 to 3 years of tamoxifen then aromatase inhibitor to year 5, recurrence RRs favored aromatase inhibitors significantly during years 0 to 1 (RR, 0.74; 0.62–0.89) but not while both groups received aromatase inhibitors during years 2 to 4, or thereafter; overall in these trials there were fewer recurrences with 5 years of aromatase inhibitors than with tamoxifen then aromatase inhibitors (RR, 0.90; 0.81–0.99; $2P = .045$), although the breast cancer mortality reduction was not significant (RR, 0.89; 0.78–1.03; $2P = .11$). In the comparison of 2 to 3 years of tamoxifen then aromatase inhibitor to year 5 versus 5 years of tamoxifen, recurrence RRs favored aromatase inhibitors significantly during years 2 to 4 (RR, 0.56; 0.46–0.67) but not subsequently, and 10-year breast cancer mortality was lower with switching to aromatase inhibitors than with remaining on tamoxifen (8.7% vs 10.1%; $2P = .015$). Aggregating all 3 types of comparison, recurrence RRs favored aromatase inhibitors during periods when treatments differed (RR, 0.70; 0.64–0.77), but not significantly thereafter (RR, 0.93; 0.86–1.01; $2P = .08$). Breast cancer mortality was reduced while treatments differed (RR, 0.79; 0.67–0.92), and also subsequently (RR, 0.89; 0.81–0.99), and for all periods combined (RR, 0.86; 0.80–0.94; $2P = .0005$). All-cause mortality was also reduced (RR, 0.88; 0.82–0.94; $2P = .0003$). RRs differed little by age, body mass index, stage, grade, progesterone receptor status, or HER2 status. There were fewer endometrial cancers with aromatase inhibitors than with tamoxifen (10-year incidence, 0.4% vs 1.2%; RR, 0.33; 0.21–0.51) but more bone fractures (5-year risk, 8.2% vs 5.5%; RR, 1.42; 1.28–1.57); non–breast cancer mortality was similar.

Interpretation
Aromatase inhibitors reduce recurrence rates by about 30% (proportionately) compared with tamoxifen while treatments differ, but not thereafter. Five years of an aromatase inhibitor reduces 10-year breast cancer mortalities by about

15% compared with 5 years of tamoxifen, hence by about 40% (proportionately) compared with no endocrine treatment.

Editorial comments Aromatase inhibitors are superior to tamoxifen or combination of the two. There were fewer recurrences with 5 years of aromatase inhibitors than with tamoxifen followed by aromatase inhibitors or tamoxifen alone. There was less endometrial cancer but more bone fractures. Aromatase inhibitors are favored in postmenopausal patients without bone disease. Because more women die of the osteoporosis than breast cancer, tamoxifen should be considered in that setting.

Early Breast Cancer Trialists' Collaborative Group (EBCTCG), Coleman R, Powles T, Paterson A, et al. Adjuvant bisphosphonate treatment in early breast cancer: meta-analyses of individual patient data from randomised trials. Lancet 2015;386(10001):1353–61.[37]

Hypothesis

Bisphosphonates, through modification of osteoclastic activity, could reduce the excess production of growth factors in bone, thereby decreasing metastasis, and therefore could improve disease-free survival.

Published Abstract

Background
Bisphosphonates have profound effects on bone physiology, and could modify the process of metastasis. The study undertook collaborative meta-analyses to clarify the risks and benefits of adjuvant bisphosphonate treatment in breast cancer.

Methods
The study sought individual patient data from all unconfounded trials in early breast cancer that randomized between bisphosphonate and control. Primary outcomes were recurrence, distant recurrence, and breast cancer mortality. Primary subgroup investigations were site of first distant recurrence (bone or other), menopausal status (postmenopausal [combining natural and artificial] or not), and bisphosphonate class (aminobisphosphonate [eg, zoledronic acid, ibandronate, pamidronate] or other [ie, clodronate]). Intention-to-treat log-rank methods yielded bisphosphonate versus control first-event RRs.

Findings
The study received data on 18,766 women (18,206 [97%] in trials of 2–5 years of bisphosphonate) with median follow-up 5.6 woman-years, 3453 first recurrences, and 2106 subsequent deaths. Overall, the reductions in recurrence (RR, 0.94; 95% CI, 0.87–1.01; $2P = .08$), distant recurrence (0.92; 0.85–0.99; $2P = .03$), and breast cancer mortality (0.91; 0.83–0.99; $2P = .04$) were of only borderline significance, but the reduction in bone recurrence was more definite (0.83; 0.73–0.94; $2P = .004$). Among premenopausal women, treatment had no apparent effect on any outcome, but among 11,767 postmenopausal women it produced highly significant reductions in recurrence (RR, 0.86; 95% CI, 0.78–0.94; $2P = .002$), distant recurrence (0.82; 0.74–0.92; $2P = .0003$), bone recurrence (0.72; 0.60–0.86; $2P = .0002$), and breast cancer mortality (0.82; 0.73–0.93; $2P = .002$). Even for bone recurrence, the heterogeneity of benefit was barely significant by menopausal status ($2P = .06$ for trend with menopausal status) or age ($2P = .03$), and it was nonsignificant by bisphosphonate class, treatment schedule, ER status, nodes, tumor grade, or concomitant chemotherapy. No differences were seen in non–breast cancer mortality. Bone fractures were reduced (RR, 0.85; 95% CI, 0.75–0.97; $2P = .02$).

Interpretation
Adjuvant bisphosphonates reduce the rate of breast cancer recurrence only in the bone and improve breast cancer survival. There is definite benefit only in women who were postmenopausal when treatment began.

Editorial interpretation Bisphosphonates improve DFS by decreasing metastasis to the bone. This decrease was independent of the type or schedule of bisphosphonate, the ER status or stage, and the use of adjuvant systemic chemotherapy. This report should lead to the routine use of bisphosphates in early breast cancer in menopausal patients.

Margolese RG, Cecchini RS, Julian TB, et al. Anastrozole versus tamoxifen is postmenopausal women with ductal carcinoma in situ undergoing lumpectomy plus radiotherapy (NSABP B-35): a randomized, double-blind, phase 3 clinical trial. Lancet 2016;387:849–56.[38]

Hypothesis

Anastrozole is superior to tamoxifen in DFS when treating patients with DCIS.

Published Abstract

Background
DCIS is currently managed with excision, radiotherapy, and adjuvant hormone therapy, usually tamoxifen. The study postulated that an aromatase inhibitor would be safer and more effective. The study therefore undertook this trial to compare anastrozole versus tamoxifen in postmenopausal women with DCIS undergoing lumpectomy plus radiotherapy.

Methods
The double-blind, randomized, phase 3 NSABP B-35 trial was done in 333 participating NSABP centers in the United States and Canada. Postmenopausal women with hormone-positive DCIS treated by lumpectomy with clear resection margins and whole-breast irradiation were enrolled and randomly assigned (1:1) to receive either oral tamoxifen 20 mg/d (with matching placebo in place of anastrozole) or oral anastrozole 1 mg/d (with matching placebo in place of tamoxifen) for 5 years. Randomization was stratified by age (<60 vs ≥60 years) and patients and investigators were masked to treatment allocation. The primary outcome was breast cancer–free interval, defined as time from randomization to any breast cancer event (local, regional, or distant recurrence, or contralateral breast cancer, invasive disease, or DCIS), analyzed by intention to treat. This study is registered with ClinicalTrials.gov, number NCT00053898, and is complete.

Findings
Between January 1, 2003, and June 15, 2006, 3104 eligible patients were enrolled and randomly assigned to the 2 treatment groups (1552 to tamoxifen and 1552 to anastrozole). As of February 28, 2015, follow-up information was available for 3083 patients for OS and 3077 for all other disease-free end points, with median follow-up of 9.0 years (IQR, 8.2–10.0). In total, 212 breast cancer–free interval events occurred: 122 in the tamoxifen group and 90 in the anastrozole group (HR, 0.73; 95% CI, 0.56–0.96; $P = .0234$). A significant time-by-treatment interaction ($P = .0410$) became evident later in the study. There was also a significant interaction between treatment and age group ($P = .0379$), showing that anastrozole is superior only in women younger than 60 years of age. Adverse events did not differ between the groups, except for thrombosis or

embolism (a known side effect of tamoxifen), for which there were 17 grade 4 or worse events in the tamoxifen group versus 4 in the anastrozole group.

Interpretation
Compared with tamoxifen, anastrozole treatment provided a significant improvement in breast cancer–free interval, mainly in women younger than 60 years of age. This finding means that women will benefit from having a choice of effective agents for DCIS.

Editorial comments Patients in the 10-year follow-up of NSABP B-24 with ER-positive DCIS receiving adjuvant tamoxifen after standard therapy showed significant reductions in subsequent breast cancer.[39] This study shows that anastrozole improves on DFS. However, when side effects are intolerable, tamoxifen is a good alternative. It is the treatment of choice for premenopausal women with DCIS.[40]

LEVEL IA EVIDENCE: PROSPECTIVE RANDOMIZED TRIALS AND META-ANALYSES ADDRESSING THE ROLE OF BIOMARKERS IN BREAST CANCER PREVENTION AND TREATMENT

Millar EK, Graham PH, O'Toole SA, et al. Prediction of local recurrence, distant metastases, and death after breast-conserving therapy in early-stage invasive breast cancer using a five-biomarker panel. J Clin Oncol 2009;27(28):4701–8.[41]

Hypothesis

Intrinsic tumor biology by a 5-biomarker panel would predict disease-free survival in patients with breast cancer undergoing BCS.

Published Abstract

Purpose
To determine the clinical utility of intrinsic molecular phenotype after BCT with lumpectomy and whole-breast irradiation with or without a cavity boost.

Patients and methods
Four-hundred and ninety-eight patients with invasive breast cancer were enrolled into a randomized trial of BCT with or without a tumor bed radiation boost. Tumors were classified by intrinsic molecular phenotype as luminal A or B, HER-2, basal-like, or unclassified using a 5-biomarker panel: ER, progesterone receptor, HER-2, CK5/6, and epidermal growth factor receptor. Kaplan-Meier and Cox proportional hazards methodology were used to ascertain relationships to IBTR, locoregional recurrence, distant DFS (DDFS), and death from breast cancer.

Results
Median follow-up was 84 months. Three-hundred and ninety-four patients were classified as luminal A, 23 were luminal B, 52 were basal, 13 were HER-2, and 16 were unclassified. There were 24 IBTR (4.8%), 35 locoregional recurrence (7%), 47 distant metastases (9.4%), and 37 breast cancer deaths (7.4%). The overall 5-year disease-free rates for the whole cohort were IBTR, 97.4%; locoregional recurrence, 95.6%; DDFS, 92.9%; and breast cancer–specific death, 96.3%. A significant difference was observed for survival between subtypes for locoregional recurrence ($P = .012$), DDFS ($P = .0035$), and breast cancer–specific death ($P = .0482$), but not for IBTR ($P = .346$).

Conclusions

The 5-year and 10-year survival rates varied according to molecular subtype. Although this approach provides additional information to predict time to IBTR, locoregional recurrence, DDFS, and death from breast cancer, its predictive power is less than that of traditional pathologic indices. This information may be useful in discussing outcomes and planning management with patients after BCT.

Editorial comments Tumor molecular subtype identifies groups with divergent rates of local regional recurrence, DFS, and OS. However, such classification was not better than traditional pathology variables such as tumor size, grade, hormonal status, lymph node status, lymphatic vascular invasion, and positive margins. The rate of positive margins in this study was very low (2.4%), as was the rate of local recurrence, which would make it difficult to assess the predictive value of any tumor attribute. The Oncotype 21-gene assay is both predictive of recurrence and prognostic for benefit of chemotherapy and survival.[42] This test was validated retrospectively on 2 prospective NSABP trials (B-14 and B-20). The TAILORX trial, which has completed accrual, will prospectively validate the assay. Recurrence score generated from the Oncotype assay is now commonly used and is included in the new staging American Joint Committee on Cancer guidelines, and has significantly decreased the use of chemotherapy. Similarly, prospective-retrospective trials with Oncotype on DCIS have shown that the DCIS score can predict risk of recurrence without XRT.[43,44]

Wang C, Zhu H, Zhou Y, et al. Prognostic value of PD-L1 in breast cancer: a meta-analysis. Breast J 2017. http://dx.doi.org/10.1111/tbj.12753.[45]

Hypothesis

PD-L1 is of prognostic significant in breast cancer.

Published Abstract

Programmed cell death 1 ligand 1 (PD-L1) is a promising therapeutic target for cancer immunotherapy. However, the correlation between PD-L1 and breast cancer survival remains unclear. This study presents the first meta-analysis to investigate the prognostic value of PD-L1 in breast cancer. The study searched PubMed, Embase, and Cochrane Central Register of Controlled Trials databases for relevant studies evaluating PD-L1 expression and breast cancer survival. Fixed-effect and random-effect meta-analyses were conducted based on heterogeneity of included studies. Publication bias was evaluated by funnel plot and Begg test. Overall, 9 relevant studies with 8583 patients were included. PD-L1 overexpression was found in 25.8% of patients with breast cancer. PD-L1 (+) associated with several high-risk prognostic indicators, such as ductal cancer ($P = .037$), high tumor grade ($P = .000$), ER negativity ($P = .000$), PR negativity ($P = .000$), HER2 positivity ($P = .001$), and aggressive molecular subtypes (HER2 rich and Basal-like; $P = .000$). PD-L1 overexpression had no significant impact on metastasis-free survival (HR, 0.924; 95% CI, 0.747–1.141; $P = .462$), DFS (HR, 1.122; 95% CI, 0.878–1.434; $P = .357$), and overall specific survival (HR, 0.837; 95% CI, 0.640–1.093; $P = .191$), but significantly correlated with shortened OS (HR, 1.573; 95% CI, 1.010–2.451; $P = .045$). PD-L1 overexpression in breast cancer associates with multiple clinicopathologic parameters that indicate poor outcome, and may increase the risk for mortality. Further standardization of PD-L1 assessment assay and well-controlled clinical trials are warranted to clarify its prognostic and therapeutic value.

Editorial comment

In the new era of checkpoint inhibitors, the findings of these studies were significantly heterogeneous; the results should be interpreted cautiously. Phase I prospective trials using PD-LI monoclonal antibodies show response rates from 4% to 14% with various drugs, which is higher in aggressive subtypes (HER2+ or triple negative) and with an acceptable safety profile.[46] The higher response rates are thought to be secondary to the higher percentage of expression of the PD-L1 that is seen in the more aggressive subtypes (triple negative and Her2+).

REFERENCES

1. Litiere S, Werutsky G, Fentiman IS, et al. Breast conserving therapy versus mastectomy for stage I-II breast cancer: 20 year follow-up of the EORTC 10801 phase 3 randomized trial. Lancet Oncol 2012;13(4):412–9.
2. Fisher B, Anderson S, Bryant J, et al. Twenty-year follow-up of a randomized trial comparing total mastectomy, lumpectomy, and lumpectomy plus irradiation for the treatment of invasive breast cancer. N Engl J Med 2002; 347:1233–41.
3. Veronesi U, Cascinelli N, Mariani L, et al. Twenty-year follow-up of a randomized study comparing breast-conserving surgery with radical mastectomy for early breast cancer. N Engl J Med 2002;347:1227–32.
4. Cowher MS, Camp L, Mamounas EP, et al. Mastery of surgery: clinical trials and follow-up for breast cancer. 2016.
5. Crago AM, Azu M, Tierney S, et al. Randomized clinical trials in breast cancer. Surg Oncol Clin North Am 2010;19:33–58.
6. Black DM, Hunt KK, Mittendorf EA. Long term outcomes reporting the safety of breast conserving therapy compared to mastectomy: 20-year results of EORTC 10801. Gland Surg 2013;2(3):120–3.
7. Krag DN, Anderson SJ, Julian TB, et al. Sentinel-lymph-node resection compared with conventional axillary-lymph-node dissection in clinically node-negative patients with breast cancer: overall survival findings from the NSABP B-32 randomized phase 3 trial. Lancet Oncol 2010;11:927–33.
8. Giuliano AE, Ballman K, McCall L, et al. Locoregional recurrence after sentinel lymph node dissection with or without axillary dissection in patients with sentinel lymph node metastases: long-term follow-up from the American College of Surgeons Oncology Group (Alliance) ACOSOG Z0011 randomized trial. Ann Surg 2016;264(3):413–20.
9. Galimberti V, Cole BF, Zurrida S, et al. Axillary dissection versus no axillary dissection in patients with sentinel lymph-node micrometastases (IBCSG 23-01): a phase 3 randomised controlled trial. Lancet Oncol 2013; 14:297–305.
10. Donker M, van Tienhoven G, Straver ME, et al. Radiotherapy or surgery of the axilla after a positive sentinel node in breast cancer (EORTC 10981-22023 AMAROS): a randomized, multicenter, open-label phase 3 non-inferiority trial. Lancet Oncol 2014;15(12):1303–10.
11. Boughey JC, Suman VJ, Mittendorf EA, et al. Sentinel lymph node surgery after neoadjuvant chemotherapy in patients with node-positive breast cancer: the ACOSOG Z1071 (Alliance) clinical trial. JAMA 2013;310:1455–61.
12. Boughey JC, Suman VJ, Mittendorf EA. Factors affecting sentinel lymph node identification rate after neoadjuvant chemotherapy for breast cancer patients enrolled in ACOSOG Z1071 (Alliance). Ann Surg 2015;261(3):547–52.

13. Boughey JC, Ballman KV, Le-Petross HT. Identification and resection of clipped node decreases the false-negative rate of sentinel lymph node surgery in patients presenting with node-positive breast cancer (T0-T4, N1-N2) who receive neoadjuvant chemotherapy: results from ACOSOG Z1071 (Alliance). Ann Surg 2016; 263(4):802–7.

14. Kuehn T, Bauerfeind I, Fehm T, et al. Sentinel-lymph-node biopsy in patients with breast cancer before and after neoadjuvant chemotherapy (SENTINA): a prospective, multicenter cohort study. Lancet Oncol 2013;14:609–18.

15. Schwentner L, Helms G, Nekljudova V, et al. Using ultrasound and palpation for predicting axillary lymph node status following neoadjuvant chemotherapy - Results from the multi-center SENTINA trial. Breast 2017;31:202–7.

16. Wapnir IL, Dignam JJ, Fisher B, et al. Long-term outcomes of invasive ipsilateral breast tumor recurrences after lumpectomy in NSABP B-17 and B-24 randomized clinical trials for DCIS. J Natl Cancer Inst 2011;103(6):478–88.

17. Hughes KS, Schnaper LA, Bellon JR, et al. Lumpectomy plus tamoxifen with or without irradiation in women age 70 years or older with early breast cancer: long-term follow-up of GALGB 9343. J Clin Oncol 2013;31(19):2382–7.

18. Early Breast Cancer Trialists' Collaborative Group (EBCTCG), Darby S, McGale P, Correa C, et al. Effect of radiotherapy after breast-conserving surgery on 10-year recurrence and 15-year breast cancer death: meta-analysis of individual patient data for 10 801 women in 17 randomised trials. Lancet 2011;378(9804):1707–16.

19. Early Breast Cancer Trialists' Collaborative Group (EBCTCG), McGale P, Taylor C, Correa C, et al. Effect of radiotherapy after mastectomy and axillary surgery on 10-year recurrence and 20-year breast cancer mortality: meta-analysis of individual patient data for 8135 women in 22 randomised trials. Lancet 2014;383(9935): 2127–35.

20. Whelan TJ, Olivotto IA, Parulekar WR, et al. Regional nodal irradiation in early-stage breast cancer. N Engl J Med 2015;373(4):307–16.

21. Poortmans PM, Collette S, Kirkove C, et al. Internal mammary and medial supraclavicular irradiation in breast cancer. N Engl J Med 2015;373(4):317–27.

22. Karlsson P, Cole BF, Price KN, et al. Timing of radiation therapy and chemotherapy after breast-conserving surgery for node-positive breast cancer: long-term results from International Breast Cancer Study Group trials VI and VII. Int J Radiat Oncol Biol Phys 2016;96:273–9.

23. Vaidya JS, Wenz F, Bulsara M. Risk-adapted targeted intraoperative radiotherapy versus whole-breast radiotherapy for breast cancer: 5-year results for local control and overall survival from the TARGIT-A randomised trial. Lancet 2014; 383(9917):603–13.

24. Veronesi U, Orecchia R, Maisonneuve P, et al. Intraoperative radiotherapy versus external radiotherapy for early breast cancer (ELIOT): a randomised controlled equivalence trial. Lancet Oncol 2013;14:1269–77.

25. Slamon D, Eirmann W, Robert N, et al. Adjuvant trastuzumab in HER2-positive breast cancer. N Engl J Med 2011;365(14):1273–83.

26. Perez EA, Romond EX, Suman VJ, et al. Four-year follow-up of trastuzumab plus adjuvant chemotherapy for operable human epidermal growth factor receptor 2-positive breast cancer: joint analysis of data from NCCTG N9831 and NSABP B-31. J Clin Oncol 2011;29:3366–73.

27. Perez EA, Barrios C, Eiermann W, et al. Trastuzumab emtansine with or without pertuzumab versus trastuzumab plus taxane for human epidermal growth factor receptor 2- positive, advanced breast cancer: primary results from the Phase II MARIANNE Study. J Clin Oncol 2017;35(2):141–8.

28. Mendes D, Alves C, Afonso N, et al. The benefit of HER2-targeted therapies on overall survival of patients with metastatic HER2-positive breast cancer – a systematic review. Breast Cancer Res 2015;17:140.

29. Kuler I, Tuxen MK, Nielsen DL. A systematic review of dual targeting in HER2-positive breast cancer. Cancer Treat Rev 2014;40:259–70.

30. Swain SM, Kim SB, Cortés J, et al. Overall survival benefit with pertuzumab, trastuzumab, and docetaxel for HER2-positive metastatic breast cancer in CLEOPATRA, a randomised Phase 3 study. Lancet Oncol 2013;1(6):461–71.

31. Perez EA, Lopez-Vega JM, Petit T, et al. Safety and efficacy of vinorelbine in combination with pertuzumab and trastuzumab for first-line treatment of patients with HER2-positive locally advanced or metastatic breast cancer: VELVET Cohort 1 final results. Breast Cancer Res 2016;18(1):126–40.

32. Rugo HS, Olopade OI, DeMichele A, et al. Adaptive randomization of veliparib-carboplatin treatment in breast cancer. N Engl J Med 2016;375(1):23–34.

33. Early Breast Cancer Trialists' Collaborative Group (EBCTCG), Peto R, Davies C, Godwin J, et al. Comparisons between different polychemotherapy regimens for early breast cancer: meta-analyses of long-term outcome among 100,000 women in 123 randomised trials. Lancet 2012;379(9814):432–44.

34. Davies C, Pan H, Godwin J, et al. Long-term effects of continuing adjuvant tamoxifen to 10 years versus stopping at 5 years after diagnosis of oestrogen receptor-positive breast cancer: ATLAS, a randomised trial. Lancet 2013; 381(9869):805–16.

35. Early Breast Cancer Trialists' Collaborative Group (EBCTCG), Davies C, Godwin J, Gray R, et al. Relevance of breast cancer hormone receptors and other factors to the efficacy of adjuvant tamoxifen: patient-level meta-analysis of randomized trials. Lancet 2011;378(9793):771–84.

36. Early Breast Cancer Trialists' Collaborative Group (EBCTCG), Dowsett M, Forbes JF, Bradley R, et al. Aromatase inhibitors versus tamoxifen in early breast cancer: patient-level meta-analysis of the randomised trials. Lancet 2015; 386(10001):1341–52.

37. Early Breast Cancer Trialists' Collaborative Group (EBCTCG), Coleman R, Powles T, Paterson A, et al. Adjuvant bisphosphonate treatment in early breast cancer: meta-analyses of individual patient data from randomised trials. Lancet 2015;386(10001):1353–61.

38. Margolese RG, Cecchini RS, Julian TB, et al. Anastrozole versus tamoxifen is postmenopausal women with ductal carcinoma in situ undergoing lumpectomy plus radiotherapy (NSABP B-35): a randomized, double-blind, phase 3 clinical trial. Lancet 2016;387:849–56.

39. Allred DC, Anderson SJ, Paik S, et al. Adjuvant tamoxifen reduces subsequent breast cancer in women with estrogen receptor-positive ductal carcinoma in situ: a study based on NSABP protocol B-24. J Clin Oncol 2012;30(12): 1268–73.

40. Ganz PA, Cecchini RS, Julian TB, et al. Patient-reported outcomes with anastrozole versus tamoxifen for postmenopausal patients with ductal carcinoma in situ treated with lumpectomy plus radiotherapy (NSABP B-35): a randomised, double-blind, phase 3 clinical trial. Lancet 2016;387:857–65.

41. Millar EK, Graham PH, O'Toole SA, et al. Prediction of local recurrence, distant metastases, and death after breast-conserving therapy in early-stage invasive breast cancer using a five-biomarker panel. J Clin Oncol 2009; 27(28):4701–8.

42. Partin JF, Mamounas EP. Impact of the 21-gene recurrence score assay compared with standard clinicopathologic guidelines in adjuvant therapy selection for node-negative, estrogen receptor-positive breast cancer. Ann Surg Oncol 2011;18(12):2299–406.

43. Solin LJ, Gray R, Baehner FL, et al. A multigene expression assay to predict local recurrence risk for ductal carcinoma in situ of the breast. J Natl Cancer Inst 2013; 105(10):701–10.

44. Mele A, Mehta P, Slanetz PJ, et al. Breast-conserving surgery alone for ductal carcinoma in situ: factors associated with increased risk of local recurrence. Ann Surg Oncol 2016;24(5):1221–6.

45. Wang C, Zhu H, Zhou Y, et al. Prognostic value of PD-L1 in breast cancer: a meta-analysis. Breast J 2017. http://dx.doi.org/10.1111/tbj.12753.

46. Nanda R, Chow L, Claire D, et al. Pembrolizumab in patients with advanced triple-negative breast cancer: phase Ib KEYNOTE-012 study. J Clin Oncol 2016;34(21):2460–7.

An Update on Randomized Clinical Trials in Gastric Cancer

Jennifer Tseng, MD[a],*, Mitchell C. Posner, MD[b,c]

KEYWORDS

- Esophageal cancer • Randomized clinical trial • Surgery • Chemotherapy
- Neoadjuvant therapy • Adjuvant therapy • Lymphadenectomy

KEY POINTS

- There is no difference in oncologic outcomes comparing transhiatal with transthoracic esophagectomy.
- Nasogastric tubes assist in decreasing perioperative complications.
- Preoperative chemotherapy trials are difficult to evaluate because studies have examined squamous cell carcinoma versus adenocarcinoma and inconsistently included gastro-esophageal junction and gastric cardia tumors.
- Standard of care in Europe includes preoperative cisplatin and 5-fluoracil; however, ongoing studies are needed to study the subgroups of patients who benefit most from neoadjuvant chemotherapy.
- Randomized trials of preoperative radiation therapy have not increased resectability rates; a few recent trials show variable results in survival and pathologic complete responses with preoperative chemoradiotherapy.

SURGICAL MANAGEMENT

The surgical approach to esophageal cancer involves either transhiatal or transthoracic esophagectomy. Hulscher and colleagues[1] randomized 220 patients with middle or distal esophageal cancer to either transhiatal or transthoracic esophagectomy. Original results revealed no difference in R0 resection rates, although the lymph node retrieval was significantly higher in the transthoracic group (31 vs 16; $P<.001$).

Disclosures: None.
[a] Department of Surgery, University of Chicago Medicine, 5841 South Maryland Avenue, Room G209, MC 5094, Chicago, IL 60637, USA; [b] Surgical Oncology, Section of General Surgery, Department of Surgery, UCM Comprehensive Cancer Center, University of Chicago Medicine, 5841 South Maryland Avenue, Room G209, MC 5094, Chicago, IL 60637, USA; [c] Department of Radiation and Cellular Oncology, UCM Comprehensive Cancer Center, University of Chicago Medicine, 5841 South Maryland Avenue, Room G209, MC 5094, Chicago, IL 60637, USA
* Corresponding author.
E-mail address: jennifer.tseng@uchospitals.edu

Postoperative pulmonary complications and hospital duration of stay were higher in patients who underwent transthoracic esophagectomy. However, there were no differences in the perioperative mortality rates. Additionally, there were no differences in local or distant recurrence rates. Five-year survival analysis was comparable (34% and 36%; $P = .71$). Three other phase III trials prospectively examined the outcomes of patients assigned to transhiatal and transthoracic esophagectomy, but no definitive conclusions could be reached owing to small sample sizes.[2–4]

Various reconstructive techniques have been addressed by 3 prospective, randomized, controlled trials. Gupta and colleagues[5] found a lower leak rate of 4.3% versus 20.8% ($P = .03$) and stricture rate of 8.5% versus 29.2% ($P = .02$) after a "novel" hand-sewn esophagogastric anastomosis compared with a standard hand-sewn anastomosis. Bhat and colleagues[6] found the anastomotic leak rate to be dramatically reduced after omental wrap of the esophagogastric anastomosis versus standard anastomosis (3.09% vs 14.43%; $P = .005$). Tabira and colleagues[7] found no difference in anastomotic leak or postoperative nutritional status at 6 and 12 months after use of a slender gastric tube for reconstruction after esophagectomy when compared with a more generous gastric tube. Nederlof and colleagues[8] studied using an end-to-end (ETE) versus an end-to-side (ETS) esophagogastrostomy after esophageal cancer resection. This Dutch trial found the anastomotic stricture rate to be higher with the ETE anastomosis, but that the anastomotic leak rate, pulmonary complications, and duration of hospital stay were greater with an ETS anastomosis.

A number of trials addressed other surgical technique issues. A comparison of the Ivor-Lewis and Sweet esophagectomy techniques was performed for esophageal squamous cell carcinoma in 2015 by Li and colleagues[9] Operative morbidity was higher with the Sweet technique, and Ivor-Lewis esophagectomy led to higher lymph node yield. A small institutional randomized trial also found that in prone versus decubitus positioning for minimally invasive esophagectomy, the prone positioning may decrease surgeon workload and lead to better ergonomic results.[10] A multicenter, open-label, randomized, controlled trial by Biere and colleagues[11] evaluated open esophagectomy versus minimally invasive esophagectomy. Short-term pulmonary complications were better with the minimally invasive technique, suggesting the usefulness of the minimally invasive approach over open esophagectomy in clinical practice and as an area for further research into long-term outcomes.

PERIOPERATIVE OUTCOMES

Shackcloth and colleagues[12] completed a well-planned and executed study addressing the most appropriate use of nasogastric tubes (NGT) in the first 48 hours after esophagectomy. Thirty-four patients were randomized to NGT with continuous sump suction, single-lumen NGT with 4-hourly aspirations, or no NGT. The patients receiving continuous suction via the sump system spent significantly less time with a pH of less than 5.5 than either of the other 2 groups (4.3% vs 39.7% vs 40.3% [$P = .007$]). Patients randomized to no NGT had significantly more pulmonary complications, 7 of 12 versus 4 of 22 ($P = .02$), and required an NGT to be inserted in 7 of 12 cases. This study argues for the use of sump NGT in patients in the immediate perioperative period. A follow-up study by Mistry and colleagues[13] hypothesized that early removal of NGT would not adversely affect major pulmonary complications and anastomotic leak rates. This was confirmed in their single-center, parallel-group, open-label randomized trial of 150 patients.

Other recent trials have focused on perioperative interventions. The safety analysis of the Japan Clinical Oncology Group 9907 trial compared preoperative and postoperative chemotherapy in 330 patients and found that operative and postoperative complications were similarly low.[14] Eicosapentaenoic acid (EPA)-enriched enteral nutrition (EN) was compared with standard EN and found to preserve fat-free mass better than standard nutrition and significantly attenuated stress response.[15] Several studies have shown that ghrelin can improve postoperative outcomes and minimize adverse events, even during the time of chemotherapy.[16–18] Synbiotics were similarly studied and found to decrease the inflammatory response after surgery.[19,20] Shyamsundar and colleagues[21] also looked at simvastatin as a method of decreasing biomarkers of inflammation, and they discovered that simvastatin was associated with the reduction of pulmonary and systemic injury after esophagectomy. Method of endoscopic resectional technique,[22] extent of lymph node resection,[23] thoracotomy versus thoracoscopy,[24] antibiotic bowel decontamination,[25] and prostaglandin E1 infusion[26] have been reported in "1c" trials without differences noted in primary endpoints.

ADJUVANT THERAPY
Preoperative Chemotherapy

There are several challenges in evaluating preoperative chemotherapy trials for esophageal cancer, because studies have variably examined squamous cell carcinoma versus adenocarcinoma and inconsistently included gastroesophageal junction and gastric cardia tumors.

A study by Boonstra and colleagues[27] studied 171 patients with squamous cell carcinoma administered cisplatin and etoposide neoadjuvant chemotherapy. Overall survival was more favorable in the chemotherapy arm compared with patients who immediately went to surgery (5-year survival 26% vs 17%; $P = .03$). The US Intergroup 0113 trial[28] randomized patients to receive perioperative cisplatin and 5-fluoracil (5-FU) or surgery alone. There were no differences in overall median or 3-year survival. Long-term follow-up confirmed these results, although a subgroup analysis revealed that patients with R1 resection seemed to benefit from postoperative chemoradiotherapy.[29] In contrast with the Intergroup trial, the Medical Research Council Oesophageal Working Group[30,31] found that preoperative cisplatin and 5-FU (at a lesser cisplatin dose of 160 mg/m^2 compared with the 450 mg/m^2 used in the Intergroup trial) conferred a survival advantage (23% vs 17%; $P = .03$), likely from an increased rate of R0 resections (60% vs 54%). The Medical Research Council study had a larger sample size of 467 patients and a greater number of patients who received chemotherapy going on to surgery (92% vs 80% in the Intergroup trial). The Medical Research Council preliminarily reported the results of neoadjuvant randomized trial OEO5, comparing 2 cycles of cisplatin and 5-FU with 4 cycles of epirubicin, cisplatin, and capecitabine in 897 patients. There was no survival benefit with more chemotherapy.[32]

Several key trials grouped together distal esophagus, gastroesophageal junction, and gastric cancers in their studies. The Cunningham trial[33] (of which 26% of patients had distal esophagus or gastroesophageal junction tumors) randomized patients to perioperative epirubicin, cisplatin, and 5-FU or surgery alone. Chemotherapy improved 5-year overall survival (36% vs 23%; $P = .009$). Yehou and colleagues[34] randomized 234 patients to immediate surgery or to perioperative cisplatin and 5-FU. The 5-year survival (38% vs 24%; $P = .02$) and R0 resection rates (84% vs 73%, $P = .04$) were better in the chemotherapy group. However, a European Organisation for Research and Treatment of Cancer trial by Schuhmacher and colleagues[35] found almost equivalent 2-year overall survival rates (70% for surgery alone vs 73% for cisplatin and 5-FU) in T3 and T4 tumors.

The standard of care in Europe for the management of esophageal cancer includes preoperative cisplatin and 5-FU. However, ongoing studies are needed to study the subgroups of patients who benefit most from neoadjuvant chemotherapy.

Preoperative Radiotherapy and Chemoradiotherapy

Randomized trials of preoperative radiation therapy alone have not increased resectability rates.[36–41] Mei and colleagues[36] reported no difference in the local failure rate, although Gignoux and colleagues[37] noticed a lower local failure rate with preoperative radiation (46% vs 67%; P = .045). Nygaard and colleagues[38] observed an improvement in 3-year survival (18% vs 5%; P = .009); however, some of these patients received chemotherapy. Therefore, preoperative radiation therapy alone has not been shown to improve survival endpoints consistently.

There are a few recent randomized trials that show variable results in survival and pathologic complete responses with preoperative chemoradiotherapy. These trials were limited by low statistical power, inadequacy of chemotherapy doses delivered, or unusually high postoperative mortality.[42–49] The CROSS trial (Chemoradiotherapy for Oesophageal Cancer Followed by Surgery Study) by van Hagen and colleagues[50] established preoperative chemoradiotherapy as standard of care in Western countries. The study randomized 366 patients with esophageal or gastroesophageal junction squamous cell carcinoma or adenocarcinoma to carboplatin at an area under the curve of 2 mg/mL per minute and paclitaxel 50 mg/m^2 once weekly for 5 weeks with concurrent radiotherapy (1.8 Gy daily to 41.4 Gy in 23 fractions) followed by surgery or surgery alone. There were no differences in perioperative outcomes (including postoperative mortality, <4%), and grade 3 or 4 toxicity was only seen in 13% of patients. R0 resection rates were achieved in 92% of patients versus 69% of patients in the surgery group (P<.001). Median survival increased from 24 to 49 months (hazard ratio, 0.0657; P = .003).

Postoperative Chemotherapy

The Japanese Oncology Group has evaluated postoperative chemotherapy in several randomized trials and found no survival benefit.[51–53] However, Iizuka and colleagues[52] noticed a trend toward, though not statistically significant, improvement in disease-free survival for node-positive patients who received adjuvant chemotherapy (53% vs 35%; P = .06). Hence, survival may be prolonged in patients who had an R0 resection and lymph node–positive disease, but data are limited.

Postoperative Radiotherapy and Chemoradiotherapy

No improvement in survival was noticed in 2 randomized trials of adjuvant radiotherapy. Teniere and colleagues[54] gave 221 patients with squamous cell carcinoma 45 to 55 Gy and observed no impact on survival. Fok and colleagues[55] administered radiation to patients with squamous cell carcinomas and adenocarcinomas undergoing curative or palliative resections; there was no improvement in local control or median survival. Additionally, 20% of the Intergroup 0116 trial's[56] 603 patients had gastroesophageal junction adenocarcinoma. Patients who received postoperative chemoradiation had an increase in overall survival (50% vs 41%; P = .005), especially the group of patients who were HER2 status negative.[57]

Definitive Radiotherapy and Chemoradiotherapy Versus Surgery

There are only 2 trials that directly compare nonoperative treatment (one with radiation alone and another with chemoradiation) with surgery.[58,59] It is difficult to draw conclusions about these 2 studies because they are limited by low statistical power and short follow-up.

Radiotherapy Versus Chemoradiotherapy

There are 6 randomized trials comparing radiation with chemoradiation.[38,60–66] However, these trials are difficult to compare because they include variable doses of radiation and systemic chemotherapy with different sequencing of therapies. An analysis of the pooled data[67] from these trials reported a significant local control and survival benefit at 1 year for chemoradiation over radiation alone, although chemoradiation predictably increased side effects. The Eastern Cooperative Oncology Group's EST-1282 trial[65] also demonstrated a median overall survival benefit (15 months vs 9 months; $P = .04$) for patients receiving chemoradiation; however, there was no improvement in 5-year overall survival. This study was confounded by 50% of the patients in each arm undergoing surgery after radiation therapy by individual investigator's choice. The Radiation Therapy Oncology Group 85-01 Intergroup Trail reported by Herskovic and colleagues[61] and Al-Sarraf and colleagues[63] examined patients who received cisplatin and 5-FU chemotherapy with 50 Gy radiation compared with patients receiving 64 Gy radiation alone. There was improved 5-year survival in patients who received chemoradiation (27% vs 0%; $P<.0001$).[49]

Surgery After Chemoradiotherapy

A French study and a separate German study examined whether surgery is required after chemoradiotherapy. In the FFCD 9102 trial(Fédération Francaise de Cancérologie Digestive 9102),[68,69] 444 patients with clinically resectable T3 or T4 N0 or 1 and M0 esophageal squamous cell carcinoma or adenocarcinoma all received 5-FU, cisplatin, and 46 Gy at 2 Gy per day or a split course with 15 Gy in weeks 1 and 3. Those patients who demonstrated a partial response were randomized to surgery versus additional chemoradiation. There was no difference in 2-year survival (34% vs 40%; $P = .44$) or median survival (17.7 months vs 19.3 months). These data suggest that patients with squamous cell carcinoma do not benefit from surgical intervention in lieu of continuing chemoradiation. A separate analysis showed that standard course radiation improved 2-year progression free survival compared with split course radiation (77% vs 57%; $P = .002$).

The German trial also did not show an improvement in survival in uT3 or T4 N0 or N1 and M0 disease.

Patients with squamous cell carcinoma of the esophagus undergoing surgery after definitive chemoradiation.[70] The German Oesophageal Cancer Study Group compared preoperative chemoradiation (3 cycles of 5-FU, leucovorin, etoposide, and cisplatin, followed by concurrent etoposide, cisplatin, plus 40 Gy followed by surgery vs the same chemotherapy regimen with 60–65 Gy with or without brachytherapy). The 3-year survival (31% vs 24%) was not significantly different. These 2 trials confirm that it is reasonable from an oncologic perspective to treatment patients with squamous cell carcinoma with definitive chemoradiation.

SUMMARY OF LEVEL IA EVIDENCE
Randomized, Controlled Trials in Esophageal Cancer

Clinical study 1
Li B, Xiang J, Zhang Y, et al. Comparison of Ivor-Lewis vs Sweet esophagectomy for esophageal squamous cell carcinoma: a randomized clinical trial. JAMA Surg 2015;150(4):292–8.

No. Patients Randomized	Study Groups	Stratification	Significance Demonstrated	% Change Identified in Trial
300	Ivor Lewis, N = 150 Sweet, N = 150	None	Yes, operative morbidity	30% vs 41.3% (P = .04)

Hypothesis To determine whether Ivor-Lewis esophagectomy is associated with increased postoperative complications compared with the Sweet procedure.

Published abstract

Background Sweet esophagectomy is performed widely in China, whereas the Ivor-Lewis procedure, with potential benefit of an extended lymphadenectomy, is limitedly conducted owing to concern for a higher risk for morbidity. Thus, the role of the Ivor-Lewis procedure for thoracic esophageal cancer needs further investigation.

Methods A randomized clinical trial was conducted from May 2010 to July 2012 at Fudan University Shanghai Cancer Center, Shanghai, China, of 300 patients with resectable squamous cell carcinoma in the middle and lower thirds of the thoracic esophagus. An intent-to-treat analysis was performed. Patients were assigned randomly to undergo either the Ivor-Lewis (n = 150) or Sweet (n = 150) esophagectomy. The primary outcome of this clinical trial was operative morbidity (any surgical or nonsurgical complications). Secondary outcomes included oncologic efficacy (number of lymph nodes resected and positive lymph nodes), postoperative mortality (30-day and in-hospital mortality), and patient discharge.

Results Resection without macroscopic residual (R0/R1) was achieved in 149 of 150 patients in each group. Although there was no difference between the 2 groups regarding the incidence of each single complication, a significantly higher morbidity rate was found in the Sweet group (62 of 150 [41.3%]) than in the Ivor-Lewis group (45 of 150 [30%]; P = .04). More patients in the Sweet group (8 of 150 [5.3%]) underwent reoperations than in the Ivor-Lewis group (1 of 150 [0.7%]) (P = .04). The median duration of hospital stay was 18 days in the Sweet group versus 16 days in the Ivor-Lewis group (P = .002). Postoperative mortality rates in the Ivor-Lewis (1 of 150) and Sweet (3 of 150) groups were 0.7% and 2.0%, respectively (P = .25). More lymph nodes were removed during Ivor-Lewis esophagectomy than during the Sweet procedure (22 vs 18; P<.001).

Conclusions The early results of this study demonstrate that the Ivor-Lewis procedure can be performed with lower rates of postoperative complications and more lymph node retrieval. Ivor-Lewis and Sweet esophagectomies are both safe procedures with low operative mortalities.

Editor's summary and comments This clinical trial evaluated 2 techniques for esophagectomy, Ivor-Lewis compared with the Sweet procedure. Higher morbidity was found with the Sweet group (41.3% vs 30%; P = .04). The Sweet group had more reoperations, greater duration of stay, and fewer lymph nodes removed. This study leads to a recommendation of Ivor-Lewis esophagectomy to reduce postoperative complications and increase lymph node retrieval.

Clinical study 2

Takata A, Takiguchi S, Miyazaki Y, et al. Randomized phase II study of the anti-inflammatory effect of ghrelin during the postoperative period of esophagectomy. Ann Surg 2015;262(2):230–6.

No. Patients Randomized	Study Groups	Stratification	Significance Demonstrated	% Change Identified in Trial
40	Ghrelin, n = 20 Placebo, n = 20	None	Yes, systemic inflammatory response syndrome duration	3.0 d vs 6.7 d (*P* = .0062)

Hypothesis Ghrelin reduces systemic inflammatory response syndrome (SIRS) duration after esophagectomy.

Published abstract

Background Esophagectomy for esophageal cancer is highly invasive and leads to prolonged SIRS duration and postoperative complications. Ghrelin has multiple effects, including antiinflammatory effects.

Methods Forty patients undergoing esophagectomy were assigned randomly to either the ghrelin group (n = 20), which received continuous infusion of ghrelin (0.5 µg/kg/h) for 5 days, or the placebo group (n = 20), which received pure saline for 5 days. The primary endpoint was SIRS duration. The secondary endpoints were the incidence of postoperative complications, time of a negative nitrogen balance, changes in body weight and composition, and levels of inflammatory markers, including C-reactive protein and interleukin (IL)-6.

Results The ghrelin group had a shorter SIRS duration and lower C-reactive protein and IL-6 levels than did the placebo group. The incidence of pulmonary complications was lower in the ghrelin group than in the placebo group, whereas other complications did not differ between the groups. Although time of the negative nitrogen balance was shorter in the ghrelin group than in the placebo group, changes in total body weight and lean body weight did not differ significantly.

Conclusions Postoperative ghrelin administration was effective for inhibiting inflammatory mediators and improving the postoperative clinical course of patients with esophageal cancer.

No. Patients Randomized	Study Groups	Stratification	Significance Demonstrated	% Change Identified in Trial
67	Decubitus, n = 32 Prone, n = 35	None	Yes Symptom scale	6.29 vs 3.13 (*P*<.001)

Editor's summary and comments This prospective, randomized, placebo-controlled phase II institutional study from Japan studied the postoperative benefit of ghrelin administration. The duration of SIRS was significantly shorter with ghrelin administration. Studies with larger sample sizes and long-term outcomes will be of benefit to clarifying the full impact of ghrelin in postesophagectomy patients.

Clinical study 3
Shen Y, Feng M, Tan L, et al. Thoracoscopic esophagectomy in prone versus decubitus position: ergonomic evaluation from a randomized and controlled study. Ann Thorac Surg 2014;98(3):1072–8.

Hypothesis Prone positioning may provide better ergonomics.

Published abstract
  Background The prone position (PP) and decubitus position (DP) have both been used for thoracoscopic esophagectomy. However, which of these positions is ergonomically better for the operating surgeon is unknown. In this randomized, controlled trial (NCT01144325), we aimed to assess the surgeon's physical and mental stress in operating on patients in the PP compared with that in the DP.

  Methods From October 2012 to June 2013, 67 consecutive patients who underwent a 3-stage, minimally invasive esophagectomy were assigned randomly to the DP or the PP during the thoracic stage. The same senior surgeon performed all operations. Objectively, the surgeon's spontaneous eye blink rate was recorded during thoracoscopic esophagectomy. Subjectively, the physician's musculoskeletal symptoms were rated on a scale ranging from 1 (uninfluenced) to 10 (maximum fatigue). Clinical characteristics, including patient demographics and operative features of the 2 patient groups, were compared statistically.

  Results There were 35 patients in the PP group and 32 in the DP group. The 2 groups were comparable in patient demographics. The thoracic stage of the operation was longer in the DP group than in the PP group (87 ± 24 minutes vs 68 ± 22 minutes; $P<.001$), and the volume of blood loss was higher (89 ± 18 mL vs 67 ± 16 mL; $P<.001$). The surgeon's eye blink rate at the end of thoracic stage decreased more from baseline in the DP group than in the PP group (3.0 ± 1.4 blinks/min vs 1.2 ± 0.9 blinks/min; $P<.001$), and the surgeon's symptom scale score was higher after operation with the patient in the DP than in the PP (6.29 ± 1.54 vs 3.13 ± 2.82; $P<.001$). No conversion to open thoracotomy was recorded in either group.

  Conclusions Thoracoscopic esophagectomy in the PP provided less workload and better ergonomic results than the DP. Further study based on a larger number of patients is required to confirm these findings.

Editor's summary and comments This small, institutional, randomized trial of prone versus decubitus positioning for esophagectomy was designed to evaluate the surgeon's mental and physical stress with each position. The musculoskeletal symptom scale was significantly higher with decubitus over prone positioning, suggesting PP may decrease surgeon workload and lead to better ergonomic results.

No. Patients Randomized	Study Groups	Stratification	Significance Demonstrated	% Change Identified in Trial
42	Synbiotics, n = 21 Control, n = 21	None	Yes Mesenteric lymph node samples Bacteremia	Mesenteric lymph node microorganisms: 3 vs 10 ($P = .035$) Bacteremia: 4 vs 12 ($P = .025$)

Clinical study 4
Yokoyama Y, Nishigaki E, Abe T, et al. Randomized clinical trial of the effect of perioperative synbiotics versus no synbiotics on bacterial translocation after oesophagectomy. Br J Surg. 2014;101(3):189–99.

Hypothesis Perioperative synbiotics reduce postoperative bacteremia.

Published abstract

Background The impact of perioperative synbiotics on bacterial translocation and subsequent bacteremia after esophagectomy is unclear. This study investigated the effect of perioperative synbiotic administration on the incidence of bacterial translocation to mesenteric lymph nodes (MLNs) and the occurrence of postoperative bacteremia.

Methods Patients with esophageal cancer were randomized to receive perioperative synbiotics or no synbiotics (control group). MLNs were harvested from the jejunal mesentery before dissection (MLN-1) and after the restoration of digestive tract continuity (MLN-2). Blood and feces samples were taken before and after operation. Microorganisms in each sample were detected using a bacterium-specific ribosomal RNA-targeted reverse transcriptase-quantitative polymerase chain reaction method.

Results Some 42 patients were included. There was a significant difference between the 2 groups in detection levels of microorganisms in the MLN-1 samples. Microorganisms were more frequently detected in MLN-2 samples in the control group than in the synbiotics group (10 of 18 vs 3 of 18; $P = .035$). In addition, bacteremia detected using reverse transcriptase-quantitative polymerase chain reaction 1 day after surgery was more prevalent in the control group than in the synbiotics group (12 of 21 vs 4 of 21; $P = .025$). Neutrophil counts on postoperative days 1, 2, and 7 were all significantly higher in the control group than in the synbiotics group.

Conclusion Perioperative use of synbiotics reduces the incidence of bacteria in the MLNs and blood. These beneficial effects probably contribute to a reduction in the inflammatory response after esophagectomy.

Editor's summary and comments This small, randomized trial studied the impact of perioperative synbiotics in patients with esophageal cancer after esophagectomy. The detection of microorganisms in MLNs and bacteremia were significantly less in the group that received synbiotics, suggesting a future role for future studies of synbiotics in the reduction of inflammatory response after esophagectomy.

Clinical study 5

Shyamsundar M, McAuley DF, Shields MO, et al. Effect of simvastatin on physiological and biological outcomes in patients undergoing esophagectomy: a randomized placebo-controlled trial. Ann Surg 2014;259(1):26–31.

No. Patients Randomized	Study Groups	Stratification	Significance Demonstrated	% Change Identified in Trial
31	Simvastatin, n = 15 Placebo, n = 16	None	Yes, pulmonary dead space at 6 h after esophagectomy	94.7 h vs 113.9 h

Hypothesis Simvastatin improves physiologic and biological outcomes in patients undergoing esophagectomy.

Published abstract

Background Single-lung ventilation during esophagectomy is associated with inflammation, alveolar epithelial and systemic endothelial injury, and the development of acute lung injury. Statins that modify many of the underlying processes are a potential therapy to prevent acute lung injury.

Methods We conducted a randomized, double-blind, placebo-controlled trial in patients undergoing esophagectomy. Patients received simvastatin 80 mg or placebo enterally for 4 and 7 days postoperatively. The primary endpoint was pulmonary dead space (Vd/Vt) at 6 hours after esophagectomy or before extubation. Inflammation was assessed by plasma cytokines and intraoperative exhaled breath condensate pH; alveolar type 1 epithelial injury was assessed by plasma receptor for advanced glycation end products and systemic endothelial injury by the urine albumin-creatinine ratio.

Results Thirty-nine patients were randomized; 8 patients did not undergo surgery and were excluded. Fifteen patients received simvastatin and 16 received placebo. There was no difference in Vd/Vt or other physiologic outcomes. Simvastatin resulted in a significant decrease in plasma monocyte chemoattractant protein 1 on day 3 and reduced exhaled breath condensate acidification. Plasma receptor for advanced glycation end products was significantly lower in the simvastatin-treated group, as was the urine albumin-creatinine ratio on postoperative day 7. Acute lung injury developed in 4 patients in the placebo group and no patients in the simvastatin group, although this difference was not statistically significant ($P = .1$).

Conclusions In this proof-of-concept study, pretreatment with simvastatin in esophagectomy decreased biomarkers of inflammation as well as pulmonary epithelial and systemic endothelial injury.

Editor's summary and comments In this multicenter, randomized, double-blind, placebo-controlled trial from Japan, the effect of daikenchuto was studied in patients recovering from total gastrectomy. The mean time to bowel movement was significantly shorter in the daikenchuto group (94.7 hours vs 113.9 hours; $P = .051$). This finding suggests a potential role for daikenchuto in the postoperative bowel recovery of total gastrectomy patients.

Clinical study 6
van Hagen P, Hulshof MC, van Lanschot JJ, et al. Preoperative chemoradiotherapy for esophageal or junctional cancer. N Engl J Med 2012;366(22):2074–84.

No. Patients Randomized	Study Groups	Stratification	Significance Demonstrated	% Change Identified in Trial
366	Chemoradiation + surgery, n = 178 Surgery alone, n = 188	None	Yes, complete resection Median overall survival	Complete resection: 92% vs 69% (*P*<.001) Median overall survival: 49.4 mo vs 24.0 mo (*P* = .003)

Hypothesis Chemoradiation improves outcomes in resectable esophageal and junctional cancer.

Published abstract

Background The role of neoadjuvant chemoradiotherapy in the treatment of patients with esophageal or esophagogastric junction cancer is not well-established. We compared chemoradiotherapy followed by surgery with surgery alone in this patient population.

Methods We randomly assigned patients with resectable tumors to receive surgery alone or weekly administration of carboplatin (doses titrated to achieve an area under the curve of 2 mg/mL/min) and paclitaxel (50 mg/m^2 body surface area) for 5 weeks and concurrent radiotherapy (41.4 Gy in 23 fractions, 5 days per week), followed by surgery.

Results From March 2004 through December 2008, we enrolled 368 patients, 366 of whom were included in the analysis: 275 (75%) had adenocarcinoma, 84 (23%) had squamous cell carcinoma, and 7 (2%) had large-cell undifferentiated carcinoma. Of the 366 patients, 178 were randomly assigned to chemoradiotherapy followed by surgery, and 188 to surgery alone. The most common major hematologic toxic effects in the chemoradiotherapy–surgery group were leukopenia (6%) and neutropenia (2%); the most common major nonhematologic toxic effects were anorexia (5%) and fatigue (3%). Complete resection with no tumor within 1 mm of the resection margins (R0) was achieved in 92% of patients in the chemoradiotherapy–surgery group versus 69% in the surgery group ($P<.001$). A pathologic complete response was achieved in 47 of 161 patients (29%) who underwent resection after chemoradiotherapy. Postoperative complications were similar in the 2 treatment groups, and in-hospital mortality was 4% in both. Median overall survival was 49.4 months in the chemoradiotherapy–surgery group versus 24.0 months in the surgery group. Overall survival was significantly better in the chemoradiotherapy–surgery group (hazard ratio, 0.657; 95% CI, 0.495–0.871; $P = .003$).

Conclusions Preoperative chemoradiotherapy improved survival among patients with potentially curable esophageal or esophagogastric junction cancer. The regimen was associated with acceptable adverse-event rates. (Funded by the Dutch Cancer Foundation [KWF Kankerbestrijding]; Netherlands Trial Register number, NTR487.)

Editor's summary and comments In this randomized trial, chemoradiotherapy (carboplatin, paclitaxel, and 41.4 Gy concurrent radiotherapy) followed by surgery was compared with surgery alone in patients with esophageal or esophagogastric junction cancer. The median overall survival was significantly better with preoperative chemoradiation compared with surgery alone.

Clinical study 7
Biere SS, van Berge Henegouwen MI, Maas KW, et al. Minimally invasive versus open oesophagectomy for patients with oesophageal cancer: a multicentre, open-label, randomised controlled trial. Lancet 2012;379(9829):1887–92.

No. Patients Randomized	Study Groups	Stratification	Significance Demonstrated	% Change Identified in Trial
105	Minimally invasive surgery, n = 59 Open, n = 56	None	Yes, pulmonary infection	34% vs 12% ($P = .005$)

Hypothesis Minimally invasive esophagectomy reduces morbidity compared with open esophagectomy.

Published abstract

Background Surgical resection is regarded as the only curative option for resectable esophageal cancer, but pulmonary complications occurring in more than one-half of patients after open esophagectomy are a great concern. We assessed whether minimally invasive esophagectomy reduces morbidity compared with open esophagectomy.

Methods We conducted a multicenter, open-label, randomized, controlled trial at 5 study centers in 3 countries between June 1, 2009, and March 31, 2011. Patients aged 18 to 75 years with resectable cancer of the esophagus or gastroesophageal junction were randomly assigned via a computer-generated randomization sequence to undergo either open transthoracic or minimally invasive transthoracicoesophagectomy. Randomization was stratified by center. Patients, and investigators undertaking interventions, assessing outcomes, and analyzing data, were not masked to group assignment. The primary outcome was pulmonary infection within the first 2 weeks after surgery and during the whole stay in hospital. Analysis was by intention to treat. This trial is registered with the Netherlands Trial Register, NTR TC 2452.

Results We randomly assigned 56 patients to the open esophagectomy group and 59 to the minimally invasive esophagectomy group. In the open esophagectomy group, 16 patients (29%) had a pulmonary infection in the first 2 weeks compared with 5 (9%) in the minimally invasive group (relative risk, 0.30; 95% CI, 0.12–0.76; $P = .005$). In the open esophagectomy group, 19 patients (34%) had pulmonary infection in-hospital compared with 7 (12%) in the minimally invasive group (relative risk, 0.35; 95% CI, 0.16–0.78; $P = .005$). For in-hospital mortality, 1 patient in the open esophagectomy group died from anastomotic leakage and 2 in the minimally invasive group from aspiration and mediastinitis after anastomotic leakage.

Conclusions These findings provide evidence for the short-term benefits of minimally invasive esophagectomy for patients with resectable esophageal cancer.

Editor's summary and comments In this multicenter, open-label, randomized, controlled trial, patients were assigned to open esophagectomy or minimally invasive esophagectomy. Short-term pulmonary complications were better with the minimally invasive technique, suggesting that the usefulness of this the minimally invasive approach over open esophagectomy.

No. Patients Randomized	Study Groups	Stratification	Significance Demonstrated	% Change Identified in Trial
64	Synbiotics, n = 30 Control, n = 34	None	Yes, infection	Infection: 10% vs 29.4% ($P = .0676$)

Clinical study 8

Tanaka K, Yano M, Motoori M, et al. Impact of perioperative administration of synbiotics in patients with esophageal cancer undergoing esophagectomy: a prospective randomized controlled trial. Surgery 2012;152(5):832–42.

Hypothesis Preoperative synbiotics are clinically beneficial.

Published abstract

Background The clinical value of synbiotics in patients undergoing esophagectomy remains unclear. This study investigated the effects of synbiotics on intestinal micro-flora and surgical outcomes in a clinical setting.

Methods We studied 70 patients with esophageal cancer who were scheduled to undergo esophagectomy. They were randomly allocated to 2 groups: 1 group received synbiotics before and after surgery, and the other did not. Fecal microflora and organic acid concentrations were determined. Postoperative infections, abdominal symptoms, and duration of SIRS were recorded.

Results Of the patients, 64 completed the trial (synbiotics, 30; control, 34). The counts of beneficial bacteria and harmful bacteria in the group given synbiotics were significantly larger and smaller, respectively, than those in the control group on postoperative day 7. The concentrations of total organic acid and acetic acid were higher in the synbiotics group than in the control group ($P<.01$), and the intestinal pH in the synbiotics group was lower than that in the control ($P<.05$) on postoperative day 7. The rate of infections was 10% in the synbiotics group and 29.4% in the control group ($P = .0676$). The duration of SIRS in the synbiotics group was shorter than in the control group ($P = .0057$). The incidence of interruption or reduction of EN by abdominal symptoms was 6.7% in the synbiotics group and 29.4% in the control group ($P = .0259$).

Conclusion Perioperative administration of synbiotics in patients with esophagectomy is useful because they suppress excessive inflammatory response and relieve uncomfortable abdominal symptoms through the adjustment of the intestinal microfloral environment.

Editor's summary and comments In this small, randomized trial, patients who received synbiotics had significantly reduced rates of infections, SIRS duration, and interruption or reduction of EN by abdominal symptoms. This study indicates the short-term benefits of synbiotics in the postoperative period after esophagectomy.

No. Patients Randomized	Study Groups	Stratification	Significance Demonstrated	% Change Identified in Trial
42	Ghrelin, n = 21	None	Yes, oral calorie	18.2 kcal/kg/d vs
	Placebo, n = 21		intake	12.7 kcal/kg/d ($P = .001$)

Clinical study 9
Hiura Y, Takiguchi S, Yamamoto K, et al. Effects of ghrelin administration during chemotherapy with advanced esophageal cancer patients: a prospective, randomized, placebo-controlled phase 2 study. Cancer 2012;118(19):4785–94.

Hypothesis Ghrelin administration minimizes side effects of cisplatin-based chemotherapy in patients with esophageal cancer.

Published abstract

Background Cisplatin reduces plasma ghrelin levels through the 5-hydroxytryptamine receptor. This may cause cisplatin-induced gastrointestinal disorders and hinders the continuation of chemotherapy. The authors of this report conducted a prospective, randomized phase II trial to evaluate the effects of exogenous ghrelin during cisplatin-based chemotherapy.

Methods Forty-two patients with esophageal cancer who were receiving cisplatin-based neoadjuvant chemotherapy were assigned to either a ghrelin group (n = 21) or a placebo group (n = 21). They received either intravenous infusions of synthetic human ghrelin (3 µg/kg) or saline twice daily for 1 week with cisplatin administration. The primary endpoint was changes in oral calorie intake, and the secondary endpoints were chemotherapy-related adverse events; appetite visual analog scale scores; changes in gastrointestinal hormones and nutritional status, including rapid turnover proteins, and quality of life estimated with the European Organization for Research and Treatment of Cancer Quality of Life core questionnaire.

Results Two patients were excluded from the final analysis: 1 patient suspended ghrelin administration because of excessive diaphoresis and another patient in the placebo group failed to monitor the self-questionnaire. Food intake and appetite visual analog scale scores were significantly higher in the ghrelin group than in the placebo group (18.2 ± 5.2 kcal/kg/d vs 12.7 ± 3.4 kcal/kg/d [P = .001] and 6.2 ± 0.9 vs 4.1 ± 0.9 [P<.0001], respectively). Patients in the ghrelin group had fewer adverse events during chemotherapy related to anorexia and nausea than patients in the control group. Significant deterioration was noted after chemotherapy in the placebo group in quality of life scores, appetite, nausea and vomiting, and global health status.

Conclusions Short-term administration of exogenous ghrelin at the start of cisplatin-based chemotherapy stimulated food intake and minimized adverse events.

Editor's summary and comments Cisplatin reduces plasma ghrelin levels through the 5-hydroxytryptamine receptor. Forty-two patients undergoing neoadjuvant cisplatin-based chemotherapy were randomized to receive ghrelin versus placebo. Patients receiving ghrelin were found to have a significantly higher caloric intake. This study suggests the importance of ghrelin in minimizing cisplatin-based chemotherapy side effects.

No. Patients Randomized	Study Groups	Stratification	Significance Demonstrated	% Change Identified in Trial
195	Omeage-3 fatty acids, n = 66 Standard enteral nutrition, n = 63 Control, N = 66	None	No	None

Clinical study 10
Sultan J, Griffin SM, Di Franco F, et al. Randomized clinical trial of omega-3 fatty acid-supplemented enteral nutrition versus standard enteral nutrition in patients undergoing oesophagogastric cancer surgery. Br J Surg 2012;99(3):346–55.

Hypothesis Perioperative omega-3 fatty acid (O3-FA)–supplemented EN improves clinical outcomes.

Published abstract
Background Esophagogastric cancer surgery is immunosuppressive. This may be modulated by O-3FAs. The aim of this study was to assess the effect of perioperative O-3FAs on clinical outcome and immune function after surgery for esophagogastric cancer.

Methods Patients undergoing subtotal esophagectomy and total gastrectomy were recruited and allocated randomly to an O-3FA enteral immunoenhancing diet (IED) or standard enteral nutrition for 7 days before and after surgery, or to postoperative supplementation alone (control group). Clinical outcome, fatty acid concentrations, and HLA-DR expression on monocytes and activated T lymphocytes were determined before and after operation.

Results Of 221 patients recruited, 26 were excluded. Groups (IED, 66; standard enteral nutrition, 63; control, 66) were matched for age, malnutrition, and comorbidity. There were no differences in morbidity ($P = .646$), mortality ($P = 1.000$), or duration of hospital stay ($P = .701$) between the groups. The O-3FA concentrations were higher in the IED group after supplementation ($P<.001$). The ratio of omega-6 fatty acid to O-3FA was 1.9:1, 4.1:1 and 4.8:1 on the day before surgery in the IED, standard enteral nutrition, and control groups, respectively ($P<.001$). There were no differences between the groups in HLA-DR expression in either monocytes ($P = .538$) or activated T lymphocytes ($P = .204$).

Conclusion Despite a significant increase in plasma concentrations of O-3FA, immunonutrition with O-3FA did not affect overall HLA-DR expression on leukocytes or clinical outcome after surgery for esophagogastric cancer.

Editor's summary and comments The aim of this 3-arm, randomized study was to assess the effect of perioperative O-3FAs on clinical outcome and immune function after esophageal cancer surgery. Immunonutrition with O-3FAs did not affect clinical outcomes.

Clinical study 11
Hirao M, Ando N, Tsujinaka T, et al. Influence of preoperative chemotherapy for advanced thoracic oesophageal squamous cell carcinoma on perioperative complications. Br J Surg 2011;98(12):1735–41.

No. Patients Randomized	Study Groups	Stratification	Significance Demonstrated	% Change Identified in Trial
330	Postoperative, n = 166	None	No	None
	Preoperative, n = 164			

Hypothesis Preoperative chemotherapy does not increase postoperative complications.

Published abstract
Background The Japan Clinical Oncology Group 9907 trial has changed the standard of care for advanced thoracic esophageal cancer in Japan from postoperative chemotherapy to preoperative chemotherapy. The impact of preoperative chemotherapy on the risk of developing postoperative complications remains controversial. This article reports the safety analysis of Japan Clinical Oncology Group 9907, focusing on risk factors for postoperative complications.

Methods Patients were potentially randomized to either postoperative or preoperative chemotherapy followed by transthoracic esophagectomy with D2-3 lymphadenectomy. Chemotherapy consisted of 2 cycles of cisplatin and 5-FU. Clinical baseline data, intraoperative complications, postoperative complications, and in-hospital mortality, collected on the case report forms in a predetermined format, were analyzed. Univariable and multivariable analyses were used to explore the risk of postoperative complications in relation to treatment group, age, sex, tumor depth, nodal metastasis, stage, and location.

Results Of 330 patients randomized, 166 were assigned to receive postoperative chemotherapy and 164 preoperative chemotherapy; 162 and 154 patients, respectively, underwent surgery. The incidence of intraoperative complications, postoperative complications and in-hospital mortality was similarly low in both groups. Multivariable analysis showed that age, sex, and tumor location were associated independently with an increase in postoperative complications, but preoperative chemotherapy was not.

Conclusion Preoperative chemotherapy does not increase the risk of complications or hospital mortality after surgery for advanced thoracicoesophageal cancer.

Editor's summary and comments This is the safety analysis of the Japan Clinical Oncology Group 9907 trial, comparing postoperative and preoperative chemotherapy in 330 randomized patients. Operative and postoperative complications were similarly low, indicating that preoperative chemotherapy does not affect short-term outcomes.

No. Patients Randomized	Study Groups	Stratification	Significance Demonstrated	% Change Identified in Trial
128	End-to-end anastomosis, n = 64 End-to-side anastomosis, n = 64	None	Yes, anastomotic stricture	End-to-end anastomosis 40% vs End-to-side anastomosis 18% (P<.01)

Clinical study 12
Nederlof N, Tilanus HW, Tran TC, et al. End-to-end versus end-to-side esophagogastrostomy after esophageal cancer resection: a prospective randomized study. Ann Surg 2011;254(2):226–33.

Hypothesis To compare single-layered hand-sewn cervical ETS anastomosis with ETE anastomosis in a prospective, randomized fashion.

Published abstract
Background The preferred organ used for reconstruction after esophagectomy for cancer is the stomach. Previous studies attempted to define the optimal site of anastomosis and anastomotic techniques. However, anastomotic stricture formation and leakage remain an important clinical problem.

Methods From May 2005 to September 2007, 128 patients (64 in each group) were randomized between ETE and ETS anastomosis after esophagectomy for cancer with gastric tube reconstruction. Routine contrast swallow studies and endoscopy were performed. Anastomotic stricture within 1 year, requiring dilatation, was the primary endpoint. Secondary endpoints were anastomotic leak rate and mortality.

Results Ninety-nine men and 29 women underwent esophagectomy and gastric tube reconstruction. Benign stenosis of the anastomosis, for which dilatation was required, occurred more often in the ETE group (40% vs ETS 18%; *P*<.01) after 1 year of follow-up. The overall (clinical and radiologic) anastomotic leak rate was lower in the ETE group (22% vs ETS 41%; *P* = .04). Patients with an ETE anastomosis suffered less often from pneumonia (ETE 17% vs ETS 44%; *P* = .002) and had subsequently significantly shorter in-hospital duration of stay (15 days vs 22 days, *P* = .02). In-hospital mortality did not differ between the groups.

Conclusion ETS anastomosis is associated with a lower anastomotic stricture rate, compared with ETE anastomosis. However, prevention of stricture formation was at high costs with increased anastomotic leakage and longer in-hospital stay. This study is registered with the Dutch Trial Registry and carries the ID number OND1317772.

Editor's summary and comments This Dutch trial compared ETE versus ETS esophagogastrostomy. The primary outcome was anastomotic stricture with secondary endpoints being anastomotic leak rate and mortality. Although anastomotic stricture rate was higher in the ETE group, the anastomotic leak rate, pneumonia and hospital stay duration were lower. Thus, each surgeon will have to evaluate the use of each technique in context for individual patients to minimize short- and long-term complications.

No. Patients Randomized	Study Groups	Stratification	Significance Demonstrated	% Change Identified in Trial
20	Ghrelin, n = 10 Placebo, n = 10	None	Yes, caloric intake	874 kcal/d vs 605 kcal/d (*P* = .015)

Clinical study 13
Yamamoto K, Takiguchi S, Miyata H, et al. Randomized phase II study of clinical effects of ghrelin after esophagectomy with gastric tube reconstruction. Surgery 2010;148(1):31–8.

Hypothesis Ghrelin ameliorates the postoperative decrease of oral food intake and body weight.

Published abstract
Background Ghrelin is a peptide hormone with pleiotropic functions, including stimulation of growth hormone secretion and appetite, and its levels decrease after esophagectomy. The aim of this study was to evaluate whether exogenous ghrelin administration can ameliorate the postoperative decrease of oral food intake and body weight, which are serious complications after esophagectomy.

Methods This prospective, randomized, placebo-controlled clinical trial assigned a total of 20 patients with thoracic esophageal cancer who underwent radical operation into either a ghrelin (n = 10) or placebo (n = 10) group. Synthetic human ghrelin (3 μg/kg) or 0.9% saline placebo was administered intravenously twice daily for 10 days from the day after the start of food intake. The primary endpoint was calories of food intake. Comparison of appetite and changes in weight and body composition were also made between the 2 groups.

Results Intake of food calories was greater in ghrelin group than placebo group (mean 874 kcal/d vs 605 kcal/d; *P* = .015). The appetite score tended to be greater in ghrelin group than placebo group (*P* = .094). Loss of weight was less in ghrelin group (−1% vs −3%; *P* = .019) and this attenuation was due largely to a decrease of lean body weight loss (0% vs −4%; $P = .012$). No side effects were observed in either groups.

Conclusion These preliminary results suggest that the administration of ghrelin after esophagectomy increased oral food intake and attenuated weight loss together with maintenance of lean body weight.

Editor's summary and comments This prospective, randomized, placebo-controlled clinical trial assigned a total of 20 patients with thoracic esophageal cancer after esophagectomy to receive ghrelin or placebo. Preliminary results suggest that ghrelin increases caloric intake and attenuates weight loss.

No. Patients Randomized	Study Groups	Stratification	Significance Demonstrated	% Change Identified in Trial
79	Twice daily proton pump inhibitors, n = 39 Placebo, n = 40	None	Yes, anastomotic stricture	13% vs 45% (P = .001)

Clinical study 14
Johansson J, Oberg S, Wenner J, et al. Impact of proton pump inhibitors on benign anastomotic stricture formations after esophagectomy and gastric tube reconstruction: results from a randomized clinical trial. Ann Surg 2009;250(5):667–73.

Hypothesis The use of proton pump inhibitors (PPIs) reduced the prevalence of benign anastomotic strictures after uncomplicated esophagectomies with gastric tube reconstruction and circular stapled anastomoses.

Published abstract
Background Benign anastomotic strictures are associated with anastomotic leaks or conduit ischemia. Also, patients without those complications develop benign anastomotic strictures. We hypothesize that patients without postoperative anastomotic complications may develop benign anastomotic strictures owing to exposure of acid gastric tube contents to the anastomotic area, and that the formation of such strictures may be reduced by prophylactic use of PPIs.

Methods Eighty patients without preoperative chemotherapy or radiotherapy and without clinical or radiologic signs of anastomotic leaks were included in this clinical trial. The patients were randomized to twice daily PPIs or no treatment for 1 year. Benign anastomotic strictures were defined as anastomotic narrowing not allowing a standard diagnostic endoscope to pass without dilatation. The study was registered in the EudraCT database (2009-009997-28) for clinical trials.

Results Seventy-nine patients were evaluated. Benign anastomotic strictures developed in 5 of 39 patients (13%) in the PPI group and in 18 of 40 (45%) in the control group (relative risk, 5.6; 95% CI, 2.0–15.9; $P = .001$). The use of a narrower 25-mm cartridge as compared with a wider 28- or 31-mm cartridge significantly increased stricture formations (relative risk, 2.9; 95% CI, 1.1–7.6; $P = .025$).

Conclusions Prophylactic PPI treatment reduced the prevalence of benign anastomotic strictures after esophagectomy with gastric tube reconstruction and circular stapled anastomoses. Larger sized circular staple cartridges additionally reduced the stricture prevalence.

Editor's summary and comments This randomized clinical trial studied whether twice daily PPI use may decrease the risk of benign anastomotic strictures. Twice daily PPI use had a lower rate of stricture formation, as was using a wide 28- or 31-mm cartridge instead of the narrower 25-mm cartridge.

No. Patients Randomized	Study Groups	Stratification	Significance Demonstrated	% Change Identified in Trial
53	Eicosapentaenoic acid enriched, N = 28 Standard, n = 25	None	Yes, fat-free mass	0 kg vs 1.9 kg (P = .030)

Clinical study 15
Ryan AM, Reynolds JV, Healy L, et al. Enteral nutrition enriched with eicosapentaenoic acid (EPA) preserves lean body mass following esophageal cancer surgery: results of a double-blinded randomized controlled trial. Ann Surg 2009;249(3):355–63.

Hypothesis EPA-enriched EN preserves lean body mass better than standard EN.

Published abstract

Background Esophagectomy represents an exemplar of controlled major trauma, with marked metabolic, immunologic, and physiologic changes as well as an associated high incidence of complications. EPA-enriched EN modulates immune function and limits catabolism in patients with advanced cancer, but its impact in the perioperative period is unclear.

Objectives To examine the effects of perioperative EPA-enriched EN on the metabolic, nutritional, and immunoinflammatory response to esophagectomy, and on postoperative complications.

Methods In a double-blind design, patients were randomized to a standard EN formula or a formula enriched with 2.2 g EPA per day for 5 days preoperatively (orally) and 21 days postoperatively (jejunostomy). Segmental bioelectrical impedance analysis was performed preoperatively and on postoperative day 21. Postoperative complications were monitored, as well as the acute phase response, coagulation markers, and serum cytokines.

Results Fifty-three patients (28 EPA, 25 standard) completed the study, and both groups were well matched. Serum and peripheral blood mononuclear cell membrane EPA levels were increased significantly in the EPA group. There was no difference in the incidence of major complications. The EPA group maintained all aspects of body composition postoperatively, whereas patients in the standard EN group lost significant amounts of fat-free mass (1.9 kg; $P = .030$) compared with the EPA group (leg, 0.3 kg [$P = .05$]; arm, 0.17 kg [$P = .01$]; and trunk, 1.44 kg [$P = .03$]). The EPA group had a significantly ($P < .05$) attenuated stress response for tumor necrosis factor alpha, IL-10, and IL-8 compared with the standard group.

Conclusions EPA-supplemented early EN is associated with preservation of lean body mass after esophagectomy compared with a standard EN. These properties may merit longer-term study to address its impact on recovery of function and quality of life in models of complex surgery or multimodal cancer treatment regimens.

Editor's summary and comments EPA-enriched EN was compared with standard EN and found to preserve fat-free mass better than standard nutrition and significantly attenuated stress response.

Clinical study 16
Mistry RC, Vijayabhaskar R, Karimundackal G, et al. Effect of short-term versus prolonged nasogastric decompression on major postesophagectomy complications: a parallel-group, randomized trial. Arch Surg 2012;147(8):747–51.

No. Patients Randomized	Study Groups	Stratification	Significance Demonstrated	% Change Identified in Trial
150	Nasogastric tube removed after 6–10 d, n = 75 Early removal of the nasogastric tube, n = 75	None	Yes, pulmonary complications, anastomotic leaks	13% vs 45% (P = .001)

Hypothesis Early removal of the NGT would not adversely affect major pulmonary complications and anastomotic leak rates.

Published abstract
Background Controversy exists over the need for prolonged nasogastric decompression after esophagectomy. We hypothesized that early removal of the NGT would not adversely affect major pulmonary complications and anastomotic leak rates.

Methods This single-center, parallel-group, open-label trial randomized participants 1:1 at a tertiary referral cancer center with high esophagectomy volume. One hundred fifty patients undergoing esophagectomy with gastric tube reconstruction were included. Patients were randomized to conventional nasogastric decompression for 6 to 10 days (75 patients) or early removal (48 hours) of NGT (75 patients) with stratification for pyloric drainage and anastomotic technique. The primary (composite) endpoint was the occurrence of major pulmonary complications and anastomotic leaks. Secondary endpoints were the need for NGT reinsertion and patient discomfort scores. Analysis was performed on an intent-to-treat basis.

Results No differences were seen in the occurrence of the composite primary endpoint of major pulmonary and anastomotic complications between the delayed (14 of 75 patients [18.7%]) and early (16 of 75 patients [21.3%]) removal groups, respectively (P = .84). NGT reinsertion was required more often (early 23 of 75 patients [30.7%] vs late 7 of 75 patients [9.3%]) in the early group (P = .001). Mean patient discomfort scores were significantly higher in the delayed (+1.3; 95% CI, 0.4–2.2; P = .006) than in the early removal group. Significantly more patients in the delayed removal group (26 of 75 patients [34.7%] vs 10 of 75 patients [13.3%] in the early removal group; P = .002) identified the NGT as the tube causing the most discomfort.

Conclusions Early removal of the NGT does not increase pulmonary or anastomotic complications after esophagectomy. Patient discomfort can be reduced significantly by early removal of the NGT.

Editor's summary and comments Early removal of NGT does not increase pulmonary or anastomotic complications. Removal at 48 hours is a feasible choice in the postoperative setting for patient comfort.

REFERENCES

1. Hulscher JB, van Sandick JW, deBoer AG, et al. Extended transthoracic resection compared with limited transhiatal resection for adenocarcinoma of the esophagus. N Engl J Med 2002;347:1662-9.

2. Goldminc M, Maddern G, LePrise E, et al. Oesophagectomy by a transhiatal approach or thoracotomy: a prospective randomized trial. Br J Surg 1993;80: 367-70.

3. Jacobi CA, Zieren HU, Muller JM, et al. Surgical therapy of esophageal carcinoma: the influence of surgical approach and esophageal resection on cardiopulmonary function. Eur J Cardiothorac Surg 1997;11:32-7.

4. Chu KM, Law SY, Fok M, et al. A prospective randomized comparison of transhiatal and transthoracic resection for lower-third esophageal carcinoma. Am J Surg 1997;174:320-4.

5. Gupta NM, Gupta R, Rao MS, et al. Minimizing cervical esophageal anastomotic complications by a modified technique. Am J Surg 2001;181:534.

6. Bhat MA, Dar MA, Lone GN, et al. Use of pedicled omentum in esophagogastric anastomosis for prevention of anastomotic leak. Ann Thorac Surg 2006;82:1857.

7. Tabira Y, Sakaguchi T, Kuhara H, et al. The width of a gastric tube has no impact on outcome after esophagectomy. Am J Surg 2004;187:417.

8. Nederlof N, Tilanus HW, Tran TC, et al. End-to-end versus end-to-side esophagogastrostomy after esophageal cancer resection: a prospective randomized study. Ann Surg 2011;254(2):226-33.

9. Li B, Xiang J, Zhang Y, et al. Comparison of Ivor-Lewis vs Sweet esophagectomy for esophageal squamous cell carcinoma: a randomized clinical trial. JAMA Surg 2015;150(4):292-8.

10. Shen Y, Feng M, Tan L, et al. Thoracoscopic esophagectomy in prone versus decubitus position: ergonomic evaluation from a randomized and controlled study. Ann Thorac Surg 2014;98(3):1072-8.

11. Biere SS, van Berge Henegouwen MI, Maas KW, et al. Minimally invasive versus open oesophagectomy for patients with oesophageal cancer: a multicentre, open-label, randomised controlled trial. Lancet 2012;379(9829):1887-92.

12. Shackcloth MJ, McCarron E, Kendall J, et al. Randomized clinical trial to determine the effect of nasogastric drainage on tracheal acid aspiration following oesophagectomy. Br J Surg 2006;93:547.

13. Mistry RC, Vijayabhaskar R, Karimundackal G, et al. Effect of short-term vs prolonged nasogastric decompression on major postesophagectomy complications: a parallel-group, randomized trial. Arch Surg 2012;147(8):747-51.

14. Hirao M, Ando N, Tsujinaka T, et al. Influence of preoperative chemotherapy for advanced thoracic oesophageal squamous cell carcinoma on perioperative complications. Br J Surg 2011;98(12):1735-41.

15. Ryan AM, Reynolds JV, Healy L, et al. Enteral nutrition enriched with eicosapentaenoic acid (EPA) preserves lean body mass following esophageal cancer surgery: results of a double-blinded randomized controlled trial. Ann Surg 2009; 249(3):355-63.

16. Takata A, Takiguchi S, Miyazaki Y, et al. Randomized Phase II Study of the Anti-inflammatory Effect of Ghrelin During the Postoperative Period of Esophagectomy. Ann Surg 2015;262(2):230–6.

17. Hiura Y, Takiguchi S, Yamamoto K, et al. Effects of ghrelin administration during chemotherapy with advanced esophageal cancer patients: a prospective, randomized, placebo-controlled phase 2 study. Cancer 2012;118(19):4785–94.

18. Yamamoto K, Takiguchi S, Miyata H, et al. Randomized phase II study of clinical effects of ghrelin after esophagectomy with gastric tube reconstruction. Surgery 2010;148(1):31–8.

19. Yokoyama Y, Nishigaki E, Abe T, et al. Randomized clinical trial of the effect of perioperative synbiotics versus no synbiotics on bacterial translocation after oesophagectomy. Br J Surg 2014;101(3):189–99.

20. Tanaka K, Yano M, Motoori M, et al. Impact of perioperative administration of synbiotics in patients with esophageal cancer undergoing esophagectomy: a prospective randomized controlled trial. Surgery 2012;152(5):832–42.

21. Shyamsundar M, McAuley DF, Shields MO, et al. Effect of simvastatin on physiological and biological outcomes in patients undergoing esophagectomy: a randomized placebo-controlled trial. Ann Surg 2014;259(1):26–31.

22. May A, Gossner L, Behrens A, et al. A prospective randomized trial of two different endoscopic resection techniques for early stage cancer of the esophagus. Gastrointest Endosc 2003;58:167.

23. Nagatani S, Shimada Y, Kondo M, et al. A strategy for determining which thoracic esophageal cancer patients should undergo cervical lymph node dissection. Ann Thorac Surg 1881;80:2005.

24. Nakatsuchi T, Otani M, Osugi H, et al. The necessity of chest physical therapy for thoracoscopic oesophagectomy. J Int Med Res 2005;33:434.

25. Farran L, Llop J, Sans M, et al. Efficacy of enteral decontamination in the prevention of anastomotic dehiscence and pulmonary infection in esophagogastric surgery. Dis Esophagus 2008;21:159.

26. Miyazaki T, Kuwano H, Kato H, et al. Predictive value of blood flow in the gastric tube in anastomotic insufficiency after thoracic esophagectomy. World J Surg 2002;26:1319.

27. Boonstra JJ, Kok TC, Wijnhoven BPL, et al. Chemotherapy followed by surgery versus surgery alone in patients with resectable oesophageal squamous cell carcinoma: long-term results of a randomized trial. BMC Cancer 2011;11:181.

28. Kelsen DP, Ginsberg R, Pajak RF, et al. Chemotherapy followed by surgery compared with surgery alone for localized esophageal cancer. N Engl J Med 1998;339:1979–84.

29. Kelsen DP, Winter KA, Gunderson LL, et al. Long-term results of RTOG Trial 8911 (USA Intergroup 113): a random assignment trial comparison of chemotherapy followed by surgery compared with surgery alone for esophageal cancer. J Clin Oncol 2007;25:3719–25.

30. Medical Research Council Oesophageal Cancer Working Group. Surgical resection with or without preoperative chemotherapy in oesophageal cancer: a randomised controlled trial. Lancet 2002;359:1727–33.

31. Allum WH, Stenning SP, Bancewicz J, et al. Long term results of a randomized trial of surgery with or without preoperative chemotherapy in esophageal cancer. J Clin Oncol 2009;27:5062–7.

32. Anderson D, Langley RE, Nankivell MG, et al. Neoadjuvant chemotherapy for resectable oesophageal and junctional adenocarcinoma: results form the UK Medical Research Council randomized OEO5 trial. 2015 ASCO Annual Meeting.

Available at: http://meetinglibrary.asco.org/content/149773-156. Accessed January 1, 2017.

33. Cunningham D, Allum W, Stenning SP, et al. Perioperative chemotherapy versus surgery alone for resectable gastroesophageal cancer. N Engl J Med 2006;355: 11–20.

34. Yehou M, Boige V, Pignon JP, et al. Perioperative chemotherapy compared with surgery alone for resectable gastroesophageal adenocarcinoma: an FNLCC and FFCF multicenter phase III trial. J Clin Oncol 2011;29:1715–21.

35. Schuhmacher C, Gretschel S, Lordick F, et al. Neoadjuvant chemotherapy compared with surgery alone for locally advanced cancer of the stomach and cardia: European Organization for Research and Treatment of Cancer randomized Trial 40954. J Clin Oncol 2010;28:5210–8.

36. Mei W, Xian-Zhi G, Weibo Y, et al. Randomized clinical trial on the combination of preoperative irradiation and surgery in the treatment of esophageal carcinoma: report on 206 patients. Int J Radiat Oncol Biol Phys 1989;16:325–7.

37. Gignoux M, Roussel A, Paillot B, et al. The value of preoperative radiotherapy in esophageal cancer: results of a study of the EORTC. World J Surg 1987;11: 426–32.

38. Nygaard K, Hagen S, Hansen JS, et al. Pre-operative radiotherapy prolongs survival in operable esophageal carcinoma: a randomized, multicenter study of preoperative radiotherapy and chemotherapy. The second Scandinavian trial in esophageal cancer. World J Surg 1992;16:1104–10.

39. Launois B, Delaru D, Campion JP, et al. Preoperative radiotherapy for carcinoma of the esophagus. Surg Gynecol Obstet 1981;153:690–2.

40. Arnott SJ, Duncan W, Kerr GR, et al. Low dose preoperative radiotherapy for carcinoma of the oesophagus: results of a randomized clinical trial. Radiother Oncol 1993;24:108–13.

41. Huang GJ, Gu XZ, Wang LJ, et al. Combined preoperative irradiation and surgery for esophageal carcinoma. In: Delalrue NC, editor. International trends in general thoracic surgery. St Louis (MO): Mosby; 1988. p. 315.

42. Walsh TN, Noonan N, Hollywood D, et al. A comparison of multimodal therapy and surgery for esophageal adenocarcinoma. N Engl J Med 1996;335:462–7.

43. Walsh TN, Grennell M, Mansoor S, et al. Neoadjuvant treatment of advanced stage esophageal adenocarcinoma increases survival. Dis Esophagus 2002; 15:121–4.

44. Tepper J, Krasna MJ, Niedzwiecki D, et al. Phase III trial of trimodality therapy with cisplatin, fluorouracil, radiotherapy, and surgery compared with surgery alone for esophageal cancer: CALGB 9781. J Clin Oncol 2008;26:1086–92.

45. Urba SG, Orringer MB, Turrisi A, et al. Randomized trial of preoperative chemoradiation versus surgery alone in patients with locoregional esophageal carcinoma. J Clin Oncol 2001;19:305–13.

46. Bosset JF, Gignoux M, Triboulet JP, et al. Chemoradiotherapy followed by surgery compared with surgery alone in squamous cell cancer of the esophagus. N Engl J Med 1997;337:161–7.

47. Burmeister BH, Smithers BM, Gebski V, et al. Surgery alone versus chemoradiotherapy followed by surgery for resectable cancer of the oesophagus: a randomised controlled phase III trial. Lancet Oncol 2005;6:659–68.

48. Mariette C, Dahan L, Mornex F, et al. Surgery alone vs chemoradiotherapy followed by surgery for stage I and II esophageal cancer. J Clin Oncol 2014; 32(23):2416–22.

49. Stahl M, Walz MK, Stuschke M, et al. Phase III comparison of preoperative chemotherapy compared with chemoradiotherapy in patients with locally advanced adenocarcinoma of the esophagogastric junction. J Clin Oncol 2009; 27:851–6.

50. Van Hagen P, Hulshof MC, van Lanschot JJ, et al. Preoperative chemoradiotherapy for esophageal or junctional cancer. N Engl J Med 2012;366:2074–84.

51. A comparison of chemotherapy and radiotherapy as adjuvant treatment to surgery for esophageal carcinoma. Japanese Esophageal Oncology Group. Chest 1993;104:203–7.

52. Iizuka AT, Isono KK, Watanabe H, et al. A randomized trial comparing surgery to surgery plus postoperative chemotherapy for localized squamous carcinoma of the thoracic esophagus: the Japan Clinical Oncology Study Group (JCOG) study. Proc Am Soc Clin Oncol 1998;17:282a.

53. Ando N, Iizuka T, Kakegawa T, et al. A randomized trial of surgery with and without chemotherapy for localized squamous carcinoma of the thoracic esophagus: the Japan Clinical Oncology Group Study. J Thorac Cardiovasc Surg 1997; 114:205–9.

54. Teniere P, Hay JM, Fingerhut A, et al. Postoperative radiation therapy does not increase survival after curative resection for squamous cell carcinoma of the middle and lower esophagus as shown by a multicenter controlled trial. French University Association for Surgical Research. Surg Gynecol Obstet 1991;173: 123.

55. Fok M, Sham JS, Choi D, et al. Postoperative radiotherapy for carcinoma of the esophagus: a prospective, randomized controlled study. Surgery 1993;113: 138–47.

56. MacDonald J, Benedetti J, Smalley S, et al. Chemoradiation of resected gastric cancer: a 10-year follow-up of the phase III trial INT 0116 (SWOG 9008). Proc Am Soc Clin Oncol 2009;27:205s.

57. Gordon MA, Gundacker HM, Benedetti J, et al. Assessment of HER2 gene amplification in adenocarcinomas of the stomach or gastroesophageal junction in the INT-0116/SWOG9008 clinical trial. Ann Oncol 2013;24:1754–61.

58. Yu J, Ren R, Sun X, et al. A randomized clinical study of surgery versus radiotherapy in the treatment of resectable esophageal cancer. Proc Am Soc Clin Oncol 2006;24:181s.

59. Chiu PWY, Chan ACW, Leung SF, et al. Multicenter prospective randomized trial comparing standard esophagectomy with chemoradiotherapy for treatment of squamous esophageal cancer: early results from the Chinese University Research Group for Esophageal Cancer (CURE). J Gastrointest Surg 2005;9:794.

60. Cooper JS, Guo MD, Herskovic A, et al. Chemoradiotherapy of locally advanced esophageal cancer: long-term follow-up of a prospective randomized trial (RTOG 85–01). Radiation Therapy Oncology Group. JAMA 1999;281:1623–7.

61. Herskovic A, Martz K, Al-Sarraf M, et al. Combined chemotherapy and radiotherapy compared with radiotherapy alone in patients with cancer of the esophagus. N Engl J Med 1992;326:1593–8.

62. Roussel A, Jacob JH, Jung GM, et al. Controlled clinical trial for the treatment of patients with inoperable esophageal carcinoma: a study of the EORTC Gastrointestinal Tract Cancer Cooperative Group. In: Schlag P, Hohenberger P, Metzger U, editors. Recent results in cancer research. Berlin: Springer-Verlag; 1988. p. 21.

63. Al-Sarraf M, Martz K, Herskovic A, et al. Progress report of combined chemora-diotherapy versus radiotherapy alone in patients with esophageal cancer: an Intergroup study. J Clin Oncol 1997;15:277–84.

64. Slabber CF, Nel JS, Schoeman L, et al. A randomized study of radiotherapy alone versus radiotherapy plus 5-fluorouracil and platinum in patients with inoperable, locally advanced squamous cancer of the esophagus. Am J Clin Oncol 1998;21: 462–5.

65. Smith TJ, Ryan LM, Douglass HO, et al. Combined chemoradiotherapy vs. radio-therapy alone for early stage squamous cell carcinoma of the esophagus: a study of the Eastern Cooperative Oncology Group. Int J Radiat Oncol Biol Phys 1998; 42:269–76.

66. Araujo C, Souhami L, Gil R, et al. A randomized trial comparing radiation therapy versus concomitant radiation therapy and chemotherapy in carcinoma of the thoracic esophagus. Cancer 1991;67:2258–61.

67. Wong RK, Malthaner RA, Zuraw L, et al. Combined modality radiotherapy and chemotherapy in nonsurgical management of localized carcinoma of the esoph-agus: a practice guideline. Int J Radiat Oncol Biol Phys 2003;55:930–42.

68. Bedenne L, Michel P, Bouche O, et al. Chemoradiation followed by surgery compared to chemoradiation alone in squamous cancer of the esophagus: FFCD 9102. J Clin Oncol 2007;25:1160–8.

69. Crehange G, Maingon P, Peignaux K, et al, Federation Francophone de Cancer-ologie Digestive 9102. Phase III trial of protracted compared with split-course chemoradiation for esophageal cancer: Federation Francophone de Cancerolo-gie Digestive 9102. J Clin Oncol 2007;25:4895–901.

70. Stahl M, Stuschke M, Lehmann N, et al. Chemoradiation with and without surgery in patients with locally advanced squamous cell carcinoma of the esophagus. J Clin Oncol 2005;23:2310–7.

An Update on Randomized Clinical Trials in Hepatocellular Carcinoma

Hao-Wen Sim, BMedSci, FRACP[a], Jennifer Knox, MD, MSc, FRCPC[a], Laura A. Dawson, MD, FRCPC[b],*

KEYWORDS

- Hepatocellular carcinoma • Randomized trials • Review • Evidence-based medicine
- Management

KEY POINTS

- Choice of treatment modality relies on consideration of tumor stage, liver function, performance status, and comorbidities.
- There has been no definitive comparison of transplantation, surgical resection, and local ablation.
- Radiofrequency ablation is currently the preferred technique for local ablation.
- Transarterial chemoembolization is currently the preferred technique for regional therapy, and confers survival benefit compared with best supportive care.
- For advanced disease, the standard of care in the first-line setting is sorafenib. Regorafenib has recently shown survival benefit in the second-line setting.

INTRODUCTION

The management of hepatocellular carcinoma (HCC) remains challenging on several accounts. First, most patients harbor background liver cirrhosis, which complicates treatment choice due to risk of liver failure. Second, HCC is driven by a variety of causes, including viral hepatitis, alcohol, and fatty liver disease, which may explain variation in the underlying biological mechanisms and treatment responses in different populations. Third, there are numerous treatment options to choose from. The Barcelona Clinic Liver Cancer classification provides a framework for treatment selection.[1] Early-stage disease is usually amenable to curative approaches, such as liver

Disclosure Statement: The authors have nothing to disclose.
[a] Department of Medical Oncology and Hematology, Princess Margaret Cancer Centre, University Health Network, 610 University Avenue, Toronto, Ontario M5G 2M9, Canada; [b] Radiation Medicine Program, Princess Margaret Cancer Centre, University Health Network, 610 University Avenue, Toronto, Ontario M5G 2M9, Canada
* Corresponding author.
E-mail address: Laura.Dawson@rmp.uhn.on.ca

transplantation, surgical resection, and local ablation. Noncurative approaches include regional, radiation, and systemic therapy. Ultimately, treatment choice requires careful consideration of tumor extent, performance status, and underlying liver function, and is commonly determined by multidisciplinary team consensus.

This article reviews the evidence from randomized clinical trials that lay the foundation for contemporary HCC management. A discussion of prevention and screening trials, followed by the supporting data for the aforementioned treatment modalities are presented. Much of the literature remains controversial because many randomized trials are small and underpowered, with varying selection criteria, and are often single-institution studies based on specific populations. The emphasis is on those randomized clinical trials that have defined the current treatment algorithm.

PREVENTION AND SCREENING

Screening for HCC has become standard practice for high-risk patients, such as those with established cirrhosis or viral hepatitis. The key evidence supporting this comes from a large randomized trial conducted in China in the early 1990s.[2] A total of 18,816 subjects with known hepatitis B infection were randomly assigned to either screening with 6-monthly alpha-fetoprotein testing and ultrasonography, or no screening. Despite low compliance with screening, there was a significant reduction in mortality from HCC in the screened group (83.2 per 100,000) compared with controls (131.5 per 100,000), corresponding to a statistically significant mortality ratio of 0.63. This mortality reduction was attributed to the detection of HCC at an earlier stage in the screened group, in which tumors were still amenable to a curative approach.

Beyond screening of infected hepatitis B patients, it has been demonstrated that antiviral suppression significantly reduces the incidence of HCC. In the seminal trial evaluating the efficacy of lamivudine for chronic hepatitis B, 651 subjects were randomly assigned to either lamivudine or placebo for a maximum of 5 years.[3] HCC occurred in 4% of the lamivudine group versus 7% of the placebo group (hazard ratio [HR] 0.49, $P = .047$). There was a similar reduction in hepatic decompensation events. Previous prevention studies in hepatitis B were inconclusive but were based on less effective interferon therapy. Based on these data, antiviral therapy is used to delay progression of liver disease and reduce complications such as HCC.

For patients with hepatitis C, treatment has historically consisted of pegylated interferon and ribavirin. Multiple studies have assessed treatment effect on HCC risk. Meta-analysis of pooled data from 20 studies, including 4 randomized controlled trials, revealed a favorable and statistically significant risk ratio of 0.43 in treated hepatitis C subjects.[4] Notably, this benefit was driven by the subjects who achieved sustained virologic response and there was no benefit of ongoing therapy for nonresponders. The new generation of potent direct-acting antivirals, such as ledipasvir or sofosbuvir, is expected to yield further benefits, although data are still emerging.

TREATMENT
Transplantation

With rare exceptions, HCC is the only solid organ malignancy in which curative transplantation is a treatment option. This is made possible by the propensity of early HCC to spread locally instead of distantly, and the technical capabilities of liver transplantation surgery. Transplantation affords the unique benefit of simultaneously addressing both the tumor and the underlying tumorigenic liver. Eligibility for orthotopic liver transplantation is traditionally based on Milan criteria (solitary lesion 5 cm or less, or

3 lesions each 3 cm or less).[5] Critically, availability is limited by the shortage of donor organs.

Despite transplantation, recurrence occurs in approximately 20% of cases. A large contemporary randomized trial, the Sirolimus in Liver Transplant Recipients with HCC (SiLVER) study, investigated whether recurrence risk could be reduced by using sirolimus, a mammalian target of rapamycin (mTOR) inhibitor, instead of conventional immunosuppression with a calcineurin inhibitor following transplantation.[6] This was based on the success of mTOR inhibitors in treating other cancers such as renal cell carcinoma. A total of 525 subjects were randomized 4 to 6 weeks after transplantation and followed for at least 5 years. Those treated with sirolimus had significantly longer recurrence-free survival (RFS) (3-year HR 0.70, 95% CI 0.48–1.00, $P = .050$) and overall survival (OS) (5-year HR 0.70, 95% CI 0.49–1.00, $P = .048$) during the initial period. Although this difference was not statistically significant at study end at 8 years, there was a consistent trend to improved outcomes. Toxicity and rejection episodes were comparable. Accordingly, the SiLVER study supports preferential use of mTOR-based immunosuppression pending further data in this setting.

Surgical Resection

Surgical resection has been a standard curative treatment of early HCC, particularly given the shortage of donor organs for transplantation. Even so, many patients are not suitable candidates due to the extent of underlying liver disease and medical comorbidities. Careful patient selection is necessary to minimize the risk of liver failure and ensure an adequate future functional liver remnant, incorporating Child-Pugh classification, model of end-stage liver disease score, and assessment of portal hypertension.

Regarding surgical technique, a noteworthy randomized trial investigated the optimal margin of resection.[7] A total of 169 subjects with solitary HCC were randomized to resection with the intention of either 1 cm or 2 cm resection margins. OS and RFS were significantly longer in the 2 cm group (5-year OS 75% vs 49%, $P = .008$; 5-year RFS 53% vs 41%, $P = .046$). It is conceivable that the poor outcomes in the 1 cm group were due to a high rate of inadvertent incomplete resection. There was no significant difference in operative morbidity or mortality. This suggests that the 2 cm margin of resection does not unduly compromise residual liver function, yet produces superior outcomes.

There have been no large, robust randomized trials to definitively address the comparison of surgical resection with the other curative treatment modalities (transplantation and local ablation). However, the following trials have been frequently cited. Chen and colleagues[8] randomized 180 subjects with solitary HCC less than 5 cm to either surgical resection or radiofrequency ablation (RFA). It is notable that more than 20% of the subjects assigned to RFA withdrew their consent and proceeded with surgery. Over a 4-year period, there was no significant difference in OS or RFS. Feng and colleagues[9] randomized 168 subjects with up to 2 lesions less than 4 cm to either surgical resection or RFA. Over a 3-year period, there was no significant difference in OS or RFS. Huang and colleagues[10] randomized 230 subjects with HCC within Milan criteria to either surgical resection or RFA. Over a 5-year period, OS and RFS favored surgical resection (5-year OS 76% vs 55%, $P = .001$; 5-year RFS 51% vs 29%, $P = .017$). Huang and colleagues[11] randomized 76 subjects with up to 2 lesions less than 3 cm to either surgical resection or percutaneous ethanol injection (PEI). After a mean follow-up of 3 years, there was a nonsignificant trend to improved survival with surgery, particularly for lesions larger than 2 cm. These results are conflicting, and their interpretation is hampered by small sample size and short follow-up. There are concerns regarding adherence to treatment allocation and the generalizability of results from these single-institution trials. Based on the available data, the consensus is that surgical resection and local ablation are comparable for carefully selected subjects, such as solitary lesions less than 2 cm.[12] For tumors of increasing size and number, there is uncertainty, and the standard approach of surgical resection is preferred.

Perioperative therapy

There is no standard neoadjuvant or adjuvant treatment with global acceptance for resected HCC. The most widely studied adjuvant treatment has been interferon. Two meta-analyses evaluated the same 7 randomized trials of adjuvant interferon versus placebo, with 620 subjects enrolled in total.[13,14] Both meta-analyses concluded that interferon was beneficial (2-year mortality ratio 0.65; OS HR 0.52, 95% CI 0.38–0.71, $P<.001$). However, there was significant heterogeneity in subject populations and treatment regimens, with 6 trials investigating interferon-alpha and 1 investigating interferon-beta, and treatment durations varying from 1 to 3 years. Moreover, the benefits of interferon need to be carefully weighed against the severe adverse effects, which were substantial even in these highly selected noncirrhotic patients. The benefits may also be partly explained by the effect of interferon on suppression of viral hepatitis. Interferon has yet to be evaluated in the current era of improved direct-acting antivirals. Due to these concerns, interferon has not been widely adopted in clinical practice.

Other potential adjuvant options have been examined, including systemic and transhepatic arterial chemotherapy with fluoropyrimidines, anthracyclines and platinum compounds, vitamin A and K2 analogues, and the heparanase inhibitor PI-88. Meta-analysis of 8 randomized trials of chemotherapy and 5 randomized trials of vitamin analogues did not reveal any efficacy.[14] The heparanase inhibitor PI-88 showed preliminary activity in a phase II trial,[15] but the subsequent phase III PI-88 in the Adjuvant Treatment of Patients with Hepatitis Virus-Related HCC After Surgical Resection (PATRON) trial did not meet the primary endpoint of disease-free survival at interim analysis.

More recently, the multikinase inhibitor sorafenib was investigated as a potential adjuvant treatment, based on its established efficacy in the advanced setting. In the Sorafenib as Adjuvant Treatment in the Prevention of Recurrence of HCC (STORM) trial, an international phase III randomized double-blind placebo-controlled trial, there were 1114 subjects with early HCC who had successfully undergone surgical resection or local ablation.[16] They were randomized to receive either sorafenib 400 mg orally twice a day or placebo for a maximum of 4 years. No significant difference was noted in RFS (HR 0.94, 95% CI 0.78–1.13, $P = .26$) or OS (HR 1.00, 95% CI 0.76–1.30, $P = .48$). A possible contributing factor was the relatively low-dose intensity in the sorafenib group (mean duration of treatment and daily dose were 12.5 months and 577 mg, respectively), reportedly due to a reduced acceptance of adverse events in an adjuvant compared with advanced setting, and over a protracted treatment duration. Despite these numerous studies, there is no standard adjuvant treatment of HCC.

Local Ablation

Local ablation encompasses a range of techniques, including PEI, percutaneous acetic acid injection (PAI), RFA, microwave ablation, laser ablation, and cryoablation, which are commonly used to treat small HCC with curative intent. As previously described, randomized data comparing surgical resection and local ablation have been conflicting but with a trend to greater benefit from surgery for tumors of increasing size and number. Consequently, local ablation is usually reserved for patients who are not surgical candidates.

RFA has emerged as the preferred local ablation technique. This is based on evidence from multiple small randomized trials in which RFA was compared with the historical practice of PEI or PAI. There were 3 key trials from Asia. Lin and colleagues[17] randomized 157 subjects with HCC less than 4 cm to either RFA, PEI, or high-dose PEI, defined as injection of twice the conventional dose of ethanol per session. OS was longest with RFA, relative to PEI ($P = .014$) and high-PEI ($P = .023$). In a separate study, Lin and colleagues[18] randomized 187 subjects to either RFA, PEI, or PAI. RFA was superior with respect to overall, recurrence-free and local recurrence rates (3-year OS RFA 74% vs PEI 51% vs PAI 53%, $P = .038$). Shiina and colleagues[19] randomized 232 subjects with up to 3 lesions, each less than 3 cm, with predominantly hepatitis C cirrhosis. RFA resulted in improved survival compared with PEI (4-year OS 74% vs 84%, $P = .01$), with a similar incidence of adverse events.

In Italy, Lencioni and colleagues[20] studied 102 subjects with HCC within Milan criteria, randomized to undergo either RFA or PEI. Data revealed longer RFS and a nonsignificant numerical improvement in OS with RFA (2-year RFS 64% vs 43%, $P = .012$; 2-year OS 98% vs 88%, $P = .138$). In a similar study, Brunello and colleagues[21] studied 139 subjects. After a median follow-up of 2 years, there was a small nonsignificant difference in OS favoring RFA (HR 0.88, 95% CI 0.50–1.53, $P = .640$). Giorgio and colleagues[22] studied 285 subjects with HCC less than 3 cm. Unlike previous studies, there was no suggestion of difference between RFA and PEI (5-year OS 70% vs 68%; 5-year local recurrence rate 11.7% vs 12.8%).

Meta-analyses of these collective studies concluded that RFA was the superior local ablation technique.[23–25] In particular, the effectiveness of PEI seemed to diminish when used to ablate larger tumors. Utility of RFA is limited in tumors with proximity to major biliary or vascular structures, due to respective risks of biliary injury and heat-sink effect.

There is emerging experience with newer techniques such as laser and microwave ablation. Ferrari and colleagues[26] randomized 81 subjects with HCC less than 4 cm to either laser ablation or RFA. In this small study, the difference in OS between laser ablation (5-year OS rate 23%) and RFA (41%) did not reach statistical significance ($P = .330$). For both groups, survival outcomes were improved for subjects with Child-Pugh A liver function ($P<.001$), lesions under 25 mm ($P<.001$), and solitary lesions ($P = .048$). Di Costanzo and colleagues[27] conducted a noninferiority study of laser ablation versus RFA. For 140 subjects with HCC within Milan criteria, laser ablation was statistically noninferior for all study endpoints. Shibata and colleagues[28] randomized 72 subjects to either microwave ablation or RFA, and found that local progression was not statistically significantly different. Survival endpoints were not reported in this study. Based on these limited data, laser and microwave ablation may be comparable techniques, but larger studies are needed before they can be widely adopted.

Finally, there has been interest in the combination of RFA and transarterial chemoembolization (TACE), with the intent of extending the effective ablation zone to deal with larger tumors. A recent meta-analysis included 6 randomized trials between 2005 and 2013 enrolling 534 subjects in total.[29] Combination therapy resulted in longer OS (HR 0.62, 95% CI 0.49–0.78, $P<.001$) and RFS (HR 0.55, 95% CI 0.40–0.76, $P<.001$) compared with RFA alone. It was notable that tumor size was a significant prognostic factor and that subjects with HCC up to 7 cm were included, which is beyond the usual criteria for local ablation. Seemingly, the benefit of combination therapy was greatest in subjects with intermediate-sized HCC. The utility of this approach relative to other modalities such as surgical resection and transplantation remains unclear.

Regional Therapy

Even though HCC has a reduced propensity for extrahepatic spread, patients with bulky multifocal or bilobar liver involvement may no longer be amenable to the local curative treatments previously described. However, there is a good rationale for regional hepatic-directed therapies for disease control, in which there is selective intravascular delivery of embolizing agents, chemotherapy, or radioactive particles into the hepatic arterial branches supplying the tumor.

Phase III studies have shown that TACE is associated with a survival benefit compared with best supportive care. Llovet and colleagues[30] carefully selected a group of subjects with HCC not suitable for curative treatment because of multifocality, with Child-Pugh A liver function and good performance status. Only 112 of 903 HCC subjects fulfilled these inclusion criteria. They were randomized to bland embolization, doxorubicin chemoembolization, or supportive care. The trial was stopped early due to an interim analysis showing a substantial OS benefit of chemoembolization over supportive care (HR 0.47, 95% CI 0.25–0.91, $P = .025$). Direct comparison between the 2 embolization arms was not possible because of the early study termination. In a similar manner, Lo and colleagues[31] selected 80 out of 279 Asian subjects with newly diagnosed HCC. Subjects were randomized to either cisplatin chemoembolization or supportive care. OS was significantly longer in the chemoembolization group (3-year OS 26% vs 3%, $P = .002$).

A meta-analysis of multiple small randomized trials of chemoembolization corroborated these findings.[32] Relative to supportive care, there was a significant OS benefit in 4 trials of 323 subjects treated with doxorubicin-based or cisplatin-based chemoembolization (OR 0.42, 95% CI 0.20–0.88). A Cochrane systematic review of 9 trials with 645 subjects showed a nonsignificant numerical benefit only (HR 0.88, 95% CI 0.71–1.10).[33] However, the results from chemoembolization and bland embolization trials were pooled together, and several favorable trials were excluded due to methodological limitations. On the whole, TACE is recommended for patients with intermediate-stage HCC, that is, tumors that are no longer amenable to curative treatment, but lacking major vascular invasion or extrahepatic spread. An important caveat is that subjects were carefully selected for these trials, which precludes the extrapolation of findings to those with a higher degree of liver dysfunction or more advanced disease.

The optimal regimen of embolic materials and chemotherapy for transarterial therapy has not been defined. A systematic review of multiple small randomized and nonrandomized studies found that no chemotherapeutic agent was superior.[34] Studies included disparate patient populations, with varying tumor burdens and degrees of cirrhosis, and used a diverse repertoire of treatment regimens. The most common chemotherapeutic agents were doxorubicin, cisplatin, and epirubicin.

Regarding the comparison of chemoembolization with bland embolization, 2 recent randomized trials suggested similar outcomes. Meyer and colleagues[35] randomized 86 subjects to either cisplatin chemoembolization or bland embolization. Over a median follow-up of 2 years, median OS and progression-free survival (PFS) were 17.3 and 16.3 months ($P = .74$), and 7.2 and 7.5 months ($P = .59$), respectively. Brown and colleagues[36] randomized 101 subjects to either doxorubicin drug-eluting bead chemoembolization or bland embolization. Over a median follow-up of 3 years, median OS and PFS were 19.6 and 20.8 months ($P = .64$), and 6.2 and 2.8 months ($P = .11$), respectively. Regrettably, because these studies were underpowered and it is conceivable that a relevant difference in efficacy could be overlooked, chemoembolization remains the usual practice.

A drug-eluting bead delivery system has been developed with the intention of enhancing chemotherapy delivery to the tumor while minimizing systemic absorption. When comparing drug-eluting beads with conventional TACE, small studies suggested similar efficacy, with a possible improvement in toxicity profile. Lammer and colleagues[37] randomized 212 subjects to either doxorubicin drug-eluting beads or conventional doxorubicin-based TACE. There was no significant difference in the primary endpoint of tumor response. However, reductions in liver toxicity ($P<.001$) and systemic side-effects ($P<.001$) were noted. Sacco and colleagues[38] made the same comparison in a randomized trial of 67 subjects, with no observed difference in efficacy but a decreased rate of transaminitis ($P = .007$). Golfieri and colleagues[39] randomized 177 subjects to either doxorubicin drug-eluting beads or conventional epirubicin-based TACE. One-year and 2-year survival rates were 86% versus 57%, and 84% versus 55%, respectively ($P = .949$). The only apparent advantage of drug-eluting bead therapy was reduced postprocedural abdominal pain.

Several trials have examined the combination of TACE followed by systemic therapy. The Sorafenib or Placebo in Combination with TACE for Intermediate-Stage HCC (SPACE) study was a randomized, double-blind, placebo-controlled Italian trial enrolling 307 subjects with intermediate-stage HCC, Child-Pugh A liver function, and Eastern Cooperative Oncology Group (ECOG) 0 performance status.[40] Subjects underwent TACE with doxorubicin drug-eluting beads, followed by either sorafenib 400 mg orally twice a day or placebo, continued indefinitely until progression, toxicity, or subject withdrawal. The primary endpoint of time to progression was not meaningfully different for sorafenib versus placebo (median 169 vs 166 days, HR 0.80, $P = .072$). Similar phase III trials have been conducted in Japan[41] and Europe[42] with negative findings. It is possible that the low sorafenib dose intensity in the treatment groups contributed to the negative findings in these trials, in a manner analogous to the adjuvant STORM study. The multikinase inhibitor brivanib was also evaluated in combination with TACE in the Brivanib Studies in HCC Patients at Risk (BRISK)- TACE study, but this study was terminated early due to disappointing findings in related trials of brivanib in the advanced setting.[43]

An emerging alternative to TACE is transarterial radioembolization (TARE). Yttrium-90 (^{90}Y) beads are incorporated into glass (TheraSphere, Nordion Inc, Ottawa) or resin microspheres (SIRTex, Sirtex Medical Limited, Sydney) and delivered as transarterial brachytherapy. A meta-analysis of retrospective studies showed no significant difference between TARE and TACE in terms of complication profile and survival rates (OS HR 1.06, 95% CI 0.81–1.46, $P = .567$).[44] In terms of the only available randomized data, there was recent publication of a phase II trial of ^{90}Y TARE versus conventional TACE.[45] A total of 179 subjects were identified as suitable candidates for transarterial therapy. Of these, 24 were randomized to ^{90}Y TARE and 21 to conventional TACE. Although the trial was underpowered for efficacy assessment, there was a promising improvement in median time to progression with TARE (>26 vs 6.8 months, $P = .001$) and comparable median OS (17.7 vs 18.6 months, $P = .99$). These findings are preliminary and, at present, TACE remains the evidence-based preference for regional therapy.

Radiation Therapy

Radiotherapy was traditionally limited to the palliation of extrahepatic metastases. However, technological advances in treatment planning and delivery now permit the administration of therapeutic doses to the primary tumor, while sufficiently sparing surrounding liver parenchyma to mitigate radiation-induced liver disease. Radiotherapy also potentially overcomes some of the technical limitations of RFA because there is no heat sink effect and no tumor size limitation. As such, stereotactic body radiation therapy (SBRT) has become a viable option for patients with localized HCC who do not meet criteria for the aforementioned treatments.

To date, the results of several randomized phase III trials are still awaited. The RTOG (Radiation Therapy Oncology Group) 1112 trial (NCT01730937) is accruing subjects with intermediate-stage or advanced-stage HCC, Child-Pugh A liver function, and good performance status, yet who are unsuitable for transplantation, surgical resection, local ablation or regional therapy. Subjects are randomized to either SBRT followed by sorafenib or sorafenib alone for a maximum duration of 5 years. The primary endpoint is OS, with expected study completion in 2020. Other upcoming randomized trials include TACE followed by SBRT versus TACE alone (NCT02470533; NCT02794337), SBRT versus TACE as bridging therapy for transplantation (NCT02182687), and SBRT versus repeat TACE after incomplete response to TACE (NCT02323360). Owing to the lack of supporting phase III data, SBRT has yet to become an accepted standard of care in most international guidelines.

Systemic Therapy

First-line treatment

Despite advances in chemotherapeutics, HCC has remained notoriously resistant to systemic therapy. Numerous clinical trials have evaluated cytotoxic, hormonal, targeted and immunotherapy agents (**Table 1**), yet few have resulted in meaningful improvements.

Historically, doxorubicin was considered to be the agent of choice. Lai and colleagues[46] conducted a prospective randomized trial in the 1980s, in which 106 subjects with advanced HCC received either doxorubicin 60 to 75 mg/m^2 every 3 weeks or no treatment. OS was dismal in both groups but improved from a median of 7.5 to 10.6 weeks with use of doxorubicin ($P = .036$), suggesting antitumor activity. This benefit was offset by unacceptable rates of sepsis and cardiotoxicity, which conferred high mortality at that time.

In subsequent decades, doxorubicin was used as the comparator in trials of cytotoxic chemotherapy. Yeo and colleagues[47] compared PIAF (cisplatin 20 mg/m^2 Days D1-4, interferon-alpha 5 MU/m^2 D1-4, doxorubicin 40 mg/m^2 D1, 5-fluorouracil 400 mg/m^2 D1-4 every 3 weeks) versus doxorubicin 60 mg/m^2 every 3 weeks. Of the 94 subjects in each treatment arm, median OS was 8.7 and 6.8 months, respectively ($P = .83$). This improvement was not statistically significant and PIAF (cisPlatin, Interferon-alpha, doxorubicin (Adriamycin), 5-Fluorouracil) was associated with severe myelosuppression. Gish and colleagues[48] evaluated nolatrexed, a novel thymidylate synthase inhibitor, in a multicenter randomized phase III trial of 445 subjects. Subjects received either nolatrexed 800 mg/m^2 D1-5 as a continuous infusion every 3 weeks or doxorubicin 60 mg/m^2 every 3 weeks. Median OS was 22.3 and 32.3 weeks, respectively ($P = .007$), in favor of doxorubicin. Due to these findings, development of nolatrexed was discontinued. In the FOLFOX4 versus doxorubicin as palliative chemotherapy in advanced hepatocellular carcinoma patients (EACH) study, 371 Asian subjects were randomized to either 5-fluorouracil 400 mg/m^2 bolus followed by 600 mg/m^2 as a continuous infusion D1-2, leucovorin 200 mg/m^2 D1-2, oxaliplatin 85 mg/m^2 D1 (FOLFOX4) every 2 weeks or doxorubicin 50 mg/m^2 every 3 weeks.[49,50] There was a trend to OS improvement with FOLFOX4 (median 6.4 vs 5.0 months, respectively; $P = .07$), which reached statistical significance in a post hoc subgroup analysis of the 279 of 371 subjects from China ($P = .03$).

Hormonal agents were studied on the basis that HCC occasionally expressed sex hormone and/or somatostatin receptors. Unfortunately, several well-conducted randomized phase III trials of tamoxifen versus placebo,[51-54] megestrol acetate versus

Table 1
First-line randomized trials for advanced hepatocellular carcinoma

Study, Year	Design	Number of Subjects	Intervention	Control	Results
Cytotoxic chemotherapy					
Lai et al,[46] 1988	Prospective randomized trial Single institution	106	Doxorubicin 60–75 mg/m^2 q3wk	No treatment	mOS: 2.4 m vs 1.7 m, $P = .036^a$
Yeo et al,[47] 2005	Phase III Single institution	188	PIAF (cisplatin 20 mg/m^2 D1-4, interferon α-2b 5 MU/m^2 D1-4, doxorubicin 40 mg/m^2 D1, 5-fluorouracil 400 mg/m^2 D1-4 q3wk)	Doxorubicin 60 mg/m^2 q3wk	mOS: 8.7 m vs 6.8 m, HR 0.97 (95% CI 0.71–1.32), $P = .83$
Gish et al,[48] 2007	Phase III Multicenter (North America, Europe, South Africa)	445	Nolatrexed 800 mg/m^2 D1-5 q3wk	Doxorubicin 60 mg/m^2 q3wk	mOS: 5.1 m vs 7.4 m, HR 1.33, $P = .007^b$
EACH study, Qin et al,[49] 2013	Phase III Multicenter (Asia)	371	5-fluorouracil 400 mg/m^2 bolus, then 600 mg/m^2 infusion D1-2, leucovorin 200 mg/m^2 D1-2, oxaliplatin 85 mg/m^2 D1 (FOLFOX4) q2wk	Doxorubicin 50 mg/m^2 q3wk	mOS: 6.4 m vs 5.0 m, HR 0.80 (95% CI 0.63–1.02), $P = .07$
Hormonal agents					
CLIP-01 study, CLIP group,[51] 1998	Prospective randomized trial Multicenter (Italy)	477	Tamoxifen 40 mg daily	No treatment	mOS: 15m vs 16m, HR 1.07 (95% CI 0.83–1.39), $P = .54$
Barbare et al,[53] 2005	Phase III Multicenter (France)	420	Tamoxifen 20 mg daily	No treatment	mOS: 4.8 m vs 4.0 m, $P = .25$
Chow et al,[54] 2002	Phase III Multicenter (Asia)	329	1. Tamoxifen 120 mg daily 2. Tamoxifen 60 mg daily	Placebo	mOS: 2.2 m vs 2.1 m vs 2.7 m, $P = .011^b$
Chow et al,[55] 2011	Phase III Multicenter (Asia)	204	Megestrol acetate 320 mg daily	Placebo	mOS: 1.9 m vs 2.1 m, HR 1.25 (95% CI 0.92–1.71), $P = .16$

(continued on next page)

Table 1
(continued)

Study, Year	Design	Number of Subjects	Intervention	Control	Results
Barbare et al,[56] 2009	Phase III Multicenter (France)	272	Long-acting octreotide 30 mg q4wk	Placebo	mOS: 6.5 m vs 7.0 m, HR 1.14 (95% CI 0.88–1.45), $P = .34$
HECTOR study, Becker et al,[57] 2007	Prospective randomized trial Multicenter (Germany, Switzerland)	120	Long-acting octreotide 30 mg q4wk	Placebo	mOS: 4.7 m vs 5.3 m, HR 1.11 (95% CI 0.76–1.63), $P = .59$
Dimitroulopoulos et al,[58] 2007	Prospective randomized trial Single institution Only eligible if somatostatin receptor positive	61	Long-acting octreotide 30 mg q4wk	Placebo	Mean survival: 11.3 m vs 6.4 m, $P<.01$[a]
Molecular targeted therapies					
SHARP study, Llovet et al,[59] 2008	Phase III Multicenter (Europe, Americas, Australasia)	602	Sorafenib 400 mg bid	Placebo	mOS: 10.7 m vs 7.9 m, HR 0.69 (95% CI 0.55–0.87), $P<.001$[a]
Asia-Pacific study, Cheng et al,[60] 2009	Phase III Multicenter (Asia)	271	Sorafenib 400 mg bid	Placebo	mOS: 6.5 m vs 4.2 m, HR 0.68 (95% CI 0.50–0.93), $P = .014$[a]
SUN 1170 study, Cheng et al,[61] 2013	Phase III Multicenter (Asia, Europe, North America)	1074	Sunitinib 37.5 mg daily	Sorafenib 400 mg bid	mOS: 7.9 m vs 10.2 m, HR 1.30 (95% CI 1.13–1.50), $P = .001$[b]
BRISK-FL study, Johnson et al,[62] 2013	Phase III Multicenter (Asia, Europe, Americas, Australia, Africa)	1155	Brivanib 800 mg daily	Sorafenib 400 mg bid	Noninferiority study (boundary HR 1.08) mOS: 9.5 m vs 9.9 m, HR 1.06 (95.8% CI 0.93–1.22), NS
LIGHT study, Cainap et al,[63] 2015	Phase III Multicenter (Asia, Europe, North America, Africa)	1035	Linifanib 17.5 mg daily	Sorafenib 400 mg bid	Noninferiority study (boundary HR 1.05) mOS: 9.1 m vs 9.8 m, HR 1.05 (95% CI 0.90–1.22), NS

Study	Phase/Type	N	Intervention	Control	Outcome
Hsu et al,[64] 2012	Phase II Multicenter (Taiwan)	67	1. Vandetanib 300 mg daily 2. Vandetanib 100 mg daily	Placebo	mOS: 6.0 m vs 5.8 m vs 4.3 m, NS
Palmer et al,[65] 2015	Combined analysis of 2 phase II studies (white and Asian populations)	188	Nintedanib 200 mg bid	Sorafenib 400 mg bid	mOS: 11.4 m vs 11.0 m, HR 0.91 (95% CI 0.65–1.29), NS
Cheng et al,[66] 2016	Phase II Multicenter (Asia)	165	Dovitinib 500 mg D1-5 weekly	Sorafenib 400 mg bid	mOS: 8.0 m vs 8.4 m, HR 1.27 (95% CI 0.90–1.79), NS
SEARCH study, Zhu et al,[67] 2015	Phase III Multicenter (Asia, Europe, Americas)	720	Sorafenib 400 mg bid + erlotinib 150 mg daily	Sorafenib 400 mg bid + Placebo	mOS: 9.5 m vs 8.5 m, HR 0.93 (95% CI 0.78–1.11), P = .408
CALGB 80802 study, Abou-Alfa et al,[69] 2016	Phase III Multicenter (North America)	356	Sorafenib 400 mg bid + doxorubicin 60 mg/m² q3wk	Sorafenib 400 mg bid	mOS: 8.9 m vs 10.5 m, HR 1.06 (95% CI 0.8–1.4), P = .24
Ciuleanu et al,[70] 2016	Phase II Multicenter (Europe, North America)	101	Sorafenib 400 mg + mapatumumab 30 mg/kg q3wk	Sorafenib 400 mg bid + Placebo	mOS: 10.0 m vs 10.1 m, HR 1.20 (90% CI 0–1.65), P = .78
Cheng et al,[71] 2015	Phase II Multicenter (Asia, North America)	163	1. Sorafenib 400 mg bid + tigatuzumab 6 mg/kg weekly 2. Sorafenib 400 mg bid + tigatuzumab 2 mg/kg weekly	Sorafenib 400 mg bid	mOS: 12.2 m vs 8.2 m, P = .737

Abbreviations: CALGB, Cancer and Leukemia Group B; CLIP, cancer of the liver italian program; D, days; HECTOR, hepatocellular carcinoma treatment with octreotide; mOS, median overall survival; NS, not statistically significant: SHARP, sorafenib HCC assessment randomized protocol; SUN 1170, Sunitinib 1170 study.
a Statistically significant in favor of intervention.
b Statistically significant in favor of control.

placebo,[55] and octreotide versus placebo[56,57] consistently demonstrated lack of efficacy in unselected subjects with advanced HCC. Dimitroulopoulos and colleagues[58] screened 127 subjects with advanced HCC, and identified 61 with positive uptake on octreotide scintigraphy. They were randomized to either octreotide or placebo. In this small study, mean survival time was longer in the octreotide group (49 vs 28 weeks, P<.01), suggesting a possible benefit in selected subjects.

On the whole, cytotoxic and hormonal agents have been disappointing, with limited efficacy and often significant toxicity concerns. In the new era of molecular targeted therapies, sorafenib became the first agent to show consistent survival benefit in advanced HCC. Sorafenib is a small molecule multikinase inhibitor which blocks Raf, vascular endothelial growth factor (VEGF) and platelet-derived growth factor (PDGF) signaling, thereby disrupting tumor growth and angiogenesis. Two major trials were pivotal to the adoption of sorafenib as the standard first-line treatment of advanced HCC. The Sorafenib HCC Assessment Randomized Protocol (SHARP) study was a randomized, double-blind, placebo-controlled phase III trial of 602 advanced HCC subjects with Child-Pugh A liver function.[59] Subjects were accrued between March 2005 and April 2006 from multiple centers throughout Europe, America, and Australasia. The main causes of underlying liver disease were hepatitis C and alcoholic cirrhosis. Subjects received either sorafenib 400 mg orally twice a day or placebo. Median OS was 10.7 months in the sorafenib group and 7.9 months in the placebo group (HR 0.69, 95% CI 0.55–0.87, P<.001). A second randomized trial was conducted in the Asia-Pacific region of predominantly hepatitis B subjects with advanced HCC and Child-Pugh A liver function.[60] A total of 271 subjects were randomized between September 2005 and January 2007 in a 2:1 ratio to either sorafenib or placebo. Median OS was 6.5 months in the sorafenib group and 4.2 months in the placebo group (HR 0.68, 95% CI 0.50–0.93, P = .014), thus corroborating the positive findings of the SHARP study.

There were several noteworthy points from these trials. First, both trials enrolled a highly select group of subjects with Child-Pugh A liver function and excellent performance status (92% and 95% of subjects were ECOG 0 or 1 in the SHARP and Asia-Pacific studies, respectively). Results cannot be readily extrapolated to subjects commonly encountered in clinical practice, who may have compromised liver function or poor performance status. Second, despite being a significant advancement, the efficacy of sorafenib is modest, with median OS still less than 1 year. Third, although the relative benefit of sorafenib was similar in both trials, subjects in the Asia-Pacific study had worse prognosis overall. This may reflect differences in the underlying biology of HCC due to hepatitis B versus other causes. Finally, survival was improved in the absence of radiologic response, with no complete responses, and 2% and 5% partial response rates in the SHARP and Asia-Pacific studies, respectively. The implication is that sorafenib may be predominantly tumoristatic, making radiologic assessment a less reliable determinant of efficacy.

Newer molecular targeted therapies have been compared against or in combination with sorafenib in randomized trials. Common targets included VEGF, PDGF, fibroblast growth factor (FGF) and epidermal growth factor (EGF) signaling pathways. Sunitinib, a broad-spectrum inhibitor of VEGF, PDGF, c-KIT, and RET signaling, was compared against sorafenib in a large randomized trial involving 1074 subjects.[61] The trial was terminated early for futility and safety reasons (median OS: sunitinib 7.9 vs sorafenib 10.2 months). The BRISK–First-Line (BRISK-FL) study evaluated brivanib, an inhibitor of VEGF and FGF signaling, in a noninferiority design involving 1155 subjects.[62] The Linifanib versus Sorafenib in Subjects with Advanced HCC (LIGHT) study evaluated linifanib, an inhibitor of VEGF and PDGF signaling, in a noninferiority design involving 1035 subjects.[63] In both BRISK-FL and LIGHT, the predefined noninferiority margins were not met (median OS: brivanib 9.5 vs sorafenib 9.9 months; linifanib 9.1 vs sorafenib 9.8 months). Furthermore, brivanib and linifanib were associated with greater adverse effects and high rates of discontinuation. Randomized trials evaluating sorafenib versus vandetanib (VEGF and EGF inhibitor),[64] nintedanib (VEGF, PDGF, and FGF inhibitor),[65] and dovitinib (VEGF, PDGF, and FGF inhibitor)[66] have also been negative.

Combination trials have been negative as well. Based on 2 promising single-arm phase II trials that showed activity of erlotinib, an EGF pathway inhibitor, the Sorafenib Plus Erlotinib in Patients with Advanced HCC (SEARCH) trial randomized 720 subjects with advanced HCC to either sorafenib plus erlotinib, or erlotinib alone.[67] In this adequately powered study, OS was similar in both groups (median 9.5 vs 8.5 months, HR 0.93, $P = .408$). Abou-Alfa and colleagues[68] conducted a randomized phase II trial of 96 subjects who received either sorafenib plus doxorubicin, or sorafenib alone. Median OS was 13.7 months in the combination group and 6.5 months in the sorafenib-only group ($P = .006$). However, the subsequent phase III Cancer and Leukemia Group B (CALGB) 80802 trial failed to confirm these findings.[69] Of 356 subjects, OS was 8.9 months in the combination group and 10.5 months in the sorafenib-only group. The discordant findings may be related to improved statistical power in the phase III trial yielding more robust results. There were also differences in the study populations, with the phase III trial including a greater proportion of Asian subjects with underlying hepatitis B infection, and consisting of a more representative real-word, but less fit, subject cohort who tolerated the combination therapy poorly. Notably, throughout all these comparative studies, sorafenib demonstrated consistent efficacy across diverse populations and remains the first-line standard of care.

Going forward, novel targeted therapies and immunotherapy agents are being investigated. Mapatumumab and tigatuzumab, agonists of the proapoptotic TRAIL (TNF-related apoptosis-inducing ligand) pathway, showed insufficient activity in randomized phase II trials.[70,71] Randomized trials are currently underway for a range of immunotherapy agents, including checkpoint inhibitors such as ipilimumab, tremelimumab, nivolumab, pembrolizumab, and durvalumab (NCT01658878; NCT02576509; NCT02702401; NCT02519348); cytokine modulators, such as galunisertib (NCT02178358); and oncolytic virus therapy (NCT02562755). The particular allure of immunotherapy is that HCC is mediated by viral hepatitis in many cases and, historically, has been amenable to immune-based approaches such as interferon. Already, encouraging response rates with manageable toxicity have been reported in phase II checkpoint inhibitor trials (NCT01658878) and the results of randomized phase III trials are eagerly awaited.

For the present, sorafenib remains the only agent with demonstrable albeit modest survival benefit in treatment-naïve advanced HCC. Accordingly, in patients with suitable liver function and performance status, sorafenib is the global standard of care for first-line treatment.

Second-line treatment

There is an unmet need for effective treatments in the second-line setting. Analogous to the trials conducted in the first-line setting, many molecular targeted therapies have been evaluated without success (**Table 2**). Randomized placebo-controlled trials of brivanib (VEGF and FGF inhibitor),[72] axitinib (VEGF inhibitor),[73] everolimus (mTOR inhibitor),[74] codrituzumab (inhibitor of cell surface molecule GPC3),[75] and ADI-PEG20 (arginine depletion)[76] have failed to demonstrate OS improvement.

Recently, the potent multikinase inhibitor regorafenib was evaluated in the second-line Regorafenib for Patients with HCC Who Progressed on Sorafenib Treatment

Table 2
Second-line randomized trials for advanced hepatocellular carcinoma

Study, Year	Design	Number of Subjects	Intervention	Control	Results
BRISK-PS study, Llovet et al,[72] 2013	Phase III Multicenter (Europe, Asia, Americas)	395	Brivanib 800 mg daily	Placebo	mOS: 9.4 m vs 8.2 m, HR 0.89 (95.8% CI 0.69–1.15), $P = .331$
Kang et al,[73] 2015	Phase II Multicenter (Asia, Europe, North America)	202	Axitinib 5 mg bid	Placebo	mOS: 12.7 m vs 9.7 m, HR 0.91 (95% CI 0.65–1.27), $P = .287$
EVOLVE-1 study, Zhu et al,[74] 2014	Phase III Multicenter (Asia, Europe, North America, Australia)	546	Everolimus 7.5 mg daily	Placebo	mOS: 7.6 m vs 7.3 m, HR 1.05 (95% CI 0.86–1.27), $P = .68$
Abou-Alfa et al,[75] 2016	Phase II Multicenter (North America, Asia, Europe)	185	Codrituzumab 1600 mg q2wk	Placebo	mOS: 8.7 m vs 10m, HR 0.96 (95% CI 0.65–1.41), $P = .82$
Abou-Alfa et al,[76] 2016	Phase III Multicenter (North America, Asia, Europe)	635	ADI-PEG20 18 mg/m^2 weekly	Placebo	mOS: 7.8 m vs 7.4 m, HR 1.02 (95% CI 0.85–1.23), $P = .884$
RESORCE study, Bruix et al,[77] 2017	Phase III Multicenter (Europe, Asia, Americas)	573	Regorafenib 160 mg daily D1-21 q4wk	Placebo	mOS: 10.6 m vs 7.8 m, HR 0.63 (95% CI 0.50–0.79), $P<.001$[a]
Santoro et al,[78] 2013	Phase II Multicenter (Europe, North America)	107	Tivantinib 360 mg bid (later amended to 240 mg bid due to high neutropenia rate)	Placebo	mOS: 6.6 m vs 6.2 m, HR 0.90 (95% CI 0.57–1.40), $P = .63$ For MET-high subgroup: 7.2 m vs 3.8 m, HR 0.38 (95% CI 0.18–0.81), $P = .01$[a]
REACH study, Zhu et al,[79] 2015	Phase III Multicenter (North America, Asia)	565	Ramucirumab 8 mg/kg q2wk	Placebo	mOS: 9.2 m vs 7.6 m, HR 0.87 (95% CI 0.72–1.05), $P = .14$ For high AFP subgroup: 7.8 m vs 4.2 m, HR 0.67 (95% CI 0.51–0.90), $P = .006$

Abbreviations: ADI-PEG, pegylated arginine deiminase; REACH, Ramucirumab versus Placebo in Participants with Advanced HCC; RESORCE, Regorafenib for Patients with HCC Who Progressed on Sorafenib Treatment.
[a] Statistically significant in favor of intervention.

(RESORCE) trial.[77] This was a randomized, double-blind, placebo-controlled phase III trial enrolling 843 subjects between May 2013 and December 2015 from multiple centers (38% Asia, 62% rest of world). Eligible subjects had Child-Pugh A liver function, ECOG 0 or 1 performance status, and tolerated sorafenib well previously. This represented a highly select cohort of second-line subjects who likely had favorable tumor biology. Subjects were randomized to either regorafenib 160 mg orally daily or placebo in a 2:1 ratio, with crossover permitted following the final analysis. Remarkably, the trial demonstrated a significant survival benefit in favor of regorafenib, with median survival of 10.6 months for regorafenib versus 7.8 months for placebo (HR 0.63, 95% CI 0.50–0.79, $P<.001$). There was comparable benefit across prespecified subgroups, including geographic region, cause, and tumor extent. Regorafenib seemed to be tolerable in this subject cohort, with almost half of the regorafenib group receiving full protocol dose without reductions, and with no significant decrement in health-related quality of life. Accordingly, this trial represents an important advance in the treatment of HCC, with regorafenib likely to become a standard second-line treatment.

In terms of upcoming randomized trials, the METIV-HCC trial (NCT01755767) is comparing tivantinib (MET inhibitor) against placebo in subjects selected for high tumor MET expression, based on promising phase II data.[78] The Ramucirumab versus Placebo in Participants with Advanced HCC (REACH)-2 trial (NCT02435433) is comparing ramucirumab (VEGF inhibitor) against placebo in subjects selected for elevated baseline alpha-fetoprotein, due to findings from the REACH trial.[79] The Cabozantinib versus Placebo in Subjects with HCC Who Have Received Prior Sorafenib (CELESTIAL) trial (NCT01908426) is evaluating cabozantinib (VEGF and MET inhibitor) and has progressed beyond the first interim analysis. Checkpoint inhibitors durvalumab and tremelimumab are under investigation in NCT02519348.

SUMMARY

HCC has become a major area for research. Many clinical uncertainties remain, due to reliance on evidence from small, single-institution studies. Future randomized studies must be multicenter, adequately powered, and incorporate appropriate subject stratification. There will need to be an acceptance of tumor evaluation and tissue banking to advance understanding of the disease. In particular, it is acknowledged that the mechanisms behind liver carcinogenesis and progression of disease are complex, with heterogeneous behavior related to differences in underlying biology and etiologic factors. Advancement is required in molecular characterization of HCC to identify novel oncogenes and tumor suppressors, and to better identify subsets of patients who will most likely respond to the various treatment modalities and systemic options. Reassuringly, there are promising clinical trials encompassing the breadth of HCC management, from prevention to locoregional therapy to systemic therapy, which offer hope in ameliorating this disease.

REFERENCES

1. Llovet JM, Bru C, Bruix J. Prognosis of hepatocellular carcinoma: the BCLC staging classification. Semin Liver Dis 1999;19(3):329–38.
2. Zhang BH, Yang BH, Tang ZY. Randomized controlled trial of screening for hepatocellular carcinoma. J Cancer Res Clin Oncol 2004;130(7):417–22.
3. Liaw YF, Sung JJ, Chow WC, et al. Lamivudine for patients with chronic hepatitis B and advanced liver disease. N Engl J Med 2004;351(15):1521–31.

4. Singal AK, Singh A, Jaganmohan S, et al. Antiviral therapy reduces risk of hepatocellular carcinoma in patients with hepatitis C virus-related cirrhosis. Clin Gastroenterol Hepatol 2010;8(2):192–9.

5. Mazzaferro V, Regalia E, Doci R, et al. Liver transplantation for the treatment of small hepatocellular carcinomas in patients with cirrhosis. N Engl J Med 1996; 334(11):693–9.

6. Geissler EK, Schnitzbauer AA, Zulke C, et al. Sirolimus use in liver transplant recipients with hepatocellular carcinoma: a randomized, multicenter, open-label phase 3 trial. Transplantation 2016;100(1):116–25.

7. Shi M, Guo RP, Lin XJ, et al. Partial hepatectomy with wide versus narrow resection margin for solitary hepatocellular carcinoma: a prospective randomized trial. Ann Surg 2007;245(1):36–43.

8. Chen M-S, Li J-Q, Zheng Y, et al. A prospective randomized trial comparing percutaneous local ablative therapy and partial hepatectomy for small hepatocellular carcinoma. Ann Surg 2006;243(3):321–8.

9. Feng K, Yan J, Li X, et al. A randomized controlled trial of radiofrequency ablation and surgical resection in the treatment of small hepatocellular carcinoma. J Hepatol 2012;57(4):794–802.

10. Huang J, Yan L, Cheng Z, et al. A randomized trial comparing radiofrequency ablation and surgical resection for HCC conforming to the Milan criteria. Ann Surg 2010;252(6):903–12.

11. Huang GT, Lee PH, Tsang YM, et al. Percutaneous ethanol injection versus surgical resection for the treatment of small hepatocellular carcinoma: a prospective study. Ann Surg 2005;242(1):36–42.

12. Cucchetti A, Piscaglia F, Cescon M, et al. Systematic review of surgical resection vs radiofrequency ablation for hepatocellular carcinoma. World J Gastroenterol 2013;19(26):4106–18.

13. Breitenstein S, Dimitroulis D, Petrowsky H, et al. Systematic review and meta-analysis of interferon after curative treatment of hepatocellular carcinoma in patients with viral hepatitis. Br J Surg 2009;96(9):975–81.

14. Wang J, He XD, Yao N, et al. A meta-analysis of adjuvant therapy after potentially curative treatment for hepatocellular carcinoma. Can J Gastroenterol 2013;27(6): 351–63.

15. Liu CJ, Lee PH, Lin DY, et al. Heparanase inhibitor PI-88 as adjuvant therapy for hepatocellular carcinoma after curative resection: a randomized phase II trial for safety and optimal dosage. J Hepatol 2009;50(5):958–68.

16. Bruix J, Takayama T, Mazzaferro V, et al. Adjuvant sorafenib for hepatocellular carcinoma after resection or ablation (STORM): a phase 3, randomised, double-blind, placebo-controlled trial. Lancet Oncol 2015;16(13):1344–54.

17. Lin SM, Lin CJ, Lin CC, et al. Radiofrequency ablation improves prognosis compared with ethanol injection for hepatocellular carcinoma < or =4 cm. Gastroenterology 2004;127(6):1714–23.

18. Lin SM, Lin CJ, Lin CC, et al. Randomised controlled trial comparing percutaneous radiofrequency thermal ablation, percutaneous ethanol injection, and percutaneous acetic acid injection to treat hepatocellular carcinoma of 3 cm or less. Gut 2005;54(8):1151–6.

19. Shiina S, Teratani T, Obi S, et al. A randomized controlled trial of radiofrequency ablation with ethanol injection for small hepatocellular carcinoma. Gastroenterology 2005;129(1):122–30.

20. Lencioni RA, Allgaier HP, Cioni D, et al. Small hepatocellular carcinoma in cirrhosis: randomized comparison of radio-frequency thermal ablation versus percutaneous ethanol injection. Radiology 2003;228(1):235–40.

21. Brunello F, Veltri A, Carucci P, et al. Radiofrequency ablation versus ethanol injection for early hepatocellular carcinoma: a randomized controlled trial. Scand J Gastroenterol 2008;43(6):727–35.

22. Giorgio A, Di Sarno A, De Stefano G, et al. Percutaneous radiofrequency ablation of hepatocellular carcinoma compared to percutaneous ethanol injection in treatment of cirrhotic patients: an Italian randomized controlled trial. Anticancer Res 2011;31(6):2291–5.

23. Cho YK, Kim JK, Kim MY, et al. Systematic review of randomized trials for hepatocellular carcinoma treated with percutaneous ablation therapies. Hepatology 2009;49(2):453–9.

24. Germani G, Pleguezuelo M, Gurusamy K, et al. Clinical outcomes of radiofrequency ablation, percutaneous alcohol and acetic acid injection for hepatocellular carcinoma: a meta-analysis. J Hepatol 2010;52(3):380–8.

25. Orlando A, Leandro G, Olivo M, et al. Radiofrequency thermal ablation vs. percutaneous ethanol injection for small hepatocellular carcinoma in cirrhosis: meta-analysis of randomized controlled trials. Am J Gastroenterol 2009;104(2):514–24.

26. Ferrari FS, Megliola A, Scorzelli A, et al. Treatment of small HCC through radiofrequency ablation and laser ablation. Comparison of techniques and long-term results. Radiol Med 2007;112(3):377–93.

27. Di Costanzo GG, Tortora R, D'Adamo G, et al. Radiofrequency ablation versus laser ablation for the treatment of small hepatocellular carcinoma in cirrhosis: a randomized trial. J Gastroenterol Hepatol 2015;30(3):559–65.

28. Shibata T, Iimuro Y, Yamamoto Y, et al. Small hepatocellular carcinoma: comparison of radio-frequency ablation and percutaneous microwave coagulation therapy. Radiology 2002;223(2):331–7.

29. Wang X, Hu Y, Ren M, et al. Efficacy and safety of radiofrequency ablation combined with transcatheter arterial chemoembolization for hepatocellular carcinomas compared with radiofrequency ablation alone: a time-to-event meta-analysis. Korean J Radiol 2016;17(1):93–102.

30. Llovet JM, Real MI, Montana X, et al. Arterial embolisation or chemoembolisation versus symptomatic treatment in patients with unresectable hepatocellular carcinoma: a randomised controlled trial. Lancet 2002;359(9319):1734–9.

31. Lo CM, Ngan H, Tso WK, et al. Randomized controlled trial of transarterial lipiodol chemoembolization for unresectable hepatocellular carcinoma. Hepatology 2002;35(5):1164–71.

32. Llovet JM, Bruix J. Systematic review of randomized trials for unresectable hepatocellular carcinoma: chemoembolization improves survival. Hepatology 2003; 37(2):429–42.

33. Oliveri RS, Wetterslev J, Gluud C. Transarterial (chemo)embolisation for unresectable hepatocellular carcinoma. Cochrane Database Syst Rev 2011;(3):CD004787.

34. Marelli L, Stigliano R, Triantos C, et al. Transarterial therapy for hepatocellular carcinoma: which technique is more effective? A systematic review of cohort and randomized studies. Cardiovasc Intervent Radiol 2007;30(1):6–25.

35. Meyer T, Kirkwood A, Roughton M, et al. A randomised phase II/III trial of 3-weekly cisplatin-based sequential transarterial chemoembolisation vs embolisation alone for hepatocellular carcinoma. Br J Cancer 2013;108(6):1252–9.

36. Brown KT, Do RK, Gonen M, et al. Randomized trial of hepatic artery embolization for hepatocellular carcinoma using doxorubicin-eluting microspheres compared with embolization with microspheres alone. J Clin Oncol 2016;34(17):2046–53.

37. Lammer J, Malagari K, Vogl T, et al. Prospective randomized study of doxorubicin-eluting-bead embolization in the treatment of hepatocellular carcinoma: results of the PRECISION V study. Cardiovasc Intervent Radiol 2010; 33(1):41–52.

38. Sacco R, Bargellini I, Bertini M, et al. Conventional versus doxorubicin-eluting bead transarterial chemoembolization for hepatocellular carcinoma. J Vasc Interv Radiol 2011;22(11):1545–52.

39. Golfieri R, Giampalma E, Renzulli M, et al. Randomised controlled trial of doxorubicin-eluting beads vs conventional chemoembolisation for hepatocellular carcinoma. Br J Cancer 2014;111(2):255–64.

40. Lencioni R, Llovet JM, Han G, et al. Sorafenib or placebo plus TACE with doxorubicin-eluting beads for intermediate stage HCC: the SPACE trial. J Hepatol 2016;64(5):1090–8.

41. Kudo M, Imanaka K, Chida N, et al. Phase III study of sorafenib after transarterial chemoembolisation in Japanese and Korean patients with unresectable hepatocellular carcinoma. Eur J Cancer 2011;47(14):2117–27.

42. Meyer T, Fox R, Ma YT, et al. TACE 2: a randomized placebo-controlled, double-blinded, phase III trial evaluating sorafenib in combination with transarterial chemoembolisation (TACE) in patients with unresectable hepatocellular carcinoma (HCC). J Clin Oncol 2016;34(suppl) [abstract: 4018].

43. Kudo M, Han G, Finn RS, et al. Brivanib as adjuvant therapy to transarterial chemoembolization in patients with hepatocellular carcinoma: a randomized phase III trial. Hepatology 2014;60(5):1697–707.

44. Lobo L, Yakoub D, Picado O, et al. Unresectable hepatocellular carcinoma: radioembolization versus chemoembolization: a systematic review and meta-analysis. Cardiovasc Intervent Radiol 2016;39(11):1580–8.

45. Salem R, Gordon AC, Mouli S, et al. Y90 radioembolization significantly prolongs time to progression compared with chemoembolization in patients with hepatocellular carcinoma. Gastroenterology 2016;151(6):1155–63.e2.

46. Lai CL, Wu PC, Chan GC, et al. Doxorubicin versus no antitumor therapy in inoperable hepatocellular carcinoma. A prospective randomized trial. Cancer 1988; 62(3):479–83.

47. Yeo W, Mok TS, Zee B, et al. A randomized phase III study of doxorubicin versus cisplatin/interferon alpha-2b/doxorubicin/fluorouracil (PIAF) combination chemotherapy for unresectable hepatocellular carcinoma. J Natl Cancer Inst 2005; 97(20):1532–8.

48. Gish RG, Porta C, Lazar L, et al. Phase III randomized controlled trial comparing the survival of patients with unresectable hepatocellular carcinoma treated with nolatrexed or doxorubicin. J Clin Oncol 2007;25(21):3069–75.

49. Qin S, Bai Y, Lim HY, et al. Randomized, multicenter, open-label study of oxaliplatin plus fluorouracil/leucovorin versus doxorubicin as palliative chemotherapy in patients with advanced hepatocellular carcinoma from Asia. J Clin Oncol 2013; 31(28):3501–8.

50. Qin S, Cheng Y, Liang J, et al. Efficacy and safety of the FOLFOX4 regimen versus doxorubicin in Chinese patients with advanced hepatocellular carcinoma: a subgroup analysis of the EACH study. Oncologist 2014;19(11):1169–78.

51. Tamoxifen in treatment of hepatocellular carcinoma: a randomised controlled trial. CLIP Group (Cancer of the Liver Italian Programme). Lancet 1998;352(9121): 17–20.

52. Perrone F, Gallo C, Daniele B, et al. Tamoxifen in the treatment of hepatocellular carcinoma: 5-year results of the CLIP-1 multicentre randomised controlled trial. Curr Pharm Des 2002;8(11):1013–9.

53. Barbare JC, Bouche O, Bonnetain F, et al. Randomized controlled trial of tamoxifen in advanced hepatocellular carcinoma. J Clin Oncol 2005;23(19):4338–46.

54. Chow PK, Tai BC, Tan CK, et al. High-dose tamoxifen in the treatment of inoperable hepatocellular carcinoma: a multicenter randomized controlled trial. Hepatology 2002;36(5):1221–6.

55. Chow PK, Machin D, Chen Y, et al. Randomised double-blind trial of megestrol acetate vs placebo in treatment-naive advanced hepatocellular carcinoma. Br J Cancer 2011;105(7):945–52.

56. Barbare JC, Bouche O, Bonnetain F, et al. Treatment of advanced hepatocellular carcinoma with long-acting octreotide: a phase III multicentre, randomised, double blind placebo-controlled study. Eur J Cancer 2009;45(10):1788–97.

57. Becker G, Allgaier HP, Olschewski M, et al. Long-acting octreotide versus placebo for treatment of advanced HCC: a randomized controlled double-blind study. Hepatology 2007;45(1):9–15.

58. Dimitroulopoulos D, Xinopoulos D, Tsamakidis K, et al. Long acting octreotide in the treatment of advanced hepatocellular cancer and overexpression of somatostatin receptors: randomized placebo-controlled trial. World J Gastroenterol 2007;13(23):3164–70.

59. Llovet JM, Ricci S, Mazzaferro V, et al. Sorafenib in advanced hepatocellular carcinoma. N Engl J Med 2008;359(4):378–90.

60. Cheng AL, Kang YK, Chen Z, et al. Efficacy and safety of sorafenib in patients in the Asia-Pacific region with advanced hepatocellular carcinoma: a phase III randomised, double-blind, placebo-controlled trial. Lancet Oncol 2009;10(1):25–34.

61. Cheng AL, Kang YK, Lin DY, et al. Sunitinib versus sorafenib in advanced hepatocellular cancer: results of a randomized phase III trial. J Clin Oncol 2013;31(32): 4067–75.

62. Johnson PJ, Qin S, Park JW, et al. Brivanib versus sorafenib as first-line therapy in patients with unresectable, advanced hepatocellular carcinoma: results from the randomized phase III BRISK-FL study. J Clin Oncol 2013;31(28):3517–24.

63. Cainap C, Qin S, Huang WT, et al. Linifanib versus Sorafenib in patients with advanced hepatocellular carcinoma: results of a randomized phase III trial. J Clin Oncol 2015;33(2):172–9.

64. Hsu C, Yang TS, Huo TI, et al. Vandetanib in patients with inoperable hepatocellular carcinoma: a phase II, randomized, double-blind, placebo-controlled study. J Hepatol 2012;56(5):1097–103.

65. Palmer D, Meyer T, Chao Y, et al. Combined analysis of two randomised Phase II trials comparing the efficacy and safety of nintedanib versus sorafenib in Caucasian and Asian patients with advanced hepatocellular carcinoma. Ann Oncol 2015;26(suppl 4):iv102.

66. Cheng AL, Thongprasert S, Lim HY, et al. Randomized, open-label phase 2 study comparing frontline dovitinib versus sorafenib in patients with advanced hepatocellular carcinoma. Hepatology 2016;64(3):774–84.

67. Zhu AX, Rosmorduc O, Evans TR, et al. SEARCH: a phase III, randomized, double-blind, placebo-controlled trial of sorafenib plus erlotinib in patients with advanced hepatocellular carcinoma. J Clin Oncol 2015;33(6):559–66.

68. Abou-Alfa GK, Johnson P, Knox JJ, et al. Doxorubicin plus sorafenib vs doxorubicin alone in patients with advanced hepatocellular carcinoma: a randomized trial. JAMA 2010;304(19):2154–60.

69. Abou-Alfa GK, Niedzwieski D, Knox JJ, et al. Phase III randomized study of sorafenib plus doxorubicin versus sorafenib in patients with advanced hepatocellular carcinoma (HCC): CALGB 80802 (Alliance). J Clin Oncol 2016;34(suppl) [abstract: 4003].

70. Ciuleanu T, Bazin I, Lungulescu D, et al. A randomized, double-blind, placebo-controlled phase II study to assess the efficacy and safety of mapatumumab with sorafenib in patients with advanced hepatocellular carcinoma. Ann Oncol 2016;27(4):680–7.

71. Cheng AL, Kang YK, He AR, et al. Safety and efficacy of tigatuzumab plus sorafenib as first-line therapy in subjects with advanced hepatocellular carcinoma: a phase 2 randomized study. J Hepatol 2015;63(4):896–904.

72. Llovet JM, Decaens T, Raoul JL, et al. Brivanib in patients with advanced hepatocellular carcinoma who were intolerant to sorafenib or for whom sorafenib failed: results from the randomized phase III BRISK-PS study. J Clin Oncol 2013;31(28):3509–16.

73. Kang YK, Yau T, Park JW, et al. Randomized phase II study of axitinib versus placebo plus best supportive care in second-line treatment of advanced hepatocellular carcinoma. Ann Oncol 2015;26(12):2457–63.

74. Zhu AX, Kudo M, Assenat E, et al. Effect of everolimus on survival in advanced hepatocellular carcinoma after failure of sorafenib: the EVOLVE-1 randomized clinical trial. JAMA 2014;312(1):57–67.

75. Abou-Alfa GK, Puig O, Daniele B, et al. Randomized phase II placebo controlled study of codrituzumab in previously treated patients with advanced hepatocellular carcinoma. J Hepatol 2016;65(2):289–95.

76. Abou-Alfa GK, Qin S, Ryoo B-Y, et al. Phase III randomized study of second line ADI-peg 20 plus best supportive care versus placebo plus best supportive care in patients with advanced hepatocellular carcinoma. J Clin Oncol 2016;23(suppl) [abstract: 4017].

77. Bruix J, Qin S, Merle P, et al. Regorafenib for patients with hepatocellular carcinoma who progressed on sorafenib treatment (RESORCE): a randomised, double-blind, placebo-controlled, phase 3 trial. Lancet 2017;389(10064):56–66.

78. Santoro A, Rimassa L, Borbath I, et al. Tivantinib for second-line treatment of advanced hepatocellular carcinoma: a randomised, placebo-controlled phase 2 study. Lancet Oncol 2013;14(1):55–63.

79. Zhu AX, Park JO, Ryoo BY, et al. Ramucirumab versus placebo as second-line treatment in patients with advanced hepatocellular carcinoma following first-line therapy with sorafenib (REACH): a randomised, double-blind, multicentre, phase 3 trial. Lancet Oncol 2015;16(7):859–70.

An Update on Randomized Clinical Trials in Metastatic Colorectal Carcinoma

 CrossMark

Naruhiko Ikoma, MD, Kanwal Raghav, MD, MBBS, George Chang, MD, MS*

KEYWORDS

- Metastatic colorectal cancer • Randomized controlled trial • Chemotherapy
- Monoclonal antibody

KEY POINTS

- Combination cytotoxic chemotherapy regimens using a 5-fluorouracil backbone, such as FOLFOX (folinic acid, fluorouracil, oxaliplatin) and FOLFIRI (folinic acid, fluorouracil, irinotecan) have significantly improved the survival of patients with metastatic colorectal cancer.
- The addition of monoclonal antibodies (bevacizumab, cetuximab/panitumumab, aflibercept, ramucirumab) to chemotherapy has further improved survival outcomes.
- Novel therapies such as regorafenib and trifluridine/tipiracil have been also approved for management of refractory disease.
- Immune checkpoint inhibitors have been reported to be effective for patients with metastatic colorectal cancer with mismatch repair–deficient tumors, but have not been examined by randomized controlled trials.

INTRODUCTION

There have been remarkable advances in the treatment of metastatic colorectal cancer (mCRC) for the last 20 years. Metastasectomy has been associated with the significant survival advantage and even the potential for cure. In some patients with initially unresectable metastases who respond well to systemic therapy, it may be possible to convert to resectable disease. However, in patients with unresectable metastatic disease, advances in therapies have directly resulted in an improvement of median overall survival from approximately 11 to 12 months in the 5-fluorouracil (5-FU) single-agent era, to more than 24 months with sequential multiagent regimens in the modern era (**Fig. 1**). These advances have been a direct result of several landmark trials that have defined the current standard of care.

Disclosure: The authors have nothing to disclose.
University of Texas MD Anderson Cancer Center, Houston, TX, USA
* Corresponding author.
E-mail address: GChang@mdanderson.org

Surg Oncol Clin N Am 26 (2017) 667–687
http://dx.doi.org/10.1016/j.soc.2017.05.007

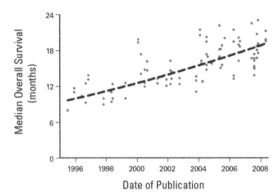

Fig. 1. Improved survival of metastatic colorectal cancer over time. (*From* Kopetz S, Chang GJ, Overman MJ, et al. Improved survival in metastatic colorectal cancer is associated with adoption of hepatic resection and improved chemotherapy. J Clin Oncol 2009;27:3678; with permission.)

Current National Comprehensive Cancer Network (NCCN) guidelines for advanced colorectal cancer or mCRC recommend use of a doublet regimen (oxaliplatin based, FOLFOX [folinic acid, fluorouracil, oxaliplatin] or CAPOX [capecitabine, oxaliplatin]; irinotecan based, FOLFIRI [folinic acid, fluorouracil, irinotecan]) with monoclonal antibody agent (anti–vascular endothelial growth factor [VEGF] agent bevacizumab or anti–epidermal growth factor receptor [EGFR] agents cetuximab or panitumumab [for RAS wild-type tumors]) as initial therapy. For appropriate patients a triplet cytotoxic backbone of 5-FU, oxaliplatin, and irinotecan (FOFOXIRI) combined with bevacizumab may be used. Following this, the patient should get a similar alternative cytotoxic agent along with a biologic agent. Anti-VEGF agents approved in this setting also include aflibercept and ramucirumab. Regorafenib or trifluridine/tipiracil are options after progression with those therapies. Anti-programmed cell death-1 (Anti-PD1) immunotherapy drugs such as nivolumab and pembrolizumab can also be used in patients with mismatch repair (MMR)-deficient mCRC. This article reviews the data from the randomized clinical trials that have contributed to the current treatment paradigms, mainly focusing on patients treated for initially inoperable metastatic disease.

Equivalence of 5-Fluorouracil and Capecitabine

Capecitabine is an oral fluoropyrimidine that gets converted to 5-FU using enzymes such as thymidine phosphorylase that are present at higher levels in tumor compared with normal tissue. Two randomized controlled trials (RCTs) have shown similar efficacy of capecitabine given daily for 14 days in every 21-day cycle and intravenous (IV) FU/leucovorin (LV) (Mayo regimen) for treatment of mCRC.[1,2] The toxicity profiles of these drugs are distinct. 5-FU is associated with more mucositis and neutropenic sepsis and capecitabine with more hyperbilirubinemia and hand-foot syndrome. In both RCTs mentioned earlier, capecitabine was compared with a bolus 5-FU regimen; it has not been compared in RCTs with infusional 5-FU, which is the more commonly used schedule. Notably, in at least 1 RCT (N = 448), an infusional regimen was associated with less toxicity and a better response rate and progression-free survival.[3] However, in a large meta-analysis of individual data from 6171 patients, oral capecitabine was equivalent to IV 5-FU in terms of overall survival.[4] These agents can be used interchangeably in combination with oxaliplatin. However, caution is advised with the use of capecitabine with irinotecan (XELIRI or CAPIRI) because of overlapping toxicity of diarrhea. In one RCT comparing CAPIRI plus bevacizumab with FOLFIRI plus bevacizumab in first-line treatment of patients with mCRC, no difference was observed in efficacy but patients in the CAPIRI-bevacizumab arm had significantly higher incidence of grade 3 or 4 diarrhea (16% vs 9%), febrile neutropenia (5% vs 0.6%), and hand-foot skin reactions (4.2% vs 1.2%).[5]

Irinotecan-Containing Regimens: 5-Flourouracil/LV with Irinotecan/Folinic Acid, Fluorouracil, Irinotecan/Capecitabine, Irinotecan

Irinotecan, a topoisomerase I inhibitor, was approved by the US Food and Drug Administration (FDA) in 1996 as a second-line treatment of patients with progressive colorectal cancer. It is effective as a monotherapy, but it is more effective in combination with 5-FU as well as with the targeted agents such as bevacizumab and cetuximab. It is most commonly administered as FOLFIRI consisting of 5-FU, leucovorin calcium (calcium folinate, LV), and irinotecan. An alternative schedule is 5-FU/LV with irinotecan (IFL), in which the FU is given as a bolus injection rather than as an infusion over 48 hours as in FOLFIRI. The survival benefit with the addition of irinotecan to conventional 5-FU/LV therapy in first line has been shown by 3 RCTs.

In France, 387 patients were randomly assigned to receive irinotecan combined with 5-FU/LV (irinotecan group) versus 5-FU/LV alone (no-irinotecan group) as first-line treatment of mCRC. The objective response rate was significantly higher (49% vs 31%; $P<.001$ for evaluable patients) and time to progression significantly longer (median 6.7 vs 4.4 months; $P<.001$) with the addition of irinotecan. Overall survival was also improved (median 17.4 vs 14.1 months; $P = .031$), and the increased frequency of treatment side effects associated with addition of irinotecan seemed manageable.[6]

The European Organisation for Research and Treatment of Cancer (EORTC) 40986 randomized 430 previously untreated patients with mCRC to FOLFIRI or 5-FU/LV alone. Patients who were treated with FOLFIRI had a higher response rate (62.2% vs 34.4%; $P<.0001$) and longer median progression-free survival (8.5 vs 6.4 months; $P<.0001$) than those treated with 5-FU/LV alone. They also had longer median overall survival (20.1 vs 16.9 months; $P = .28$), but this was not statistically significant, likely because two-thirds of the 5-FU/LV patients received irinotecan in the second-line setting.[7]

The benefit of a combination regimen of irinotecan and 5-FU/LV was also reported by Saltz and colleagues[8] from North America. The multicenter randomized controlled study of 683 patients investigating first-line treatment of mCRC compared 3 arms: bolus 5-FU/LV, bolus IFL, and irinotecan alone. The combination of irinotecan with 5-FU/LV was associated with higher response rate (39% vs 21%; $P<.001$), longer progression-free survival (median, 7.0 vs 4.3 months; $P = .004$), and longer overall survival (median, 14.8 vs 12.6 months; $P = .04$). The treatment outcomes were similar between the 5-FU/LV group and the irinotecan-alone group.

These studies proved the effectiveness of the addition of irinotecan to an FU-based regimen, and established the basic concept of doublet therapy for mCRC. Drug sequencing and method of administration are associated with frequency of toxicity. Fuchs and colleagues[9] reported a phase III study (BICC-C trial) that compared the safety and efficacy of different irinotecan-containing regimens in first-line treatment. The 3 arms included 144 patients who received FOLFIRI, 141 patients who received modified IFL, and 145 patients who received CAPIRI. Median progression-free survival was longer in the FOLFIRI group (7.6 months) compared with modified IFL (5.9 months; $P = .004$) or CAPIRI (5.8 months; $P = .15$). CAPIRI was associated with a higher rate of side effects, particularly with vomiting and diarrhea. This study showed the superiority of the FOLFIRI regimen compared with the other irinotecan-containing regimens.

Higher rates of gastrointestinal side effects associated with CAPIRI compared with FOLFIRI were also reported by other prospective studies.[5,10]

Oxaliplatin-Containing Regimens: Folinic Acid, Fluorouracil, Oxaliplatin/Capecitabine, Oxaliplatin/XELOX

Oxaliplatin, a platinum derivative agent effective for colorectal cancer, was approved by the FDA in 2002 for progressive colorectal cancer and in 2004 as an initial treatment of advanced colorectal cancer. Oxaliplatin has been shown in phase II trials to have some activity as monotherapy, but it is much more effective in combination with an FU-based regimen, likely because of a synergetic effect with FU. In RCTs, single-agent oxaliplatin had no significant activity and therefore, unlike irinotecan, oxaliplatin should not be used as a single-agent therapy in mCRC.[11] FOLFOX is now the standard regimen for mCRC. A variety of modifications of 5-FU/LV and oxaliplatin dosage have been used. Modified FOLFOX6 (mFOLFOX6) is the most commonly used, which administers 85 mg/m^2 of oxaliplatin on day 1 and FU over 2 days (400 mg/m^2 bolus on day 1, followed by 2400–3000 mg/m^2 over 46 hours).

De Gramont and colleagues[12] reported a randomized controlled study of 420 previously untreated patients with mCRC, comparing 5-FU/LV either with or without oxaliplatin. The oxaliplatin-containing regimen (FOLFOX) had a higher response rate (50.7% vs 22.3%; $P = .0001$) and longer progression-free survival (median 9.0 vs 6.2 months; $P = .0003$) than the control. Overall survival was not statistically significantly different between the groups (median, 16.2 vs 14.7 months; $P = .12$), but this was likely because crossover obscured the impact on survival.

To replace IV 5-FU with the oral agent capecitabine, multiple randomized trials were conducted comparing CAPOX (or XELOX) and 5-FU with oxaliplatin as a first-line treatment, which showed comparable efficacies but different toxicity profiles. The German Arbeitsgemeinschaft Internistische Onkologie (AIO) study group compared CAPOX with high-dose infusional 5-FU/LV and oxaliplatin (FUFOX) in a randomized controlled study of 474 patients. There were no differences between CAPOX and FUFOX in the response rate (54% vs 48%), progression-free survival (hazard ratio [HR], 1.17; 95% confidence interval [CI], 0.96–1.43; $P = .117$), or overall survival (HR, 1.12; 95% CI, 0.92–1.38; $P = .26$). Both regimens were generally well tolerated, but CAPOX was associated with a higher rate of grade 2 or 3 hand-foot syndrome (10% vs 4%; $P = .028$).[13] A recent meta-analysis of 8 RCTs including 4363 patients, comparing CAPOX and FOLFOX, showed that there were no statistically significant differences between the regimens with respect to overall survival and response rates. However, CAPOX was associated with a higher incidence of thrombocytopenia, hand-foot syndrome, and diarrhea, whereas FOLFOX was associated with a higher incidence of neutropenia.[14]

Oxaliplatin-containing regimens have been shown to be effective for second-line or third-line treatment after progression with irinotecan-containing regimens. Rothenberg and colleagues[11] reported an RCT of 463 patients with mCRC from 120 sites in North America, who progressed after IFL therapy. This study compared 5-FU/LV, oxaliplatin monotherapy, and FOLFOX4. The objective response rate was higher in the FOLFOX4 group (9.9%) compared with 5-FU/LV (0%; $P<.001$), with longer time to progression (4.6 vs 2.7 months; $P<.001$). Oxaliplatin monotherapy had a similar efficacy to 5-FU/LV. The investigators concluded that FOLFOX4 is superior treatment to 5-FU/LV as a second-line regimen.

In a randomized trial of 214 patients with progressive mCRC after 2 previous chemotherapy regimens that include irinotecan-containing but not oxaliplatin-containing regimens, patients were randomized to receive bolus and infusional

5-FU/LV with or without oxaliplatin (FOLFOX4). In this salvage setting, the objective response rate was higher with FOLFOX4 than with 5-FU/LV (13% vs 2%; $P = .0027$) and median time to progression was longer with FOLFOX4 as well (4.8 vs 2.4 months; $P<.001$). There was no overall survival difference between groups (9.9 vs 11.4 months; $P = .20$). Grade 3 and 4 toxicities were notably higher in the FOLFOX4 patients; neutropenia (42% vs 13%), diarrhea (16% vs 6%), and neuropathy (6% vs 0%).[15] The noninferiority of CAPOX to FOLFOX as second-line therapy has also been shown. In a study of 627 patients with mCRC after progression with prior irinotecan-based chemotherapy, patients were randomized to CAPOX or FOLFOX4. There was no significant difference between CAPOX and FOLFOX in median progression-free survival (4.7 vs 4.8 months), or overall survival (median, 11.9 vs 12.5 months; HR, 1.02; 95% CI, 0.86–1.21). Grade 3 and 4 adverse events were observed in 50% of CAPOX and 65% of FOLFOX4 patients. The investigators concluded that CAPOX is noninferior to FOLFOX4 as second-line therapy after progression with irinotecan-based regimens.[16]

Folinic Acid, Fluorouracil, Oxaliplatin Versus Folinic Acid, Fluorouracil, Irinotecan

The demonstrated efficacy of the combination regimens with irinotecan or oxaliplatin led to the obvious next question of the comparative efficacy of FOLFOX (or oxaliplatin-containing regimens) and FOLFIRI (or irinotecan-containing regimens). Several studies have shown that they have similarly efficacy to first-line therapy.

The GERCOR group compared patients with advanced colorectal cancer randomized to FOLFIRI followed by FOLFOX6 or the reverse sequence. A total of 230 patients were randomly assigned to either group. There were no significant differences between the FOLFIRI-first or FOLFOX-first groups in median overall survival (21.5 vs 20.6 months; $P = .99$) or median second progression-free survival (14.2 vs 10.9 months; $P = .64$). Response rates as first-line therapy were similar between FOLFIRI-first and FOLFOX-first groups (56% vs 54%; P-value was not significant). Metastasectomy was performed more frequently in the FOLFOX-first group (22% vs 9%; $P = .02$), and those patients who underwent metastasectomy achieved excellent survival. Response rates as second-line therapy were higher with FOLFOX than FOLFIRI (15% vs 4%; $P = .05$). The investigators concluded that both sequences achieved a similarly prolonged survival.[17]

A multicenter study of the Gruppo Oncologico Dell'Italia Meridionale compared first-line FOLFIRI and FOLFOX in patients with mCRC. A total of 360 patients were randomized to either group. There was no statistically significant difference between FOLFIRI and FOLFOX groups in overall response rates (31% vs 34%; $P = .60$), in median time to progression (7 vs 7 months; $P = .64$), or overall survival (14 vs 15 months; $P = .28$). Grade 3 or 4 toxicities were uncommon in either group, but the toxicity profiles were different between groups; FOLFIRI was more frequently associated with gastrointestinal symptoms and FOLFOX was more frequently associated with thrombocytopenia and neurosensorial symptoms. The investigators concluded that either FOLFIRI or FOLFOX was similarly effective as first-line therapy for patients with advanced colorectal cancer.[18]

Irinotecan and oxaliplatin were also compared in the setting of bevacizumab-containing regimens in a recent randomized controlled study from Japan (WJOG4407G) that randomized patients with mCRC to bevacizumab plus FOLFIRI or bevacizumab plus mFOLFOX6 as first-line treatment. A total of 402 patients were enrolled and no difference between FOLFIRI and FOLFOX groups was observed in median progression-free survival (12.1 vs 10.7 months; HR, 0.905; 95% CI, 0.72–1.13; $P = .003$ for noninferiority) or median overall survival (31.4 vs 30.1 months; HR, 0.99; 95% CI, 0.79–1.25), showing the equivalent efficacy of FOLFIRI and FOLFOX in combination with bevacizumab in first-line treatment.[19]

FOLFOX and FOLFIRI were compared in combination with cetuximab in a setting of unresectable liver-only metastases. The phase II CELIM trial included 111 patients with initially nonresectable liver metastases, who were randomly assigned to receive cetuximab with either FOLFOX6 or FOLFIRI. There was no difference in response rate (68% vs 57%; $P = .23$) between groups. Response rate in patients with KRAS wild-type tumor was 70% (47 out of 67), which was higher than that of patients with KRAS mutated tumors (29%; 11 out of 27; $P = .008$). R0 resection was achieved in 38% (20 out of 53) in the FOLFOX6 group, and 30% (16 out of 53) in the FOLFIRI group (P-value not provided).[20]

Oxaliplatin-Containing and Irinotecan-Containing Regimens: Oxaliplatin and Irinotecan/FOLFOXIRI

Regimens containing both oxaliplatin and irinotecan (IROX) have been investigated. IROX with the addition of a 5-FU/LV infusion is called FOLFOXIRI.

Oxaliplatin and irinotecan

With the expansion of treatment options, the US Intergroup (INT) N9741 trial investigated the efficacy of IROX.[21–23] This study randomly assigned a total of 1691 patients into one of 7 regimens containing FU, oxaliplatin, and irinotecan between 1998 and 2002. Four out of those 7 arms were discontinued because of inefficacy or toxicity. The remaining 3 arms were weekly bolus IFL, FOLFOX, and bolus IROX. The FOLFOX group had a better 5-year survival rate (9.8%) than IFL (3.7%; $P = .04$) or IROX (5.1%; $P = .128$). Median overall survival and time to progression were also longer in the FOLFOX group (20.2 months and 8.9 months, respectively) than for IFL (14.6 months and 6.1 months, respectively; $P<.001$ for both) or IROX (17.3 months and 6.7 months, respectively; $P<.001$).[23] IROX was associated with higher frequency of grade 3 or worse hematologic toxicity in patients more than 70 years of age than FOLFOX.[22] The IROX regimen is an acceptable alternative in patients who cannot receive either capecitabine or 5-FU in combination with oxaliplatin and irinotecan.

FOLFOXIRI

FOLFOXIRI contains all 3 active cytotoxic agents. In 2 Italian RCTs, progression-free survival was improved by FOLFOXIRI compared with FOLFIRI with and without bevacizumab. The first study randomized a total of 244 patients to receive FOLFOXIRI or FOLFIRI. FOLFOXIRI was associated with a longer median progression-free survival (9.8 vs 6.8 months; $P<.001$) and longer median overall survival (23.4 vs 16.7 months; $P = .026$) with higher 5-year overall survival rate (15% vs 8%) than FOLFIRI.[24] However, FOLFOXIRI was associated with higher rates of grade 2 to 3 peripheral neuropathy (19% vs 0%; $P<.001$) and grade 3 to 4 neutropenia (50% vs 28%; $P<.001$). The incidences of febrile neutropenia (5% vs 3%) and grade 3 to 4 diarrhea were not different. However, by achieving a higher response rate with FOLFOXIRI (66% vs 41%; $P = .002$), subsequent R0 metastasectomy was more frequently achieved in FOLFOXIRI-treated patients than in the control patients (15% vs 6% [$P = .033$] among all patients, and 36% vs 12% [$P = .017$] among patients with liver-only metastasis).[25]

Based on the efficacy of the FOLFOXIRI triplet cytotoxic combination, the TRIBE phase III randomized controlled study compared FOLFIRINOX plus bevacizumab with FOLFIRI plus bevacizumab. A total of 508 patients with previously untreated mCRC were randomized. The overall response rate was higher (65% vs 53%; $P = .006$) and median progression-free survival was longer (12.1 vs 9.7 months; $P = .003$) with the

FOLFOXIRI and bevacizumab group. Overall survival was not statistically different between groups (31.0 vs 25.8 months; HR, 0.79; 95% CI, 0.63–1.00; $P = .054$) and FOLFOXIRI was associated with a higher frequency of toxicity. In addition, this study did not confirm the benefit of FOLFOXIRI compared with FOLFIRI in terms of rate of successful metastasectomy; the rates of R0 resection of metastases were 15% in FOLFOXIRI group and 12% in FOLFIRI group ($P = .33$).[26]

In contrast, a report from the Hellenic Oncology Research Group in the United Kingdom did not confirm the benefit of the FOLFOXIRI regimen compared with FOLFIRI. Souglakos and colleagues[27] reported a multicenter randomized controlled study of 283 previously untreated patients with mCRC, comparing FOLFOXIRI and FOLFIRI as first-line therapy. There was no difference in response rate (43% vs 33.6%; $P = .168$), median time to progression (8.4 vs 6.9 months; $P = .17$), or median overall survival (21.5 vs 19.5 months; $P = .34$). However, the 3-drug combination of FOLFOXIRI was associated with higher frequency of toxicity, including alopecia, diarrhea, and neurosensory toxicity, compared with FOLFIRI.

There are limited available data comparing FOLFOXIRI with FOLFOX. Gruenberger and colleagues[28] reported a multinational randomized phase II trial comparing mFOLFOX6 plus bevacizumab and FOLFOXIRI plus bevacizumab as first-line treatment of patients with colorectal cancer with unresectable liver metastases (OLIVIA trial). A total of 80 patients were enrolled. Bevacizumab plus FOLFOXIRI was associated with higher response rate (81% vs 62%) and R0 resection rate (49% vs 23%) and longer median progression-free survival (18.6 vs 11.5 months) compared with bevacizumab plus FOLFOX. The FOLFOXIRI arm was associated with higher rate of grade 3 and higher toxicities of neutropenia (50% vs 35%) and diarrhea (30% vs 14%) but, because of the small sample size and type of study (phase II), statistical comparison was not made in the analysis.

The preliminary results of a phase II STEAM trial were presented at the 2016 American Society of Clinical Oncology (ASCO) Gastrointestinal Cancers Symposium.[29] This phase II trial randomized 280 unresectable previously untreated patients with mCRC to 3 treatment arms: (1) bevacizumab plus concurrent FOLFOXIRI, (2) bevacizumab plus sequential FOLFOXIRI (alternating FOLFOX and FOLFIRI), or (3) bevacizumab plus FOLFOX. The concurrent FOLFOXIRI plus bevacizumab group had a higher response rate (77% vs 54%) and higher R0 resection rate (15% vs 6%) compared with the FOLFOX plus bevacizumab group. The study was completed in March 2016, and results are pending.

In summary, although a triplet cytotoxic backbone has more activity than a doublet, it comes at the cost of increased toxicity and therefore should be used in carefully selected patients; preferably, patients who are young and have good performance status.

Monoclonal Antibody Therapy

Bevacizumab

Bevacizumab (Avastin) is a humanized monoclonal antibody targeting VEGF that inhibits angiogenesis. Bevacizumab has been shown to be effective to prolong survival when combined with a variety of first-line regimens for mCRC; however, the survival benefit of the addition of bevacizumab is modest, at most, if it is used with modern doublet regimens such as FOLFIRI and FOLFOX. In the first phase III trial comparing IFL plus bevacizumab and IFL plus placebo, 813 patients with previously untreated mCRC were randomized. The bevacizumab group had a higher response rate (44.8% vs 34.8%; $P = .004$) and longer median progression-free survival (10.6 vs 6.2 months; $P<.001$) compared with the placebo group. The addition of bevacizumab resulted in prolonged median overall survival (20.3 vs 15.6 months; $P<.001$).

Grade 3 hypertension was more commonly observed in the bevacizumab group (11.0% vs 2.3%) but it was easily manageable.[30]

The addition of bevacizumab has also been reported in combination with bolus 5-FU/LV in patients who are not optimal candidates for a first-line irinotecan-containing regimen. A randomized phase II trial compared 5-FU/LV and bevacizumab versus 5-FU/LV and placebo as first-line therapy in 209 patients with mCRC who were not considered optimal for an irinotecan-containing regimen. The addition of bevacizumab was associated with an improved response rate (26% vs 15.2%; P = .055) and longer progression-free survival (9.2 vs 5.5 months; P<.001). Overall survival was also longer in bevacizumab group, albeit statistically not significant (16.6 vs 12.9 months; P = .16).[31]

Benefit of the addition of bevacizumab has been reported in combination with FOLFIRI. The BICC-C randomized phase III study (described in more detail earlier) compared irinotecan-containing regimens with or without bevacizumab in 430 previously untreated patients with mCRC. FOLFIRI plus bevacizumab had a longer progression-free survival than modified IFL plus bevacizumab, although the difference was not statistically significant (11.2 vs 8.3 months; P = .28).[9] In a follow-up report, there was superior median overall survival for FOLFIRI plus bevacizumab compared with modified IFL plus bevacizumab (28.0 vs 19.2 months; HR, 1.79; 95% CI, 1.12–2.88; P = .037).

In contrast, a Greek RCT failed to confirm a survival benefit with bevacizumab in combination with FOLFIRI in treatment-naive patients. A total of 222 patients were enrolled, and there was no statistically significant difference between the bevacizumab versus placebo groups in response rate (37% vs 35%; P-value not provided) or median overall survival (22 vs 25 months; P = .139).[32] However, survival in the control arm with FOLFIRI was better than expected.

Bevacizumab was also studied in combination with oxaliplatin-based regimens. The TREE study randomized patients with previously untreated metastatic or recurrent colorectal cancer to receive mFOLFOX6, bolus FOL (bolus 5-FU/LV with oxaliplatin), or CAPOX at phase 1 (n = 150), and subsequently modified such that patients in phase 2 were randomized to the same regimens plus bevacizumab (n = 223). Overall response rates were improved from no-bevacizumab regimens (41%, 20%, and 27%, respectively) to bevacizumab-containing regimens (52%, 39%, and 46%, subsequently). First-line bevacizumab plus oxaliplatin-containing therapy achieved median overall survival of 23.7 months, whereas it was 18.2 months for no-bevacizumab regimens.[33]

The Eastern Cooperative Oncology Group (ECOG) E3200 study compared FOLFOX4 with and without bevacizumab as second-line therapy after progression with irinotecan-containing therapy. This study enrolled 829 patients for randomization. The addition of bevacizumab to FOLFOX4 resulted in a higher response rate and 2.1 months longer median overall survival (22.7% and 12.9 months in bevacizumab plus FOLFOX group vs 8.6% and 10.8 months in FOLFOX group, respectively; HR, 0.75; P = .001). Progression-free survival was also longer in the bevacizumab plus FOLFOX group than in the FOLFOX group (7.3 vs 4.7 months; P<.001). The addition of bevacizumab with FOLFOX4 resulted in a 14% overall increase in grade 3 and 4 toxicity, including hypertension, bleeding, and vomiting (**Table 1**).[34]

Results from another large RCT of bevacizumab in addition to oxaliplatin-based therapy did not confirm survival benefit. Saltz and colleagues[35] reported the NO16966 study, which randomized a total of 1401 patients in 2 by 2 factorial design, to CAPOX versus FOLFOX4, and then to bevacizumab versus placebo. Although the addition of bevacizumab was associated with improved progression-free survival

Table 1
Phase III clinical trials of monoclonal antibody therapies for metastatic colorectal cancer

Agents	Indication	Author, Year (Study Name)	N	Treatment	Median Survival (mo)	P-Value
Bev	First line	Hurwitz et al,[30] 2004	813	Bev + IFL vs IFL	PFS: 10.6 vs 6.2 OS: 20.3 vs 15.6	<.001 <.001
		Stathopoulos et al,[32] 2010	222	Bev + FOLFIRI vs FOLFIRI	OS: 22 vs 25	.139
		Giantonio et al,[34] 2007 (ECOG E3200)	829	Bev + FOLFOX vs FOLFOX	PFS: 7.3 vs 4.7 OS: 12.9 vs 10.8	<.001 .001
		Saltz et al,[35] 2008 (NO16966)	1401	2 × 2 factorial design CAPOX vs FOLFOX4, Bev vs placebo	(Bev vs placebo) PFS: 9.4 vs 8.0 OS: 21.3 vs 19.9	.002 .077
	Second line	Bennouna et al,[36] 2013 (ML18147)	820	Bev + chemo vs chemo (oxaliplatin or irinotecan based)	OS: 11.2 vs 9.8	.006
		Masi et al,[37] 2015 (BEBYP)	185	Bev + chemo vs chemo (mFOLFOX or FOLFIRI)	OS: 6.8 vs 5.0	.043
Aflibercept	Second line	Van Cutsem et al,[38] 2012	1226	Aflibercept + FOLFIRI vs FOLFIRI	PFS: 6.9 vs 4.7 OS: 13.5 vs 12.1	<.001 .003
Ramucirumab	Second line	Tabernero et al,[39] 2015 (RAISE)	1072	Ramucirumab + FOLFIRI vs FOLFIRI	PFS: 5.7 vs 4.5 OS: 13.3 vs 11.7	<.001 .022

(continued on next page)

Table 1
(continued)

Agents	Indication	Author, Year (Study Name)	N	Treatment	Median Survival (mo)	P-Value
Cet	Progressive disease	Jonker et al,[41] 2007; Karapetis et al,[42] 2008	572	Cet vs placebo	OS: 9.5 vs 4.8 Analysis of K-ras WT pts, n = 394	<.001
	Second line	Sobrero et al,[44] 2008 (EPIC)	1298	Cet + irinotecan vs irinotecan	PFS: 4.0 vs 2.6 OS: 10.7 vs 10.0	<.001 .71
	Second line	Cunningham et al,[45] 2004	329	Cet vs Cet + irinotecan	PFS: 4.1 vs 1.5 OS: 8.6 vs 4.9	<.001 .48
	First line	Van Cutsem et al,[46] 2009	1198	Cet + FOLFIRI vs FOLFIRI	PFS: 9.9 vs 8.7 OS: 23.5 vs 20.0 Analysis of K-ras WT pts, n = 348	.02 .009
	First line	Maughan et al,[51] 2011 (MRC COIN)	1630	Cet + chemo vs chemo (FOLFOX or CAPOX)	OS: 17.0 vs 17.9 Analysis of K-ras WT pts, n = 729	.67
	First line	Primrose et al,[52] 2014 (New EPOC)	257	Cet + chemo vs chemo (oxaliplatin based)	OS: 14.1 vs 20.5	.03
Bev vs Cet	First line	Heinemann et al,[53] 2014 (FIRE-3)	592	Bev + FOLFIRI vs Cet + FOLFIRI	OS: 25.0 vs 28.7	.017
	First line	Venook et al,[55] 2014 (CALGB/SWOG 80405, abstract)	1137	FOLFIRI or mFOLFOX6, combined with Bev or Cet	Bev group vs Cet group PFS: 10.8 vs 10.5 OS: 29.0 vs 29.9	Not reported .34
Panitumumab	First line	Douillard et al,[60] 2010 (PRIME)	1183	Pan + FOLFOX4 vs FOLFOX4	PFS: 10.0 vs 8.6 OS: 23.9 vs 19.7 Analysis of K-ras WT pts, n = 656	.01 .17

Abbreviations: Bev, bevacizumab; Cet, cetuximab; Chemo, chemotherapy; OS, overall survival; Pan, panitumumab; PFS, progression-free survival; pts, patients; WT, wild type.

(9.4 vs 8.0 months; $P = .0023$), there was no statistically significant difference between the bevacizumab group and the no-bevacizumab group in median overall survival (21.3 vs 19.9 months; $P = .077$), with similar response rates.

Continuation of bevacizumab in second-line regimens after progression with first-line bevacizumab-containing regimens has also been studied and found beneficial. A European multicenter phase III TML trial compared bevacizumab plus chemotherapy and chemotherapy alone as second-line therapy after progression with bevacizumab-containing first-line therapy. This study randomized a total of 820 patients with mCRC in this setting. Maintenance of bevacizumab in the second-line therapy was associated with longer median overall survival (11.2 vs 9.8 months; $P = .0062$).[36] The benefit of continuation of bevacizumab in second-line therapy was confirmed by the randomized BEBYP trial. This Italian study randomized a total of 185 patients with mCRC who progressed after first-line chemotherapy plus bevacizumab, to receive either mFOLFOX6 or FOLFIRI as the first-line regimen, with or without bevacizumab. Continuation of bevacizumab was associated with improved overall survival (HR, 0.77; 95% CI, 0.56–1.06; stratified log-rank, $P = .043$).[37]

Other anti–vascular endothelial growth factor agents (aflibercept and ramucirumab)
There are 2 other anti-VEGF agents approved for mCRC: aflibercept and ramucirumab.

Van Custsem and colleagues[38] reported an RCT of 1226 patients with mCRC who had progressed on or after previous treatment with an oxaliplatin-based chemotherapy regimen. Patients were randomly assigned to receive aflibercept or placebo in combination with FOLFIRI. Addition of aflibercept was associated with an improved response rate (19.8% vs 11.1%; $P<.001$), improved progression-free survival (HR, 0.76; 95% CI, 0.66–0.87; $P<.001$), and improved overall survival (HR, 0.82; 95% CI, 0.71–0.94; $P = .003$).

An international multicenter RCT showed effectiveness of ramucirumab. This trial randomly assigned 1072 patients with mCRC after disease progression during or within 6 months of the last dose of first-line therapy to receive ramucirumab or placebo in combination with FOLFIRI. There was no difference in response rate (13.4% in ramucirumab group vs 12.5% in placebo group; $P = .63$), but progression-free survival (HR, 0.79; 95% CI, 0.70–0.90; $P<.001$) and overall survival (HR, 0.84; 95% CI, 0.73–0.98; $P = .022$) were better in the ramucirumab group compared with the placebo group. The incidence of grade 3 or worse adverse events was higher in the ramucirumab group than in the placebo group (79% vs 62%; P-value not provided).[39]

Because both these studies and the TML study showed the value of continued VEGF inhibition after progression on a bevacizumab-based regimen in first-line treatment, aflibercept, ramucirumab, and bevacizumab are all reasonable agents in this setting. The toxicity profile of bevacizumab seems to be favorable and it has therefore been a more widely used agent.

Epidermal growth factor receptor inhibitors
Cetuximab (Erbitux) and panitumumab (Vectibix) are monoclonal antibodies targeting EGFR and they been proved to be effective against mCRC in patients whose tumors are associated with a mutation in KRAS. KRAS mutation status is the first predictive molecular marker for treatment response in patients with advanced disease, and patient selection based on biomarker analysis is critical because both cetuximab and panitumumab are known to be effective only on tumors with wild-type (not mutated) K-ras oncogenes, which is observed in approximately 60% of patients with mCRC.[40]

Cetuximab
Cetuximab is a mouse/human chimeric monoclonal antibody targeting EGFR. Cetuximab efficacy has been shown as monotherapy or in combination with irinotecan for

patients with K-ras wild-type tumors. A multicenter RCT of cetuximab monotherapy versus best supportive care for patients with progressive disease after FU, irinotecan, and oxaliplatin or patients with contraindications for those agents showed improved overall survival (median, 6.1 vs 4.6 months; HR, 0.77; 95% CI, 0.64–0.92; P = .005) and longer progression-free survival (HR, 0.68; 95% CI, 0.57–0.80; P<.001).[41] After further analysis, the benefit of cetuximab was found to be limited to patients with K-ras wild-type tumors. Of the tumors evaluated for K-ras mutations (n = 394), 42.3% had at least 1 mutation in exon 2 of the K-ras gene. In patients with K-ras wild-type tumors, cetuximab treatment was strongly associated with overall survival (median, 9.5 vs 4.8 months; HR, 0.55; 95% CI, 0.41–0.74; P<.001), whereas it was not in patients with K-ras–mutated tumors (HR, 0.98; P = .89).[42] Cetuximab monotherapy compared with best supportive care was also associated with improved quality of life in patients with mCRC.[43]

The EPIC phase III study showed the efficacy of cetuximab in combination with irinotecan in second-line therapy. It compared cetuximab plus irinotecan and irinotecan alone as second-line therapy, after progression with FU and oxaliplatin treatment in patients with mCRC. A total of 1298 patients were enrolled. The combination with cetuximab had longer progression-free survival than irinotecan alone (median, 4.0 vs 2.6 months; HR, 0.692; 95% CI, 0.617–0.776; P<.0001) and a higher response rate (16.4 vs 4.2%; P = .047). Overall survival was not different between groups (10.7 vs 10.0 months; P = .71), likely because 47% of the irinotecan-alone group subsequently received cetuximab. Skin rash (76 vs 5%), grade 3 to 4 diarrhea (28 vs 16%), and fatigue (8 vs 3%) were more frequently observed with combination therapy, but quality of life was reported to be better in the combination therapy group.[44]

Cetuximab monotherapy and cetuximab plus irinotecan in patients who progressed with previous irinotecan-based chemotherapy were compared in a randomized study of 329 patients with metastatic K-ras wild type colorectal cancer. The response rate was higher in the combination therapy group than the cetuximab monotherapy group (22.9% vs 10.8%; P = .007) and the time to progression was longer in the combination group as well (4.1 vs 1.5 months; P<.001). However, the difference in overall survival did not reach statistical significance (8.6 vs 4.9 months; P = .48).[45]

Cetuximab has also been investigated in first-line treatment of mCRC. The CRYSTAL multicenter phase III trial compared first-line FOLFIRI with or without cetuximab in a total of 1198 patients. The addition of cetuximab was associated with improved progression-free survival (HR, 0.85; 95% CI, 0.72–0.99; P = .048), although overall survival was not different between groups (HR, 0.93; 95% CI, 0.81–1.07; P = .31).[46] After further analysis of K-ras status (89% of patients were tested), K-ras wild-type patients were found to have improved response rate (57% vs 40%; P<.001), progression-free survival (median, 9.9 vs 8.7 months; P = .02), and overall survival (median, 23.5 vs 20.0 months; HR, 0.796; P = .009). The rate of R0 resection was also higher with cetuximab and in subgroup analysis of patients with K-ras wild-type tumors was 5.1% versus 2.0% (odds ratio, 2.65; P = .026). Toxicity was more frequently observed in the cetuximab group; grade 3 to 4 diarrhea, 16% versus 11%; skin toxicity, 19.7% versus 0.2%; and infusion reaction, 2.5% versus 0%.[47]

Addition of cetuximab has also been tested with FOLFOX as first-line therapy. The OPUS phase II trial randomized previously untreated patients with mCRC to receive FOLFOX4 with or without cetuximab.[48] In subsequent analysis with more patients tested with biomarker status (including 179 patients with wild-type K-ras status), K-ras wild-type patients who were treated with cetuximab plus FOLFOX4 had a higher response rate (57% vs 34%; P = .0027) and prolonged progression-free survival (median, 8.3 vs 7.2 months; P = .0064) than those who received FOLFOX4 alone, but the difference in overall survival did not reach statistical significance (median, 22.8 vs 18.5 months; $P = .39$).[49]

A benefit of adding cetuximab to chemotherapy was also tested in a Chinese study of a total of 138 patients with synchronous unresectable liver-only metastases. Patients with KRAS wild-type tumors were randomized after resection of the primary tumors to receive chemotherapy (FOLFOX6 or FOLFIRI) plus cetuximab or chemotherapy alone. The R0 resection rate was significantly improved with addition of cetuximab (25.7% vs 7.4%; $P<.01$), and 3-year overall survival was also improved (41% vs 18%; $P = .013$).[50]

Other studies have examined the impact of adding cetuximab to oxaliplatin-based regimens. The phase III MRC COIN trial conducted in the United Kingdom randomized 1630 patients with mCRC to either chemotherapy (either FOLFOX or CAPOX) alone or chemotherapy with cetuximab. In subset analysis of K-ras wild-type tumors (n = 729; 58%), the response rate was higher with cetuximab (64% vs 57%; $P = .049$) but there was no survival difference between groups (median overall survival, 17.9 months in the chemotherapy-alone group vs 17.0 months in the cetuximab group; $P = .67$).[51] Another study from the United Kingdom (EPOC) randomized a total of 257 patients with potentially resectable mCRC with K-ras wild-type tumors and showed inferior survival outcomes with cetuximab plus oxaliplatin-based chemotherapy compared with chemotherapy alone (median progression-free survival, 14.1 vs 20.5 months; $P = .03$).[52] Thus the results are inconclusive with respect to first-line treatment with cetuximab and an oxaliplatin-containing chemotherapy backbone (**Table 2**).

Bevacizumab versus cetuximab

Several randomized studies have attempted to compare bevacizumab and cetuximab. The FIRE-3 study is a multicenter randomized phase III trial that compared FOLFIRI plus cetuximab versus FOLFIRI plus bevacizumab as first-line therapy for patients with mCRC with K-ras wild-type tumors. This study enrolled a total of 592 patients and although response rates and progression-free survival were not different between groups, overall survival was significantly longer in the cetuximab group compared with the bevacizumab group (median, 28.7 vs 25.0 months; $P = .017$).[53] A criticism of this study is that details regarding treatment after progression with the first-line treatment have not been described. The protocol recommended second-line treatment of FOLFOX plus bevacizumab for the cetuximab group or cetuximab second-line therapy for the bevacizumab group; however, investigators were free to vary these recommendations.[54]

In the United States, another randomized controlled study compared bevacizumab and cetuximab in combination with FOLFOX or FOLFIRI in patients with K-ras wild-type metastatic colorectal metastasis (CALGB/SWOG 80405). In contrast with FIRE-3, 80405 did not show the superiority of cetuximab compared with bevacizumab. This study randomized a total of 1137 patients. In a preliminary report at the ASCO 2014 annual meeting, there were no difference between groups in either progression-free survival (median, 10.8 months in bevacizumab group vs 10.5 months in cetuximab group) or overall survival (median, 29.0 months in bevacizumab group vs 29.9 months in cetuximab group).[55]

Bevacizumab plus cetuximab

Given the efficacy of bevacizumab and of cetuximab, there was interest in a potential role for dual antibody therapy with both bevacizumab and cetuximab. However, data from the CAIRO2 study, which randomly assigned 755 patients with previously untreated K-ras wild-type mCRC to CAPOX plus bevacizumab with or without

Table 2
Phase III clinical trials of chemotherapy regimens for metastatic colorectal cancer

Regimens	Indication	Author, Year (Study Name)	N	Treatment	Median Survival (mo)	P-Value
Irinotecan regimens	First line	Douillard et al,[6] 2000	287	Irinotecan + 5-FU/LV vs 5-FU/LV	PFS: 6.7 vs 4.4 OS: 17.4 vs 14.1	<.001 .031
		Kohne et al,[7] 2005 (EORTC 40986)	430	FOLFIRI vs 5-FU/LV	PFS: 8.5 vs 6.4 OS: 20.1 vs 16.9	<.001 .28
		Fuchs et al,[9] 2007 (BICC-C)	430	FOLFIRI vs IFL vs CAPIRI	PFS: 7.6 vs 5.9 vs 5.8 OS: 23.1 vs 17.6 vs 18.9	.004[a] .09[a]
Oxaliplatin regimens	First line	De Gramont et al,[12] 2000	420	FOLFOX vs 5-FU/LV	PFS: 9.0 vs 6.2 OS: 16.2 vs 14.7	<.001 .12
		Ducreux et al,[69] 2011 (FFCD 2000-05)	205	First/second/third line 1. 5-FU + LV/FOLFOX6/FOLFIRI 2. FOLFOX6/FOLFIRI	OS: 16.2 vs 16.4	.85
		Porschen et al,[13] 2007	474	CAPOX vs FUFOX	PFS: 7.1 vs 8.0 OS: 16.8 vs 18.8	.12 .26
	Second line	Rothenberg et al,[11] 2003	463	FOLFOX4 vs 5-FU/LV vs oxaliplatin	PFS: 4.6 vs 2.7 vs 1.6	<.001[a]
		Rothenberg et al,[16] 2008	627	FOLFOX4 vs CAPOX	PFS: 4.8 vs 4.7 OS: 12.5 vs 11.9	Noninferior <.001
	Third line	Kemeny et al,[15] 2004	214	FOLFOX4 vs 5-FU/LV	PFS: 4.8 vs 2.4 OS: 9.9 vs 11.4	<.001 .20
FOLFIRI vs FOLFOX	First line	Tournigand et al,[17] 2004 (GRECOR)	230	First/second line 1. FOLFIRI/FOLFOX 2. FOLFOX/FOLFIRI	OS: 21.5 vs 20.6 Second PFS: 14.2 vs 10.9	.99 .64
		Colucci et al,[18] 2005	360	FOLFIRI vs FOLFOX	PFS: 7 vs 7 OS: 14 vs 15	.64 .28
		Yamazaki et al,[19] 2016 (WJOG4407G)	402	Bev + FOLFIRI vs Bev + mFOLFOX6	PFS: 12.1 vs 10.7 OS: 31.4 vs 30.4	Noninferior
FOLFOXIRI	First line	Falcone et al,[25] 2007	244	FOLFOXIRI vs FOLFIRI	PFS: 9.8 vs 6.8 OS: 23.4 vs 16.7	<.001 .026
		Loupakis et al,[26] 2014 (TRIBE)	508	Bev + FOLFOXIRI vs Bev + FOLFIRI	PFS: 12.1 vs 9.7 OS: 31.0 vs 25.8	.003 .054
		Souglakos et al,[27] 2006	283	FOLFOXIRI vs FOLFIRI	PFS: 8.4 vs 6.9 OS: 21.5 vs 19.5	.17 .34

[a] Comparing first 2 regimens.

cetuximab, show that the addition of cetuximab was associated with shorter progression-free survival (10.7 months in no-cetuximab group vs 9.4 months in cetuximab group; $P = .01$), whereas there was no difference in overall survival and response rate.[56]

Panitumumab

Panitumumab is a fully human monoclonal antibody specific for the extracellular domain of EGFR. Panitumumab was shown to be beneficial in K-ras wild-type tumors, either as monotherapy (vs best supportive care)[57–59] or in combination as first-line therapy.[60,61] Panitumumab was associated with a high incidence of skin toxicity (90%).[61]

The multicenter phase III PRIME trial randomized 1183 previously untreated patients with mCRC to either to receive panitumumab plus FOLFOX4 or FOLFOX4 alone.[60] In analysis of K-ras wild-type patients (n = 656), panitumumab plus FOLFOX4 was associated with prolonged progression-free survival (median, 10.0 vs 8.6 months; $P = .01$) without a significant improvement in overall survival (median, 23.9 vs 19.7 months; $P = .17$). Survival analysis showed that the panitumumab regimen was associated with improved overall survival (HR, 0.83; 95% CI, 0.70–0.98; $P = .03$).[61] The addition of panitumumab was associated with reduced progression-free survival in K-ras mutant patients (HR, 1.29; 95% CI, 1.04–1.62; $P = .02$).[60]

Regorafenib

Regorafenib and trifluridine/tipiracil are two recently approved agents for palliative therapy in patients with refractory mCRC. Regorafenib (BAY 73-4506), an orally active multikinase inhibitor that blocks several protein kinases, including receptors associated with angiogenesis (VEGF receptor [VEGFR] 1, VEGFR2, VFGFR3, and TIE2), oncogenesis (KIT, RET, RAF1, and BRAF), and the tumor microenvironment (platelet-derived growth factor receptor and fibroblast growth factor receptor). Regorafenib was approved by the FDA in 2012 for patients with mCRC who progressed after FU, oxaliplatin, and irinotecan chemotherapy, and monoclonal antibodies including anti-VEGF and (if K-ras wild type) anti-EGFR agents. Grothey and colleagues[62] reported its efficacy for patients with progressive mCRC in the phase III multicenter CORRECT trial. This study randomized a total of 760 patients in a 2:1 ratio to receive oral regorafenib or placebo. Regorafenib treatment was associated with a modest increase in median overall survival (6.4 vs 5.0 months; $P = .005$) but treatment-associated adverse events were observed more frequently in the regorafenib group (93% vs 61%), most commonly with hand-foot skin reaction (17%) and fatigue (10%).

The benefit of regorafenib compared with best supportive care was confirmed in the Asian multicenter CONCUR phase III trial. This study randomized a total of 243 patients with progressive mCRC in a 2:1 ratio to receive regorafenib or placebo. Regorafenib treatment was associated with longer median overall survival (8.8 vs 6.3 months; 1-sided $P = .00016$). Again, drug-related adverse events were observed frequently (97%) in the regorafenib group, most frequently with hand-foot skin reaction (16%).[63]

Trifluridine/Tipiracil

Trifluridine/tipiracil (TAS-102) is an orally active combination of trifluridine (a thymidine-based nucleic acid analogue) and tipiracil hydrochloride (a thymidine phosphorylase inhibitor). Trifluridine is the active cytotoxic component by being incorporated into DNA, causing strand breaks, whereas tipiracil inhibits trifluridine metabolism. TAS-102 was approved by FDA in 2015 for the same indication as for regorafenib.

The RECOURSE phase III trial proved the efficacy of TAS-102 monotherapy compared with placebo in patients with refractory mCRC. This study randomly assigned a total of 800 patients with refractory colorectal cancer, who progressed with at least previous 2 standard chemotherapy regimens, in a 2:1 ratio, to receive either TAS-102 or placebo. TAS-102 treatment was associated with improved median overall survival (7.1 vs 5.3 months; $P<.001$) compared with placebo. The most common adverse events observed in the TAS-102 group were neutropenia (38%) and leukopenia (21%).[64]

Immune Checkpoint Inhibitors

Immunotherapies have achieved remarkable discoveries for the last decade in cancer treatment, not limited to colorectal cancer. Of those recent discoveries, immune checkpoint inhibitors, such as PD-1/PD-L1 inhibitors, which were initially found to be effective against melanoma, were now reported to be potentially effective against mCRC as well, particularly in tumors with mutations in one of several DNA MMR genes.[65] Although pembrolizumab has received FDA breakthrough therapy designation for mCRC and is now included in NCCN guidelines, these immune checkpoint inhibitors have not been examined in randomized controlled studies.

Resectable Liver Metastases

With the accumulation of case series that reported excellent outcomes, with 5-year overall survival averaging 40% to 50% after surgical resection of liver metastases,[66] surgical resection is thought to offer the best chance of cure for patients with resectable liver metastases (≤4 liver lesions). However, resectability of disease and the optimal patient selection and timing for surgical resection of mCRC are not well defined.[67] The EORTC 40,983 trial was conducted to establish whether perioperative chemotherapy improves survival after resection of liver metastasis. In this phase III study, a total of 364 patients with resectable metastatic liver disease of colorectal cancer recruited from 78 hospitals internationally were randomly assigned to either perioperative FOLFOX4 or surgery alone. The perioperative therapy group received 6 cycles of chemotherapy before and after the surgery. Similar proportions of patients underwent successful resection of metastatic disease (83% in perioperative therapy group vs 84% in surgery-alone group). In the update at a median follow-up of 8.5 years, there was no difference in overall survival with the addition of perioperative chemotherapy; 5-year overall survival was 51.2% in the perioperative therapy group and 47.8% in the surgery-alone group ($P = .34$). In a subset analysis only including eligible patients (n = 342), they found an improved progression-free survival in perioperative therapy group (3-year progression-free survival 39% vs 30%; $P = .035$).[68] Because of these mixed results from this randomized trial, the benefit of perioperative therapy for resectable liver metastasis remains unclear.

SUMMARY

This article reviews the available data from randomized clinical trials in advanced mCRC. Remarkable discoveries have been made over the last 20 years that have dramatically improved survival and established the current treatment. Improved response rates to those systemic therapies have also increased the potential for identifying patients who are candidates for curative resection. Current evidence supports combination therapy such as FOLFOX plus bevacizumab as first-line therapy, but further studies are needed to define the optimal sequence of treatment regimens. Future discoveries are expected in molecularly directed monoclonal antibody therapies and for the use of immune checkpoint inhibitors to improve the prognosis of patients with mCRC.

REFERENCES

1. Hoff PM, Ansari R, Batist G, et al. Comparison of oral capecitabine versus intravenous fluorouracil plus leucovorin as first-line treatment in 605 patients with metastatic colorectal cancer: results of a randomized phase III study. J Clin Oncol 2001;19(8):2282–92.

2. Van Cutsem E, Twelves C, Cassidy J, et al. Oral capecitabine compared with intravenous fluorouracil plus leucovorin in patients with metastatic colorectal cancer: results of a large phase III study. J Clin Oncol 2001;19(21):4097–106.

3. de Gramont A, Bosset JF, Milan C, et al. Randomized trial comparing monthly low-dose leucovorin and fluorouracil bolus with bimonthly high-dose leucovorin and fluorouracil bolus plus continuous infusion for advanced colorectal cancer: a French intergroup study. J Clin Oncol 1997;15(2):808–15.

4. Cassidy J, Saltz L, Twelves C, et al. Efficacy of capecitabine versus 5-fluorouracil in colorectal and gastric cancers: a meta-analysis of individual data from 6171 patients. Ann Oncol 2011;22(12):2604–9.

5. Souglakos J, Ziras N, Kakolyris S, et al. Randomised phase-II trial of CAPIRI (capecitabine, irinotecan) plus bevacizumab vs FOLFIRI (folinic acid, 5-fluorouracil, irinotecan) plus bevacizumab as first-line treatment of patients with unresectable/metastatic colorectal cancer (mCRC). Br J Cancer 2012;106(3):453–9.

6. Douillard JY, Cunningham D, Roth AD, et al. Irinotecan combined with fluorouracil compared with fluorouracil alone as first-line treatment for metastatic colorectal cancer: a multicentre randomised trial. Lancet 2000;355(9209):1041–7.

7. Kohne CH, van Cutsem E, Wils J, et al. Phase III study of weekly high-dose infusional fluorouracil plus folinic acid with or without irinotecan in patients with metastatic colorectal cancer: European Organisation for Research and Treatment of Cancer Gastrointestinal Group Study 40986. J Clin Oncol 2005;23(22):4856–65.

8. Saltz LB, Cox JV, Blanke C, et al. Irinotecan plus fluorouracil and leucovorin for metastatic colorectal cancer. Irinotecan Study Group. N Engl J Med 2000; 343(13):905–14.

9. Fuchs CS, Marshall J, Mitchell E, et al. Randomized, controlled trial of irinotecan plus infusional, bolus, or oral fluoropyrimidines in first-line treatment of metastatic colorectal cancer: results from the BICC-C Study. J Clin Oncol 2007;25(30): 4779–86.

10. Kohne CH, De Greve J, Hartmann JT, et al. Irinotecan combined with infusional 5-fluorouracil/folinic acid or capecitabine plus celecoxib or placebo in the first-line treatment of patients with metastatic colorectal cancer. EORTC study 40015. Ann Oncol 2008;19(5):920–6.

11. Rothenberg ML, Oza AM, Bigelow RH, et al. Superiority of oxaliplatin and fluorouracil-leucovorin compared with either therapy alone in patients with progressive colorectal cancer after irinotecan and fluorouracil-leucovorin: interim results of a phase III trial. J Clin Oncol 2003;21(11):2059–69.

12. de Gramont A, Figer A, Seymour M, et al. Leucovorin and fluorouracil with or without oxaliplatin as first-line treatment in advanced colorectal cancer. J Clin Oncol 2000;18(16):2938–47.

13. Porschen R, Arkenau HT, Kubicka S, et al. Phase III study of capecitabine plus oxaliplatin compared with fluorouracil and leucovorin plus oxaliplatin in metastatic

colorectal cancer: a final report of the AIO Colorectal Study Group. J Clin Oncol 2007;25(27):4217–23.

14. Guo Y, Xiong BH, Zhang T, et al. XELOX vs. FOLFOX in metastatic colorectal cancer: an updated meta-analysis. Cancer Invest 2016;34(2):94–104.

15. Kemeny N, Garay CA, Gurtler J, et al. Randomized multicenter phase II trial of bolus plus infusional fluorouracil/leucovorin compared with fluorouracil/leucovorin plus oxaliplatin as third-line treatment of patients with advanced colorectal cancer. J Clin Oncol 2004;22(23):4753–61.

16. Rothenberg ML, Cox JV, Butts C, et al. Capecitabine plus oxaliplatin (XELOX) versus 5-fluorouracil/folinic acid plus oxaliplatin (FOLFOX-4) as second-line therapy in metastatic colorectal cancer: a randomized phase III noninferiority study. Ann Oncol 2008;19(10):1720–6.

17. Tournigand C, Andre T, Achille E, et al. FOLFIRI followed by FOLFOX6 or the reverse sequence in advanced colorectal cancer: a randomized GERCOR study. J Clin Oncol 2004;22(2):229–37.

18. Colucci G, Gebbia V, Paoletti G, et al. Phase III randomized trial of FOLFIRI versus FOLFOX4 in the treatment of advanced colorectal cancer: a multicenter study of the Gruppo Oncologico Dell'Italia Meridionale. J Clin Oncol 2005; 23(22):4866–75.

19. Yamazaki K, Nagase M, Tamagawa H, et al. Randomized phase III study of bevacizumab plus FOLFIRI and bevacizumab plus mFOLFOX6 as first-line treatment for patients with metastatic colorectal cancer (WJOG4407G). Ann Oncol 2016; 27(8):1539–46.

20. Folprecht G, Gruenberger T, Bechstein WO, et al. Tumour response and secondary resectability of colorectal liver metastases following neoadjuvant chemotherapy with cetuximab: the CELIM randomised phase 2 trial. Lancet Oncol 2010;11(1):38–47.

21. Delaunoit T, Goldberg RM, Sargent DJ, et al. Mortality associated with daily bolus 5-fluorouracil/leucovorin administered in combination with either irinotecan or oxaliplatin: results from intergroup trial N9741. Cancer 2004;101(10):2170–6.

22. Ashley AC, Sargent DJ, Alberts SR, et al. Updated efficacy and toxicity analysis of irinotecan and oxaliplatin (IROX): intergroup trial N9741 in first-line treatment of metastatic colorectal cancer. Cancer 2007;110(3):670–7.

23. Sanoff HK, Sargent DJ, Campbell ME, et al. Five-year data and prognostic factor analysis of oxaliplatin and irinotecan combinations for advanced colorectal cancer: N9741. J Clin Oncol 2008;26(35):5721–7.

24. Masi G, Vasile E, Loupakis F, et al. Randomized trial of two induction chemotherapy regimens in metastatic colorectal cancer: an updated analysis. J Natl Cancer Inst 2011;103(1):21–30.

25. Falcone A, Ricci S, Brunetti I, et al. Phase III trial of infusional fluorouracil, leucovorin, oxaliplatin, and irinotecan (FOLFOXIRI) compared with infusional fluorouracil, leucovorin, and irinotecan (FOLFIRI) as first-line treatment for metastatic colorectal cancer: the Gruppo Oncologico Nord Ovest. J Clin Oncol 2007; 25(13):1670–6.

26. Loupakis F, Cremolini C, Masi G, et al. Initial therapy with FOLFOXIRI and bevacizumab for metastatic colorectal cancer. N Engl J Med 2014;371(17):1609–18.

27. Souglakos J, Androulakis N, Syrigos K, et al. FOLFOXIRI (folinic acid, 5-fluorouracil, oxaliplatin and irinotecan) vs FOLFIRI (folinic acid, 5-fluorouracil and irinotecan) as first-line treatment in metastatic colorectal cancer (MCC): a multicentre randomised phase III trial from the Hellenic Oncology Research Group (HORG). Br J Cancer 2006;94(6):798–805.

28. Gruenberger T, Bridgewater J, Chau I, et al. Bevacizumab plus mFOLFOX-6 or FOLFOXIRI in patients with initially unresectable liver metastases from colorectal cancer: the OLIVIA multinational randomised phase II trial. Ann Oncol 2015; 26(4):702–8.

29. Bendell JC, Tan BR, Reeves JA, et al. Overall response rate (ORR) in STEAM, a randomized, open-label, phase 2 trial of sequential and concurrent FOLFOXIRI-bevacizumab (BEV) vs FOLFOX-BEV for the first-line (1L) treatment (tx) of patients (pts) with metastatic colorectal cancer (mCRC). J Clin Oncol 2016;34(4).

30. Hurwitz H, Fehrenbacher L, Novotny W, et al. Bevacizumab plus irinotecan, fluorouracil, and leucovorin for metastatic colorectal cancer. N Engl J Med 2004; 350(23):2335–42.

31. Kabbinavar FF, Schulz J, McCleod M, et al. Addition of bevacizumab to bolus fluorouracil and leucovorin in first-line metastatic colorectal cancer: results of a randomized phase II trial. J Clin Oncol 2005;23(16):3697–705.

32. Stathopoulos GP, Batziou C, Trafalis D, et al. Treatment of colorectal cancer with and without bevacizumab: a phase III study. Oncology 2010;78(5–6):376–81.

33. Hochster HS, Hart LL, Ramanathan RK, et al. Safety and efficacy of oxaliplatin and fluoropyrimidine regimens with or without bevacizumab as first-line treatment of metastatic colorectal cancer: results of the TREE study. J Clin Oncol 2008; 26(21):3523–9.

34. Giantonio BJ, Catalano PJ, Meropol NJ, et al. Bevacizumab in combination with oxaliplatin, fluorouracil, and leucovorin (FOLFOX4) for previously treated metastatic colorectal cancer: results from the Eastern Cooperative Oncology Group Study E3200. J Clin Oncol 2007;25(12):1539–44.

35. Saltz LB, Clarke S, Diaz-Rubio E, et al. Bevacizumab in combination with oxaliplatin-based chemotherapy as first-line therapy in metastatic colorectal cancer: a randomized phase III study. J Clin Oncol 2008;26(12):2013–9.

36. Bennouna J, Sastre J, Arnold D, et al. Continuation of bevacizumab after first progression in metastatic colorectal cancer (ML18147): a randomised phase 3 trial. Lancet Oncol 2013;14(1):29–37.

37. Masi G, Salvatore L, Boni L, et al. Continuation or reintroduction of bevacizumab beyond progression to first-line therapy in metastatic colorectal cancer: final results of the randomized BEBYP trial. Ann Oncol 2015;26(4):724–30.

38. Van Cutsem E, Tabernero J, Lakomy R, et al. Addition of aflibercept to fluorouracil, leucovorin, and irinotecan improves survival in a phase III randomized trial in patients with metastatic colorectal cancer previously treated with an oxaliplatin-based regimen. J Clin Oncol 2012;30(28):3499–506.

39. Tabernero J, Yoshino T, Cohn AL, et al. Ramucirumab versus placebo in combination with second-line FOLFIRI in patients with metastatic colorectal carcinoma that progressed during or after first-line therapy with bevacizumab, oxaliplatin, and a fluoropyrimidine (RAISE): a randomised, double-blind, multicentre, phase 3 study. Lancet Oncol 2015;16(5):499–508.

40. Allegra CJ, Rumble RB, Hamilton SR, et al. Extended RAS gene mutation testing in metastatic colorectal carcinoma to predict response to anti-epidermal growth factor receptor monoclonal antibody therapy: American Society of Clinical Oncology Provisional Clinical Opinion Update 2015. J Clin Oncol 2016;34(2): 179–85.

41. Jonker DJ, O'Callaghan CJ, Karapetis CS, et al. Cetuximab for the treatment of colorectal cancer. N Engl J Med 2007;357(20):2040–8.

42. Karapetis CS, Khambata-Ford S, Jonker DJ, et al. K-ras mutations and benefit from cetuximab in advanced colorectal cancer. N Engl J Med 2008;359(17): 1757–65.

43. Au HJ, Karapetis CS, O'Callaghan CJ, et al. Health-related quality of life in patients with advanced colorectal cancer treated with cetuximab: overall and KRAS-specific results of the NCIC CTG and AGITG CO.17 Trial. J Clin Oncol 2009;27(11):1822–8.

44. Sobrero AF, Maurel J, Fehrenbacher L, et al. EPIC: phase III trial of cetuximab plus irinotecan after fluoropyrimidine and oxaliplatin failure in patients with metastatic colorectal cancer. J Clin Oncol 2008;26(14):2311–9.

45. Cunningham D, Humblet Y, Siena S, et al. Cetuximab monotherapy and cetuximab plus irinotecan in irinotecan-refractory metastatic colorectal cancer. N Engl J Med 2004;351(4):337–45.

46. Van Cutsem E, Kohne CH, Hitre E, et al. Cetuximab and chemotherapy as initial treatment for metastatic colorectal cancer. N Engl J Med 2009;360(14):1408–17.

47. Van Cutsem E, Kohne CH, Lang I, et al. Cetuximab plus irinotecan, fluorouracil, and leucovorin as first-line treatment for metastatic colorectal cancer: updated analysis of overall survival according to tumor KRAS and BRAF mutation status. J Clin Oncol 2011;29(15):2011–9.

48. Bokemeyer C, Bondarenko I, Makhson A, et al. Fluorouracil, leucovorin, and oxaliplatin with and without cetuximab in the first-line treatment of metastatic colorectal cancer. J Clin Oncol 2009;27(5):663–71.

49. Bokemeyer C, Bondarenko I, Hartmann JT, et al. Efficacy according to biomarker status of cetuximab plus FOLFOX-4 as first-line treatment for metastatic colorectal cancer: the OPUS study. Ann Oncol 2011;22(7):1535–46.

50. Ye LC, Liu TS, Ren L, et al. Randomized controlled trial of cetuximab plus chemotherapy for patients with KRAS wild-type unresectable colorectal liver-limited metastases. J Clin Oncol 2013;31(16):1931–8.

51. Maughan TS, Adams RA, Smith CG, et al. Addition of cetuximab to oxaliplatin-based first-line combination chemotherapy for treatment of advanced colorectal cancer: results of the randomised phase 3 MRC COIN trial. Lancet 2011; 377(9783):2103–14.

52. Primrose J, Falk S, Finch-Jones M, et al. Systemic chemotherapy with or without cetuximab in patients with resectable colorectal liver metastasis: the New EPOC randomised controlled trial. Lancet Oncol 2014;15(6):601–11.

53. Heinemann V, von Weikersthal LF, Decker T, et al. FOLFIRI plus cetuximab versus FOLFIRI plus bevacizumab as first-line treatment for patients with metastatic colorectal cancer (FIRE-3): a randomised, open-label, phase 3 trial. Lancet Oncol 2014;15(10):1065–75.

54. O'Neil BH, Venook AP. Trying to understand differing results of FIRE-3 and 80405: does the first treatment matter more than others? J Clin Oncol 2015;33(32): 3686–8.

55. Venook AP, Niedzwiecki D, Lenz HJ, et al. CALGB/SWOG 80405: phase III trial of irinotecan/5-FU/leucovorin (FOLFIRI) or oxaliplatin/5-FU/leucovorin (mFOLFOX6) with bevacizumab (BV) or cetuximab (CET) for patients (pts) with KRAS wild-type (wt) untreated metastatic adenocarcinoma of the colon or rectum (MCRC). J Clin Oncol 2014;32(18).

56. Tol J, Koopman M, Cats A, et al. Chemotherapy, bevacizumab, and cetuximab in metastatic colorectal cancer. N Engl J Med 2009;360(6):563–72.

57. Van Cutsem E, Peeters M, Siena S, et al. Open-label phase III trial of panitumumab plus best supportive care compared with best supportive care alone in

patients with chemotherapy-refractory metastatic colorectal cancer. J Clin Oncol 2007;25(13):1658–64.

58. Van Cutsem E, Siena S, Humblet Y, et al. An open-label, single-arm study assessing safety and efficacy of panitumumab in patients with metastatic colorectal cancer refractory to standard chemotherapy. Ann Oncol 2008;19(1):92–8.

59. Amado RG, Wolf M, Peeters M, et al. Wild-type KRAS is required for panitumumab efficacy in patients with metastatic colorectal cancer. J Clin Oncol 2008; 26(10):1626–34.

60. Douillard JY, Siena S, Cassidy J, et al. Randomized, phase III trial of panitumumab with infusional fluorouracil, leucovorin, and oxaliplatin (FOLFOX4) versus FOLFOX4 alone as first-line treatment in patients with previously untreated metastatic colorectal cancer: the PRIME study. J Clin Oncol 2010;28(31):4697–705.

61. Douillard JY, Siena S, Cassidy J, et al. Final results from PRIME: randomized phase III study of panitumumab with FOLFOX4 for first-line treatment of metastatic colorectal cancer. Ann Oncol 2014;25(7):1346–55.

62. Grothey A, Van Cutsem E, Sobrero A, et al. Regorafenib monotherapy for previously treated metastatic colorectal cancer (CORRECT): an international, multicentre, randomised, placebo-controlled, phase 3 trial. Lancet 2013;381(9863): 303–12.

63. Li J, Qin S, Xu R, et al. Regorafenib plus best supportive care versus placebo plus best supportive care in Asian patients with previously treated metastatic colorectal cancer (CONCUR): a randomised, double-blind, placebo-controlled, phase 3 trial. Lancet Oncol 2015;16(6):619–29.

64. Mayer RJ, Van Cutsem E, Falcone A, et al. Randomized trial of TAS-102 for refractory metastatic colorectal cancer. N Engl J Med 2015;372(20):1909–19.

65. Le DT, Uram JN, Wang H, et al. PD-1 blockade in tumors with mismatch-repair deficiency. N Engl J Med 2015;372(26):2509–20.

66. Morris EJ, Forman D, Thomas JD, et al. Surgical management and outcomes of colorectal cancer liver metastases. Br J Surg 2010;97(7):1110–8.

67. Poston GJ, Adam R, Alberts S, et al. OncoSurge: a strategy for improving resectability with curative intent in metastatic colorectal cancer. J Clin Oncol 2005; 23(28):7125–34.

68. Nordlinger B, Sorbye H, Glimelius B, et al. Perioperative FOLFOX4 chemotherapy and surgery versus surgery alone for resectable liver metastases from colorectal cancer (EORTC 40983): long-term results of a randomised, controlled, phase 3 trial. Lancet Oncol 2013;14(12):1208–15.

69. Ducreux M, Malka D, Mendiboure J, et al. Sequential versus combination chemotherapy for the treatment of advanced colorectal cancer (FFCD 2000-05): an open-label, randomised, phase 3 trial. Lancet Oncol 2011;12(11):1032–44.

Randomized Clinical Trials in Colon and Rectal Cancer

Atif Iqbal, MD[a], Thomas J. George, MD[b],*

KEYWORDS

- Colon cancer • Rectal cancer • Colorectal cancer • Surgery • Radiation
- Chemotherapy • Adjuvant • Neoadjuvant

KEY POINTS

- Surgery remains the mainstay of curative treatment for both colon and rectal cancers.
- Colon cancer outcomes have improved with the use of laparoscopic techniques, enhanced recovery pathways, and adjuvant chemotherapy.
- Multimodality management of rectal cancer continues to evolve with total mesorectal excision being the cornerstone.
- Oncologic results from recent studies do not support the use of laparoscopic resection in patients with rectal cancer.
- Preoperative radiation for stage II or III rectal cancer has less toxicity than postoperative treatment. Long course chemoradiation offers greater tumor downstaging and improved local control.

COLON CANCER
Surgical Approach and Techniques

The feasibility of laparoscopic surgery was highlighted by more than 24 randomized, controlled trials (RCTs) including 5 level I RCTs in the previous review with mostly consistent results.[1] Only the UK CLASICC trial (Conventional Versus Laparoscopic-assisted Surgery in Patients with Colorectal Cancer), which included patients with rectal cancer, noted an insignificantly increased rate of positive circumferential margins in the laparoscopic cohort without an increase in long-term tumor recurrence.[2] Since the last review, 14 additional RCTs and metaanalyses on laparoscopic surgery for colon cancer have confirmed the short-term benefits and oncologic noninferiority to the open approach. This includes a metaanalysis (including 23 RCTs and 20

Disclosure Statement: Dr A. Iqbal has nothing to disclose. Dr T. George is a consultant for Bayer and Merck.
^a Department of Surgery, University of Florida, 1600 Southwest Archer Road, PO Box 100106, Gainesville, FL 32610-0019, USA; ^b Department of Medicine, University of Florida, 1600 Southwest Archer Road, PO Box 100278, Gainesville, FL 32610-0278, USA
* Corresponding author.
E-mail address: Thom.George@medicine.ufl.edu

systematic reviews for RCTs)[3] and the Australasian Laparoscopic Colon Cancer Study Trial.[4] In total, laparoscopic surgery compared with open surgery had been shown to be technically feasible with multiple short-term benefits (less blood loss, less narcotics use, earlier return of bowel function, and decreased duration of hospital stay), similar or noninferior oncologic outcomes (lymph node retrieval, margins, overall survival [OS], disease-free survival [DFS]), and lower rates of incisional hernia and adhesive small bowel obstruction. As such, laparoscopic colectomy for colon cancer should currently be considered an acceptable alternative to an open resection in the hands of experienced surgeons. Only 1 RCT has investigated a robotic approach compared with laparoscopic colectomy for right-sided tumors with the robotic approach providing few benefits (similar pain, hospital stay, complication rates, and pathologic outcomes) to justify the greater cost and longer duration.[5] Thus, the robotic approach does not currently have RCT data to justify use over laparoscopic surgery.

Historical RCTs[1] have demonstrated no oncologic benefit with the no-touch technique, high ligation of the inferior mesenteric artery and an increased radiologically detected leak rate with hand-sewn compared with stapled anastomosis.[1] Since the last review, an RCT compared iso-versus antiperistaltic stapled side-to-side anastomosis (SSSA) and showed no significant difference in outcomes, but was suspended after detecting increased morbidity in the isoperistaltic SSSA group (which had the only two anastomotic leaks).[6] An RCT demonstrated no difference in terms of infection rates between subcuticular and interrupted suture closure of clean-contaminated wounds after colon cancer resection.[7] Specimen extraction through the anus versus mini-laparotomy showed no significant difference in terms of operative time, blood loss or length of hospital stay with the exception of less postoperative pain and no infections in the former group.[8]

Endoscopic Stent for Colonic Obstruction

For the purposes of this review, we will focus on the role of colonic stents (SEMS) in avoiding surgery at the time of emergent bowel obstruction. The majority of literature on this subject is nonrandomized with very few RCTs and conflicting results. A systematic review of uncontrolled trials and case reports on SEMS revealed a clinical success rate of 72% when used as bridge to surgery and uncommon major complications.[9] These results were not supported by the first RCT on this topic (Stent-In 2 trial) which revealed stent-related perforations in 13%–23% of patients and a higher risk of cancer recurrence if a perforation occurred.[10] This raised long-term oncologic apprehension, but a metaanalysis of four RCT's and seven subsequent RCTs suggested similar cumulative mortality rates after stenting as a bridge to surgery versus surgery alone.[11] Interestingly, while overall stoma rates differed significantly in favor of SEMS, the permanent stoma rates were similar.

Based on the available RCT data, the use of SEMS is associated with a higher rate of a successful primary anastomosis, lower rate of short-term colostomy requirement and avoids the need for a second procedure for colostomy reversal. The length of stay for SEMS placement and elective surgery (within 1–2 weeks) is also shorter than that for emergency surgery. This makes SEMS an attractive option despite the higher than anticipated perforation rate, noting that OS is not negatively impacted.

Primary Tumor Resection in Setting of Metastatic Disease

Current guidelines limit primary tumor resection (PTR) in the presence of metastatic disease (mCRC) to symptomatic patients, which is supported by literature. However, the role of PTR in asymptomatic patients to avoid future symptoms or improve survival is controversial. No RCTs have currently addressed this topic but two trials are ongoing.[12,13] A retrospective analysis of two RCTs with a different aim[14,15] and 22 nonrandomized studies showed significantly better survival for the PTR group. However, these studies have inherent biases and are thus inconclusive. Improving survival despite decreasing incidence of PTR could be due to improved systemic therapy use. Until the ongoing RCTs conclude,[12,13] a nonoperative approach in the absence of symptoms is recommended in accordance with NCCN guidelines.

Perioperative Care/Enhanced Recovery After Surgery

These clinical pathways were developed to accelerate recovery after surgery and include perioperative interventions focusing on anesthesia, multimodal narcotic-sparing analgesia, reduction of surgical stress, goal-directed fluid therapy, prevention of nausea and ileus, thromboembolic prophylaxis, minimally invasive techniques, early nutrition and early mobilization. A total of 16 RCTs and two metaanalysis of RCTs have been published on this topic.[1,16,17] Results indicate earlier return of bowel function, shorter hospital stay, and decreased overall morbidity without an increase in readmission rates or surgical complications.[16,17] The randomized LAFA trial demonstrated sustained superiority of ERAS pathway for colon cancer patients undergoing laparoscopic surgery compared with open surgery.[18] Thus, implementation of ERAS pathways in colon cancer patients has led to shorter hospital stays (by 2–3 days) and decreased morbidity without an increase in the readmission rate and should be implemented nationwide.

Postoperative Surveillance Schedules

Prior to the last review, 5 RCTs compared surveillance strategies for early diagnosis of cancer recurrence[1] and failed to show a survival difference with intensive surveillance. Of the several large RCTs published since then, we chose three as level I evidence: FACS, CEAWatch and GILDA trials.[19–21] All of these failed to show an OS benefit with intensive regimens, despite earlier detection of recurrences that were treated with curative intent. Another RCT looking at this question is ongoing.[22] In summary, published RCTs do not demonstrate an OS advantage with intensive surveillance regimens despite DFS improvement.

Adjuvant Therapy

Prior to the last review, adjuvant chemotherapy (intravenous fluoropyrimidine {FP} monotherapy) for 6 months was associated with improved survival in patients with stage III and possibly high-risk stage II colon cancer patients. Subsequent studies tested the noninferiority of oral FP alternatives and benefit of FP-based polychemotherapy and confirmed that capecitabine is equivalent to infusional 5-fluorouracil (5-FU)[1] and that the addition of oxaliplatin to either infusional or oral FP therapy is superior to monotherapy with FP alone.[1,23,24] The role of adjuvant therapy for stage II disease remains controversial with no additional RCTs to address this issue since the last review.

Biologic-targeted therapies, cetuximab (cmab) and bevacizumab (bev) have been shown to improve outcomes when combined with chemotherapy in mCRC. However cmab added to adjuvant FOLFOX for resected stage III colon cancer failed to show a benefit, rather a trend toward harm was noted in the US NCI-based study.[25] Similarly, the addition of bev to polychemotherapy in another US NCI-based study showed no benefit.[26] Given early separation of survival curves in favor of bev, an RCT is currently testing the benefit of expanded duration anti-VEGF therapy (regorafenib) after completion of standard adjuvant therapy (NCT02664077). While 6 months of adjuvant therapy is currently the standard of care, an ongoing global study (IDEA Study) is assessing the noninferiority of 3 versus 6 months of postoperative adjuvant chemotherapy. Initial results failed to demonstrate statistical non-inferiority with continued analysis ongoing.[27]

RECTAL CANCER

Rectal cancer is managed in a multimodality fashion, with surgery continuing to be the cornerstone for cure. Total mesorectal excision (TME) continues to be the gold standard for surgical excision but has never been tested in an RCT. TME alone leads to lower rates of local recurrence (LR), now ranging from 3% to 7%, and increased DFS. However, distant recurrences remain problematic.

Surgical Approach and Techniques

The last review included several trials but the findings of the rectal cancer subset of patients in the UK-CLASICC trial who underwent TME and had a higher rate of positive circumferential margin (CRM) in the laparoscopic group is worth mentioning. However, this did not translate into significant long-term differences in rates of LR, 3-year DFS, or OS.[2] Since then, 10 RCTs have been published on this topic and four are being presented as level 1 evidence below.[27–30] Both the COREAN[30] and COLOR II trial[29] compared laparoscopic to open rectal cancer resections and showed no difference in the quality of the oncologic resection, complication rates and long-term survival outcomes. However, both trials had limitations such as nonobese population, involvement limited to 3 tertiary centers with experienced surgeons, and low complete mesorectal excision rate (73%) in the COREAN trial. Similarly, the COLOR II trial used neoadjuvant therapy in stage I patients, had low rate of pathologic complete response (pCR), high rate for CRM involvement for tumors located in the low rectum (22%) in the open group and a high permanent stoma rate (29%) in the laparoscopic group. Since the above two trials, two major well-done large RCTs have been published on this topic; ACOSOG-Z6051[28] and ALaCaRT trial[27] which are highlighted in **Table 1**. Both trials failed to show noninferiority of the laparoscopic approach compared with open surgery for pathologic outcomes. In all four trials, the laparoscopic group had significantly longer operative time, less blood loss, quicker return of bowel function and two trials demonstrated a shorter hospital stay. In summary, the available RCT data do not support the use of laparoscopic resection in patients with rectal cancer at this time. The ROLARR trial, the only large RCT, comparing robotic-assisted and laparoscopic surgery for curable rectal cancer is currently under way. At the time of the last unpublished report,[31] no significant differences were noted between groups.

A few additional RCTs have looked at various aspects of rectal cancer resection as below. The French GRECCAR III trial demonstrated higher infectious morbidity for rectal cancer surgery without mechanical bowel preparation (MBP).[32] The role of diverting loop ileostomies (DLI) with low anterior resection (LAR) has been studied in three large RCTs and a pooled analysis of RCT's.[33–35] All found a lower incidence of anastomotic leaks when DLI was performed.

Three RCTs have also explored surgical approaches to improve the quality of the distal resection in low rectal cancer. We review one of the two on sphincter saving procedures[36] and the only one on abdominoperineal resection (APR) patients below.[37] Transanal/perineal dissection of the distal LAR specimen resulted in a significant decrease in CRM positivity rate compared with laparoscopic dissection.[36] Extralevator (cylindrical) APR in prone position demonstrated a lower LR rate compared with conventional APR in a lithotomy position but also had a higher complication rate (larger defect with more pain).[37] Together, these trials highlight the need for a better surgical approach for the distal portion of the dissection. While we continue to investigate optimization of sphincter saving procedures, cylindrical APR is recommended to decrease the incidence of a positive CRM and associated morbidity.

Reconstructive Techniques

Eight RCTs (including some prior to the last review) have shown the functional superiority and decreased complication rate (leak and strictures) with colonic J-pouches (CJP) over straight anastomosis.[33,38] Three RCTs (two prior to the last review) compared CJPs to side-to-end anastomosis and found similar functional outcomes.[39–41] Comparison of 3-cm and 6-cm side limb sizes in a side-to-end anastomosis revealed no difference, but the study was underpowered.[42] Six RCTs (5 prior to last review) compared CJPs with transverse coloplasty pouches (TCPs) showing better functional outcomes with CJPs in two trials[33] but comparable outcomes in the other four trials.[33,43] This contradicts previous reports suggesting a higher leak rate with TCP. Data suggests that a straight end-to-end anastomosis has the poorest functional outcome. Due to lack of added functional benefit and ease of creation, a side-to-end anastomosis appears to be a good alternative to CJP.

Organ Preservation

The last review discussed two RCTs on this subject looking at cT1N0 and cT2N0 lesions separately.[33] Both compared transanal endoscopic microsurgery (TEM) to TME with no difference in rates of R0 resection, LR or DFS. However, both studies were underpowered with inadequate long-term follow-up considering the high rates of LR noted in multiple large retrospective data sets. Although, level 1 evidence to define the role of organ preservation is currently deficient, nonrandomized studies have shown organ preservation rates of greater than 75% with cT1-2N0 tumors and rates of 50% with cT3N0 tumors. Appropriate patient selection and follow up is critical. Of particular mention in this 'watch and wait' approach is Angelita Habr-Gama and her group in San Paulo who have published their largest and longest experience.[44] They deliver three cycles of chemotherapy after chemoradiotherapy (CRT) before reassessment at 10 weeks with a strict definition of clinical complete response (cCR). Patients with suspicious areas undergo full-thickness local excision. Only 10% to 20% of cases show a cCR (including T2-3,N0-1 lesions) with LR rates of 10% to 30% and the vast majority amenable to salvage resection. A current RCT (NCT02008656) is assessing the possibility of organ preservation in patients with cCR in the setting of total neoadjuvant therapy (TNT).

Neoadjuvant Radiotherapy

The last review highlighted eight trials showing a decrease in LR with radiotherapy (XRT) administered either preoperatively or postoperatively.[33] Of these, the Dutch trial[45] underscored the benefit of preoperative XRT even when optimal TME surgery was performed. One RCT showed an improvement in OS with preoperative XRT[46] but most studies have not replicated this finding. No RCT has added to this topic since the last review.

Prior to the last review, the CAO/ARO/AIO 94 trial randomized patients to pre- or postoperative long-course chemoradiation (LC-CRT). Results showed less toxicity and improved 5- and 10-year LR rate in the preoperative chemoradiation group with no difference in OS or DFS.[47] Another RCT compared preoperative short-course radiotherapy (SC-XRT) followed by surgery (within 7 days) to surgery with selective postoperative LC-CRT (for CRM positive patients).[48] Short- and long-term local

Table 1
Trials comparing laparoscopic and open surgery for rectal cancer patients

Trial	Inclusion Criteria/on	Primary Endpoint	Results				
			Successful Resection	Negative CRM	Clear Distal Margin	Complete or Near-Complete TME	Other
Kang et al,[30] 2010	Stage II-III tumors within 9 cm of verge/340 patients	3-y DFS rate	—	97.1% lap vs 95.9% open (P = .77)	100% lap vs 100% open (P = .54)	91.8% lap vs 88% open (P = .41)	• *3-y LR, DFS, OS:* Similar • *OR time:* 245 min lap vs 197 min open • *EBL:* 200 mL lap vs 217 mL open • *ROBF:* 38 h lap vs 60 h open • *Hospital stay:* 8 d lap vs 9 d open • *Conversion rate:* 1.5%
Van der Pas et al,[61] 2013	T1-T3 tumors within 15 cm of verge/1044 patients	3-y LR rate	—	90% lap vs 90% open (P = .85)	100% lap vs 100% open (P = .67)	97% lap vs 98% open (P = .25)	• *3-y LR, DFS, OS:* Similar • *OR time:* 240 min lap vs 188 min open • *EBL:* 200 mL lap vs 400 mL open • *ROBF:* 2 d lap vs 3 d open • *Hospital stay:* 8 d lap vs 9 d open • *Conversion rate:* 17%

Study	Population	Criteria					Conversion rate
Stevenson et al,[27] 2015	T1-T3 tumors within 15 cm of verge/475 patients	Meeting all the following criteria: Complete TME, CRM ≥1 mm and distal margin ≥1 mm	82% lap vs 89% open	93% lap vs 97% open (P = .06)	98% lap vs 98% open (P = .91)	97% lap vs 99% open (P = .06)	Conversion rate: 9%
Fleshman et al,[28] 2015	Stage II-III tumors within 12 cm of verge/248 patients	Composite of CRM >1 mm, negative distal margin and completeness of TME	81.7% lap vs 86.9% open	87.9% lap vs 92% open (P = .11)	99% lap vs 99% open (P = .67)	92% lap vs 95% open (P = .20)	Conversion rate: 11.3%

Abbreviations: CRM, circumferential margin; DFS, disease-free survival rate; EBL, estimated blood loss; lap, laparoscopic; LR, local recurrence rate; OR time, operative time; OS, overall survival rate; ROBF, return of bowel function; TME, total mesorectal excision.

control and DFS were significantly improved in the preoperative treatment group with similar OS. Neoadjuvant XRT leads to fewer LR, less toxicity and postoperative complications without an effect on survival.

Two trials have directly compared preoperative SC-XRT (surgery within 7 days) with LC-CRT (surgery in 4–6 weeks) and showed no difference in LR or long-term DFS or OS between treatment groups.[33,49] Subgroup analysis of the Trans-Tasman trial[49] revealed a significant benefit of treating low rectal cancer (<5 cm) with LC-CRT in terms of LR, which is consistent with the Dutch trial results. Another RCT revealed greater tumor downstaging with neoadjuvant LC-CRT compared with SC-XRT but with no difference in the R0 resection rates.[50] Thus, both SC-XRT and LC-CRT have similar rates of LR, DFS and OS with LC-CRT offering greater tumor downstaging. At present, SC-XRT has gained favor in Europe but not in the US, likely due to differences in practice patterns and reimbursement.

The optimal timing of surgery following neoadjuvant therapy has been evaluated in two RCTs. The Lyon trial (surgery within 6–8 weeks after neoadjuvant therapy completion) demonstrated increased clinical response and pCR rate compared with a 2 week delay.[51] However, this did not translate into improved rates of long-term LR, DFS or OS. The second trial increased the interval further by comparing surgery at either 7 or 11 weeks after LC-CRT.[52] The 11 week group had no increase in the pCR rate but had higher morbidity and more difficult surgical resection. A Polish trial compared early (7–10 days) versus delayed surgery (4–5 weeks) after SC-XRT and showed similar results with more downstaging in the delay group but no effect on rates of R0 resection, LR and OS.[53] These results are reinforced by the interim analysis of the ongoing Stockholm III trial. In total, RCTs support surgical resection more than 6 to 8 weeks after neoadjuvant XRT due to more downstaging and higher pCR rate, but a survival benefit is unproven. Moreover, the above studies use pCR as a primary endpoint, which is a poor surrogate for DFS and OS.

Chemotherapy as a Radiation Sensitizer

Previous RCTs have demonstrated that the combined modality of CRT leads to improved LR rates compared with XRT alone but does not impact OS, thus supporting the addition of FP chemotherapy (5-FU and LV) to XRT.[33,54] Several small studies have suggested a further improvement in pCR and downstaging with the addition of oxaliplatin to FP when given with neoadjuvant CRT. The NCI NSABP R-04 study formally evaluated the substitution of oral capecitabine (cape) for infusional 5-FU (CVI 5-FU) as well as intensification of radiosensitization by adding oxaliplatin.[55] Over 1500 patients were randomized into one of four neoadjuvant CRT arms. Local control, surgical downstaging and pCR rates were similar between the cape and CVI 5-FU arms. However, the addition of oxaliplatin failed to improve rates of DFS, OS, pCR, surgical downstaging or sphincter-sparing surgery. Five other RCTs confirmed that cape was an acceptable replacement for 5-FU and that adding oxaliplatin to CRT offered only toxicity. The incorporation of irinotecan, cetuximab, panitumumab and bevacizumab has been explored in small studies suggesting increased downstaging, but larger RCTs are awaited.

Chemotherapy for Systemic Disease Control

Five RTCs and a metaanalysis[56] have attempted to demonstrate a survival advantage with adjuvant chemotherapy but only one succeeded.[57] However, most studies had limitations of inconsistent clinical staging, underpowering and limited compliance with heterogenous chemotherapy regimens. A metaanalysis[56] confirmed nearly 1/3rd of patients in most RCTs did not receive intended adjuvant treatment. A 14%

increase in mortality was reported for each 4-week delay in starting adjuvant therapy, after a 4-week postoperative interval.[58] In part due to the limited data, current consensus guidelines continue to recommend 4 months of adjuvant FP-based chemotherapy either pre- or postoperatively, independent of those receiving neoadjuvant XRT. Early RCT data suggests that preoperative chemotherapy may be more effectively delivered, better tolerated without compromising surgical outcomes and possibly leads to additional downstaging for selective elimination of radiotherapy or surgery.[59,60] The NCI-NCTN PROSPECT study (NCT01515787) is an ongoing RCT testing if preoperative XRT can be excluded in some patients when objective tumor regression is seen with neoadjuvant chemotherapy alone.

   The RCTs that follow do not represent all trials that have contributed to our current knowledge of the optimal care for the patient with colon or rectal cancer. Rather, we have highlighted those trials that have helped define the standard of care in 2017. Only RCTs published in a peer-reviewed format are considered.

1. Bagshaw PF, Allardyce RA, Frampton CM, et al; Australasian Laparoscopic Colon Cancer Study Group. Long-term outcomes of the australasian randomized clinical trial comparing laparoscopic and conventional open surgical treatments for colon cancer: the Australasian Laparoscopic Colon Cancer Study trial. Ann Surg 2012;256(6):915–9. PMID: 23154392.

   This trial investigated whether the short-term benefits associated with laparoscopic-assisted colon resection (LCR) compared with open colon resection (OCR) could be achieved safely, without survival disadvantages. A total of 587 of 601 eligible patients with potentially curable colon cancer were randomized to receive LCR or OCR. Primary endpoints were 5-year OS, recurrence-free survival, and freedom from recurrence rates, compared using an intention-to-treat analysis. With 5-year confirmed follow-up data for survival and recurrence on 567 (96.6%), there were no significant differences between the LCR and OCR groups in 5-year follow-up of OS (77.7% vs 76.0%, $P = .64$), recurrence-free survival (72.7% vs 71.2%, $P = .70$), or freedom from recurrence (86.2% vs 85.6%, $P = .85$). With long-term follow-up, this study demonstrated that LCR was not inferior to OCR in direct measures of survival and disease recurrence.

2. Sloothaak DA, van den Berg MW, Dijkgraaf MG, et al; collaborative Dutch Stent-In study group. Oncological outcome of malignant colonic obstruction in the Dutch Stent-In 2 trial. Br J Surg 2014;101(13):1751–7. PMID: 25298250.

   This study randomized patients with malignant colonic obstruction to emergency surgery or stent placement as a bridge to elective surgery with an aim to compare the oncological outcomes. Of 98 patients included in the original Stent-In 2 trial, patients with benign (16) or incurable (23) disease were excluded from this analysis study, along with a patient who had withdrawn from the trial. Of the remaining 58 patients, 32 were randomized to emergency surgery (31 resection, 1 stoma only) and 26 to stenting. Unsuccessful stenting required emergency surgery in six patients owing to wire or stent perforation. Locoregional or distant disease recurrence developed in nine of 32 patients in the emergency surgery group and 13 of 26 in the stent group. DFS was worse in the subgroup with stent- or guidewire-related perforation. Five of six patients in this subgroup developed a recurrence, compared with nine of 32 in the emergency surgery group and eight of 20 who had unperforated stenting. The authors concluded that there is not enough evidence to strongly refute the approach.

3. Vlug MS, Wind J, Hollmann MW, et al; LAFA study group. Laparoscopy in combination with fast track multimodal management is the best perioperative strategy in patients undergoing colonic surgery: a randomized clinical trial (LAFA-study). Ann Surg 2011;254(6):868–75. PMID: 21597360.

This RCT investigated which perioperative treatment (fast track [FT] or standard care), is the optimal approach for patients undergoing segmental laparoscopic or open resection for colon cancer. Patients eligible for segmental colectomy were randomized to laparoscopic or open colectomy, and to FT or standard care, resulting in 4 treatment groups. Primary outcome was total postoperative hospital stay (THS). Secondary outcomes were postoperative hospital stay (PHS), morbidity, reoperation rate, readmission rate, in-hospital mortality, quality of life at 2 and 4 weeks, patient satisfaction and in-hospital costs. Median THS in the laparoscopic/FT group was 5 (interquar-tile range: 4–8) days; open/FT 7 (5–11) days; laparoscopic/standard 6 (4.5–9.5) days, and open/standard 7 (6–13) days (P<.001). Median PHS in the laparoscopic/FT group was 5 (4–7) days; open/FT 6 (4.5–10) days; laparoscopic/standard 6 (4–8.5) days and open/standard 7 (6–10.5) days (P<.001). Secondary outcomes did not differ significantly among the groups. Regression analysis showed that laparoscopy was the only independent predictive factor to reduce hospital stay and morbidity. Optimal perioperative treatment for patients requiring segmental colectomy for colon cancer is laparoscopic resection embedded in an FT program. If open surgery is performed, it is also preferentially done in FT care.

4. Verberne CJ, Zhan Z, van den Heuvel E, et al. Intensified follow-up in colorectal cancer patients using frequent Carcino-Embryonic Antigen (CEA) measurements and CEA-triggered imaging: Results of the randomized "CEAwatch" trial. Eur J Surg Oncol 2015;41(9):1188–96. PMID: 26184850.

This RCT aimed to determine the value of frequent Carcino-Embryonic Antigen (CEA) measurements and CEA-triggered imaging for detecting recurrent disease after definitive therapy for colon cancer. Participating sites were sequentially assigned an alternating change from their usual follow-up care to an intensified follow-up schedule of CEA measurements every 2 months with imaging in case of two CEA rises. The primary outcomes were the proportion of recurrences that could be treated with curative intent, recurrences with definitive curative treatment outcome, and the time to detection of recurrent disease. In the 3223 patients that were included; 243 recurrences were detected (7.5%). A higher proportion of recurrences were detected in the intervention protocol compared with the control protocol (OR = 1.80; 95%-CI: 1.33–2.50; P = .0004) as well as the proportion of recurrences that could be treated with curative intent (OR = 2.84; 95%-CI: 1.38–5.86; P = .0048) and were treated with curative treatment (OR = 3.12, 95%-CI: 1.25–6.02, P-value: 0.0145). The time to detection of recurrent disease was significantly shorter in the intensified follow-up protocol (HR = 1.45; 95%-CI: 1.08–1.95; P = .013). However, OS and DFS endpoints have not yet been reported.

5. Fleshman J, Branda M, Sargent DJ, et al. Effect of Laparoscopic-Assisted Resection versus Open Resection of Stage II or III Rectal Cancer on Pathologic Outcomes: The ACOSOG Z6051 Randomized Clinical Trial. JAMA 2015;314(13):1346–55. PMID: 26441179.

This RCT sought to determine whether laparoscopic (lap) resection is noninferior to open resection for patients with stage II or III rectal cancer as determined by gross pathologic and histologic evaluation of the resected proctectomy specimen. The trial was conducted by credentialed surgeons from 35 institutions in and comprised a total of 486 patients. The primary outcome assessing efficacy was a composite of CRM greater than 1 mm, distal margin without tumor, and completeness of TME. Surgical resections occurred in 240 patients randomized to lap and 222 with open resection. Successful resection occurred in 81.7% of lap cases (95% CI, 76.8%–86.6%) and 86.9% of open resection cases (95% CI, 82.5%–91.4%) and did not support noninferiority (difference, −5.3%; 1-sided 95% CI, −10.8% to ∞; P for noninferiority = .41). Conversion to open resection occurred in 11.3% of patients. Patients underwent LAR (76.7%) or APR (23.3%). Operative time was significantly longer for lap resections (mean, 266.2 vs 220.6 minutes; mean difference, 45.5 minutes; 95% CI, 27.7–63.4; $P < .001$) while length of stay (7.3 vs 7.0 days; mean difference, 0.3 days; 95% CI, −0.6–1.1), readmission within 30 days (3.3% vs 4.1%; difference, −0.7%; 95% CI, −4.2% to 2.7%), and severe complications (22.5% vs 22.1%; difference, 0.4%; 95% CI, −4.2% to 2.7%) did not significantly differ. The TME was complete (77%) and nearly complete (16.5%) in 93.5% of the cases. Negative CRM was observed in 90% of the overall group (87.9% laparoscopic resection and 92.3% open resection; $P = .11$) while distal margin result was negative in more than 98% of patients irrespective of type of surgery ($P = .91$). Thus, the use of lap resection compared with open resection failed to meet the criterion for noninferiority for pathologic outcomes and do not support the use of lap resection in these patients.

6. Han JG, Wang ZJ, Wei GH, et al. Randomized clinical trial of conventional versus cylindrical abdominoperineal resection for locally advanced lower rectal cancer. Am J Surg 2012;204(3):274–82. PMID: 22920402.

   This study sought to compare the outcomes of patients with rectal cancer undergoing conventional APR versus cylindrical APR (cyAPR). Between January 2008 and December 2010, sixty-seven patients with T3-T4 low rectal cancer were identified and randomized (conventional n = 32, cylindrical n = 35). Those who received cyAPR had less operative time for the perineal portion ($P<.001$), larger perineal defect ($P<.001$), less intraoperative blood loss ($P = .001$), larger total cross-sectional tissue area ($P<.001$), similar total operative time ($P = .096$), and more incidence of perineal pain ($P<.001$). The local recurrence of the cyAPR group was statistically improved ($P = .048$). The authors concluded that cyAPR in the prone jackknife position has the potential to reduce the risk of LR without increased complications when compared with conventional APR in the lithotomy position for the treatment of low rectal cancer.

7. Allegra CJ, Yothers G, O'Connell MJ, et al. Neoadjuvant 5-FU or Capecitabine Plus Radiation With or Without Oxaliplatin in Rectal Cancer Patients: A Phase III Randomized Clinical Trial. J Natl Cancer Inst 2015;107(11). PMID: 26374429

   NSABP R-04 was designed to determine whether the oral FP capecitabine (cape) could be substituted for continuous infusion (CIVI) 5-FU in the curative setting of stage II/III rectal cancer during neoadjuvant radiation therapy and whether the addition of oxaliplatin could further enhance the activity of fluoropyrimidine-sensitized radiation. This was a 2 × 2 trial design: CVI 5-FU or oral cape with or without oxaliplatin. The primary endpoint was local-regional tumor control. Among 1608 randomized patients there were no statistically significant differences between regimens using 5-FU versus cape in 3-year local-regional tumor event rates (11.2% vs 11.8%), 5-year DFS (66.4% vs 67.7%), or 5-year OS (79.9% vs 80.8%); or for oxaliplatin versus no oxaliplatin for the three endpoints of local-regional events, DFS, and OS (11.2% vs 12.1%, 69.2% vs 64.2%, and 81.3% vs 79.0%). The addition of oxaliplatin was associated with statistically significantly more overall and grade 3 to 4 diarrhea (P<.0001). Three-year rates of local-regional recurrence among patients who underwent R0 resection ranged from 3.1% to 5.1% depending on the study arm. This study established capecitabine as a standard of care in the pre-operative rectal setting while the addition of oxaliplatin failed to improve the local-regional failure rate, DFS, or OS for any patient risk group but did add toxicity.

8. Hong YS, Nam BH, Kim KP, et al. Oxaliplatin, fluorouracil, and leucovorin versus fluorouracil and leucovorin as adjuvant chemotherapy for locally advanced rectal cancer after preoperative chemoradiotherapy (ADORE): an open-label, multicentre, phase 2, randomised controlled trial. Lancet Oncol 2014;15(11):1245–53. PMID: 25201358.

This study aimed to determine the impact of adjuvant chemotherapy for patients with rectal cancer, especially when used after preoperative CRT. The RCT was designed to compare the efficacy and safety of adjuvant fluorouracil and leucovorin with that of FOLFOX in patients with locally advanced rectal cancer after preoperative CRT. Patients with postoperative pathologic stage II (ypT3-4N0) or III (ypTanyN1-2) rectal cancer after receiving neoadjuvant FP-based CRT and TME were randomized to receive 4 months of adjuvant chemotherapy with either fluorouracil and leucovorin or FOLFOX. The primary endpoint was 3-year DFS, analyzed by intention to treat. Three hundred twenty-one patients were randomly assigned to fluorouracil and leucovorin (n = 161) or FOLFOX (n = 160). Most all patients (141 [95%] of 149 patients in the fluorouracil plus leucovorin group and 141 [97%] of 146 in the FOLFOX group) completed all planned cycles of adjuvant treatment. Three-year DFS was 71·6% (95% CI 64·6–78·6) in the FOLFOX group and 62·9% (55·4–70·4) in the fluorouracil plus leucovorin group (hazard ratio 0·657, 95% CI 0·434–0·994; P = 0·047). Any grade neutropenia, thrombocytopenia, fatigue, nausea, and sensory neuropathy were significantly more common in the FOLFOX group; however, however, there were no significant differences in these grade 3 or 4 toxicities. In this patient population, the authors demonstrated that adjuvant FOLFOX improved DFS compared with fluorouracil plus leucovorin after preoperative CRT and TME.

REFERENCES

1. Neuman HB, Park J, Weiser MR. Randomized clinical trials in colon cancer. Surg Oncol Clin N Am 2010;19(1):183–204.

2. Jayne DG, Guillou PJ, Thorpe H, et al. Randomized trial of laparoscopic-assisted resection of colorectal carcinoma: 3-year results of the UK MRC CLASICC Trial Group. J Clin Oncol 2007;25:3061–8.

3. Martel G, Crawford A, Barkun JS, et al. Expert opinion on laparoscopic surgery for colorectal cancer parallels evidence from a cumulative meta-analysis of randomized controlled trials. PLoS One 2012;7(4):e35292.

4. Bagshaw PF, Allardyce RA, Frampton CM, et al. Long-term outcomes of the australasian randomized clinical trial comparing laparoscopic and conventional open surgical treatments for colon cancer: the Australasian Laparoscopic Colon Cancer Study trial. Ann Surg 2012;256(6):915–9.

5. Park JS, Choi GS, Park SY, et al. Randomized clinical trial of robot-assisted versus standard laparoscopic right colectomy. Br J Surg 2012;99(9):1219–26.

6. Matsuda A, Miyashita M, Matsumoto S, et al. Isoperistaltic versus antiperistaltic stapled side-to-side anastomosis for colon cancer surgery: a randomized controlled trial. J Surg Res 2015;196(1):107–12.

7. Tanaka A, Sadahiro S, Suzuki T, et al. Randomized controlled trial comparing subcuticular absorbable suture with conventional interrupted suture for wound closure at elective operation of colon cancer. Surgery 2014;155(3):486–92.

8. Leung AL, Cheung HY, Fok BK, et al. Prospective randomized trial of hybrid NOTES colectomy versus conventional laparoscopic colectomy for left-sided colonic tumors. World J Surg 2013;37(11):2678–82.

9. Sebastian S, Johnston S, Geoghegan T, et al. Pooled analysis of the efficacy and safety of self-expanding metal stenting in malignant colorectal obstruction. Am J Gastroenterol 2004;99(10):2051–7.

10. Sloothaak DA, van den Berg MW, Dijkgraaf MG, et al. Oncological outcome of malignant colonic obstruction in the Dutch Stent-In 2 trial. Br J Surg 2014; 101(13):1751–7.

11. Tan CJ, Dasari BV, Gardiner K. Systematic review and meta-analysis of randomized clinical trials of self-expanding metallic stents as a bridge to surgery versus emergency surgery for malignant left-sided large bowel obstruction. Br J Surg 2012;99:469–76.

12. Rahbari NN, Lordick F, Fink C, et al. Resection of the primary tumour versus no resection prior to systemic therapy in patients with colon cancer and synchronous unresectable metastases (UICC stage IV): SYNCHRONOUS—a randomised controlled multicentre trial (ISRCTN30964555). BMC Cancer 2012;12:142.

13. Lam-Boer J, Mol L, Verhoef C, et al. The CAIRO4 study: the role of surgery of the primary tumour with few or absent symptoms in patients with synchronous unresectable metastases of colorectal cancer: a randomized phase III study of the Dutch Colorectal Cancer Group (DCCG). BMC Cancer 2014;14:741.

14. Koopman M, Antonini NF, Douma J, et al. Sequential versus combination chemotherapy with capecitabine, irinotecan, and oxaliplatin in advanced colorectal cancer (CAIRO): a phase III randomised controlled trial. Lancet 2007;370(9582): 135–42.

15. Tol J, Koopman M, Rodenburg CJ, et al. A randomised phase III study on capecitabine, oxaliplatin and bevacizumab with or without cetuximab in first-line advanced colorectal cancer, the CAIRO2 study of the Dutch Colorectal Cancer Group (DCCG). An interim analysis of toxicity. Ann Oncol 2008;19(4):734–8.

16. Greco M, Capretti G, Beretta L, et al. Enhanced recovery program in colorectal surgery: a meta-analysis of randomized controlled trials. World J Surg 2014; 38(6):1531–41.

17. Spanjersberg WR, Reurings J, Keus F, et al. Fast track surgery versus conventional recovery strategies for colorectal surgery. Cochrane Database Syst Rev 2011;(2):CD007635.

18. Vlug MS, Wind J, Hollmann MW, et al. Laparoscopy in combination with fast track multimodal management is the best perioperative strategy in patients undergoing colonic surgery. Ann Surg 2011;254:868–75.

19. Rosati G, Ambrosini G, Barni S, et al. A randomized trial of intensive versus minimal surveillance of patients with resected Dukes B2-C colorectal carcinoma. Ann Oncol 2016;27(2):274–80.

20. Primrose JN, Perera R, Gray A, et al. Effect of 3 to 5 years of scheduled CEA and CT follow-up to detect recurrence of colorectal cancer: the FACS randomized clinical trial. JAMA 2014;311(3):263–70.

21. Verberne CJ, Zhan Z, van den Heuvel E, et al. Intensified follow-up in colorectal cancer patients using frequent Carcino-Embryonic Antigen (CEA) measurements and CEA-triggered imaging: results of the randomized "CEAwatch" trial. Eur J Surg Oncol 2015;41:1188–96.

22. Lepage C, Phelip JM, Cany L, et al. Effect of 5 years of imaging and CEA follow-up to detect recurrence of colorectal cancer: the FFCD PRODIGE 13 randomised phase III trial. Dig Liver Dis 2015;47:529–31.

23. Schmoll HJ, Tabernero J, Maroun J, et al. Capecitabine plus oxaliplatin compared with fluorouracil/folinic acid as adjuvant therapy for stage III Colon cancer: final results of the NO16968 randomized controlled phase III trial. J Clin Oncol 2015;33(32):3733–40.

24. Schmoll HJ, Twelves C, Sun W, et al. Effect of adjuvant capecitabine or fluoro-uracil, with or without oxaliplatin, on survival outcomes in stage III colon cancer and the effect of oxaliplatin on post-relapse survival: a pooled analysis of individual patient data from four randomised controlled trials. Lancet Oncol 2014;15(13):1481–92.

25. Alberts SR, Sargent DJ, Nair S, et al. Effect of oxaliplatin, fluorouracil, and leuco-vorin with or without cetuximab on survival among patients with resected stage III colon cancer: a randomized trial. JAMA 2012;307(13):1383–93.

26. Allegra CJ, Yothers G, O'Connell MJ, et al. Phase III trial assessing bevacizumab in stages II and III carcinoma of the colon: results of NSABP protocol C-08. J Clin Oncol 2011;29(1):11–6.

27. Stevenson AR, Solomon MJ, Lumley JW, et al. Effect of laparoscopic-assisted resection vs open resection on pathological outcomes in rectal cancer: the ALaCaRT randomized clinical trial. JAMA 2015;314(13):1356–63.

28. Fleshman J, Branda M, Sargent DJ, et al. Effect of laparoscopic-assisted resection vs open resection of stage II or III rectal cancer on pathologic outcomes: the ACOSOG Z6051 randomized clinical trial. JAMA 2015;314(13):1346–55.

29. Bonjer HJ, Deijen CL, Abis GA, et al. A randomized trial of laparoscopic versus open surgery for rectal cancer. N Engl J Med 2015;372(14):1324–32.

30. Kang SB, Park JW, Jeong SY, et al. Open versus laparoscopic surgery for mid or low rectal cancer after neoadjuvant chemoradiotherapy (COREAN trial): short-term outcomes of an open-label randomised controlled trial. Lancet Oncol 2010;11(7):637–45.

31. Pigazz A. An international, multicentre, prospective, randomised, controlled, un-blinded, parallel-group trial of robotic-assisted versus standard laparoscopic surgery for the curative treatment of rectal cancer. Oral presentation. Boston (MA), ASCRS May 30-June 3, 2015.

32. Bretagnol F, Panis Y, Rullier E, et al. Rectal cancer surgery with or without bowel preparation: the French GRECCAR III multicenter single-blinded randomized trial. Ann Surg 2010;252(5):863–8.

33. Park J, Neuman HB, Weiser MR, et al. Randomized clinical trials in rectal and anal cancers. Surg Oncol Clin N Am 2010;19(1):205–23.

34. Mrak K, Uranitsch S, Pedross F, et al. Diverting ileostomy versus no diversion after low anterior resection for rectal cancer: a prospective, randomized, multicenter trial. Surgery 2016;159(4):1129–39.

35. den Dulk M, Marijnen CA, Collette L, et al. Multicentre analysis of oncological and survival outcomes following anastomotic leakage after rectal cancer surgery. Br J Surg 2009;96(9):1066–75.

36. Denost Q, Adam JP, Rullier A, et al. Perineal transanal approach: a new standard for laparoscopic sphincter-saving resection in low rectal cancer, a randomized trial. Ann Surg 2014;260(6):993–9.

37. Han JG, Wang ZJ, Wei GH, et al. Randomized clinical trial of conventional versus cylindrical abdominoperineal resection for locally advanced lower rectal cancer. Am J Surg 2012;204(3):274–82.

38. Parray FQ, Farouqi U, Wani ML, et al. Colonic J pouch neo-rectum versus straight anastomosis for low rectal cancers. Indian J Cancer 2014;51(4):560–4.

39. Jiang JK, Yang SH, Lin JK. Transabdominal anastomosis after low anterior resection: a prospective, randomized, controlled trial comparing long-term results between side-to-end anastomosis and colonic J-pouch. Dis Colon Rectum 2005;48: 2100–8.

40. Machado M, Nygren J, Goldman S, et al. Similar outcome after colonic pouch and side-to-end anastomosis in low anterior resection for rectal cancer: a prospective randomized trial. Ann Surg 2003;238:214–20.

41. Doeksen A, Bakx R, Vincent A, et al. J-pouch vs side-to-end coloanal anastomosis after preoperative radiotherapy and total mesorectal excision for rectal cancer: a multicentre randomized trial. Colorectal Dis 2012;14(6):705–13.

42. Tsunoda A, Kamiyama G, Narita K, et al. Prospective randomized trial for determination of optimum size of side limb in low anterior resection with side-to-end anastomosis for rectal carcinoma. Dis Colon Rectum 2009;52(9):1572–7.

43. Biondo S, Frago R, Codina Cazador A, et al. Long-term functional results from a randomized clinical study of transverse coloplasty compared with colon J-pouch after low anterior resection for rectal cancer. Surgery 2013;153(3):383–92.

44. Habr-Gama A, Perez RO, Nadalin W, et al. Operative versus nonoperative treatment for stage 0 distal rectal cancer following chemoradiation therapy: long-term results. Ann Surg 2004;240(4):711–7.

45. van Gijn W, Marijnen CA, Nagtegaal ID, et al. Preoperative radiotherapy combined with total mesorectal excision for resectable rectal cancer: 12-year follow-up of the multicentre, randomised controlled TME trial. Lancet Oncol 2011;12(6):575–82.

46. Folkesson J, Birgisson H, Pahlman L, et al. Swedish Rectal Cancer Trial: longlasting benefits from radiotherapy on survival and local recurrence rate. J Clin Oncol 2005;23:5644–50.

47. Sauer R, Fietkau R, Wittekind C, et al. Adjuvant vs. neoadjuvant radiochemotherapy for locally advanced rectal cancer: the German trial CAO/ARO/AIO-94. Colorectal Dis 2003;5:406–15.

48. Sebag-Montefiore D, Stephens RJ, Steele R, et al. Preoperative radiotherapy versus selective postoperative chemoradiotherapy in patients with rectal cancer (MRC CR07 and NCIC-CTG C016): a multicentre, randomised trial. Lancet 2009; 373(9666):811–20.

49. Ngan SY, Burmeister B, Fisher RJ, et al. Randomized trial of short-course radiotherapy versus long-course chemoradiation comparing rates of local recurrence in patients with T3 rectal cancer: Trans-Tasman Radiation Oncology Group trial 01.04. J Clin Oncol 2012;30(31):3827–33.

50. Latkauskas T, Pauzas H, Gineikiene I, et al. Initial results of a randomized controlled trial comparing clinical and pathological downstaging of rectal cancer after preoperative short-course radiotherapy or long-term chemoradiotherapy, both with delayed surgery. Colorectal Dis 2012;14(3):294–8.

51. Francois Y, Nemoz CJ, Baulieux J, et al. Influence of the interval between preoperative radiation therapy and surgery on downstaging and on the rate of

sphincter-sparing surgery for rectal cancer: the Lyon R90-01 randomized trial. J Clin Oncol 1999;17(8):2396.

52. Lefevre JH, Mineur L, Kotti S, et al. Effect of Interval (7 or 11 weeks) Between Neoadjuvant Radiochemotherapy and Surgery on Complete Pathologic Response in Rectal Cancer: a Multicenter, Randomized, Controlled Trial (GREC-CAR-6). J Clin Oncol 2016;18:JCO676049.

53. Pach R, Kulig J, Richter P, et al. Randomized clinical trial on preoperative radiotherapy 25 Gy in rectal cancer–treatment results at 5-year follow-up. Langenbecks Arch Surg 2012;397(5):801–7.

54. Hofheinz RD, Wenz F, Post S, et al. Chemoradiotherapy with capecitabine versus fluorouracil for locally advanced rectal cancer: a randomised, multicentre, non-inferiority, phase 3 trial. Lancet Oncol 2012;13(6):579–88.

55. Allegra CJ, Yothers G, O'Connell MJ, et al. Neoadjuvant 5-FU or capecitabine plus radiation with or without oxaliplatin in rectal cancer patients: a phase III randomized clinical trial. J Natl Cancer Inst 2015;107(11):djv248.

56. Breugom AJ, Swets M, Bosset J-F, et al. Adjuvant chemotherapy after preoperative (chemo) radiotherapy and surgery for patients with rectal cancer: a systematic review and meta-analysis of individual patient data. Lancet Oncol 2015;16(2):200–7.

57. Hong YS, Nam BH, Kim KP, et al. Oxaliplatin, fluorouracil, and leucovorin versus fluorouracil and leucovorin as adjuvant chemotherapy for locally advanced rectal cancer after preoperative chemoradiotherapy (ADORE): an open-label, multicentre, phase 2, randomised controlled trial. Lancet Oncol 2014;15(11):1245–53.

58. Biagi JJ, Raphael MJ, Mackillop WJ, et al. Association between time to initiation of adjuvant chemotherapy and survival in colorectal cancer: a systematic review and meta-analysis. JAMA 2011;305(22):2335–42.

59. Fernández-Martos C, Pericay C, Aparicio J, et al. Phase II, randomized study of concomitant chemoradiotherapy followed by surgery and adjuvant capecitabine plus oxaliplatin (CAPOX) compared with induction CAPOX followed by concomitant chemoradiotherapy and surgery in magnetic resonance imaging–defined, locally advanced rectal cancer: grupo cáncer de recto 3 study. J Clin Oncol 2010;28(5):859–65.

60. Garcia-Aguilar J, Chow OS, Smith DD, et al. Effect of adding mFOLFOX6 after neoadjuvant chemoradiation in locally advanced rectal cancer: a multicentre, phase 2 trial. Lancet Oncol 2015;16(8):957–66.

61. Van der Pas MH, Haglind E, Cuesta MA. Laparoscopic versus open surgery for rectal cancer (COLOR II): short-term outcomes of a randomised, phase 3 trial. Lancet Oncol 2013;14(3):210–8.

Randomized Clinical Trials in Localized Anal Cancer

Clayton A. Smith, MD, PhD[a], Lisa A. Kachnic, MD[b],*

KEYWORDS

- Anal • Cancer • Radiotherapy • Chemotherapy • Chemoradiation • Randomized

KEY POINTS

- Combined chemotherapy and radiation therapy reduce rates of anal cancer recurrence, need for colostomy, and anal cancer specific survival over radiotherapy alone.
- 5-Fluoracil (5-FU) and mitomycin C (MMC) concurrent with radiation therapy provide superior disease-free and colostomy-free survival over single agent 5-FU and radiotherapy alone.
- Phase III trials of induction chemotherapy, radiation dose intensification, and maintenance chemotherapy have not been shown to improve outcomes over standard chemoradiation for anal cancer.
- Concurrent cisplatin in place of MMC may be a reasonable alternative in patients who are unable to tolerate MMC.
- Planned treatment gaps in radiotherapy may have a negative impact on disease control. Modern radiation techniques significantly reduce acute toxicity and the need for treatment breaks.

INTRODUCTION

Historically, squamous cell carcinoma of the anal canal was treated with surgical resection by abdominoperineal resection. This produced overall survival rates of approximately 50%, but resulted in a permanent colostomy and high rates of locoregional recurrence.[1,2] In an effort to reduce the rates of local recurrence after surgery, Nigro and colleagues[3] pioneered a neoadjuvant regimen combining radiation therapy (30 Gy in 15 fractions) and chemotherapy with 5-fluorouracil (5-FU; 25 mg/kg continuous infusion) and mitomycin C (MMC; 0.5 mg/kg bolus). In a report of 28 patients undergoing this regimen, 26 patients underwent either abdominoperineal resection or

Disclosure Statement: The authors have nothing to disclose.
[a] Division of Radiation Oncology, Mitchell Cancer Institute, University of South Alabama, 1660 Spring Hill Avenue, Mobile, AL 36604, USA; [b] Department of Radiation Oncology, Vanderbilt University Medical Center, 2220 Pierce Avenue, Preston Research Building B-1003, Nashville, TN 37232, USA
* Corresponding author.
E-mail address: Lisa.a.kachnic@vanderbilt.edu

Surg Oncol Clin N Am 26 (2017) 705–718
http://dx.doi.org/10.1016/j.soc.2017.05.009
1055-3207/17/© 2017 Elsevier Inc. All rights reserved.

local excision after chemoradiation.[4] Of the patients, 80% were found to have pathologic complete response. In a subsequent series of 38 patients treated with chemoradiation as definitive therapy, an 84% complete response rate was achieved.[5] After these promising results, randomized clinical trials of anal cancer treatment have sought to validate definitive chemoradiation as the primary treatment for anal cancer, to establish the optimal systemic agents, and to assess the potential benefit of adjuvant chemotherapy or increased radiation dose, with the overarching goal of providing maximal colostomy-free survival while reducing treatment-related morbidity (**Table 1**).

RADIATION VERSUS COMBINED MODALITY THERAPY
Anal Cancer Trial I

The United Kingdom Coordinating Committee on Cancer Research (UKCCCR) Anal Cancer Trial I (ACT I) was designed to compare radiation therapy alone with combined modality therapy with radiation and concurrent 5-FU and MMC.[6] There were 585 patients (51% clinical T3 disease, 20% positive nodes) accrued between 1987 to 1994 and randomized to (1) radiation therapy of 45 Gy in 20 to 25 fractions with anteroposterior-posteroanterior (AP-PA) opposed fields targeting the anus and perineum, lower pelvic nodes, and optionally inguinal nodes, or to (2) the same radiation therapy given concurrently with 5-FU 1000 mg/m^2/d continuous infusion on days 1 to 4 or 750 mg/m^2 on days 1 to 5 and MMC 12 mg/m^2 bolus on day 1 of radiation. During the final week of radiation therapy, 5-FU was given as a second cycle. Response to treatment was assessed by clinical examination 6 weeks after completion of radiation. Patients with less than 50% response were referred for surgical resection and patients with greater than 50% response received a boost to the primary site of 15 Gy in 6 fractions with external beam therapy or 25 Gy over 2.5 days by iridium-192 brachytherapy implant.

At the initial response assessment 6 weeks after completion of the primary radiation treatment, there were comparable rates of patients with greater than 50% response (92% in both arms). With a median follow-up of 42 months at first reporting, 3-year local failure was 61% in the radiation alone arm versus 39% in the combined modality arm ($P<.0001$), demonstrating significant improvement with the combination of radiation and chemotherapy. Three-year cancer-specific survival was also improved significantly by combined modality therapy (72% vs 61% in patients treated with radiation alone; $P = .02$); however, there was no difference in 3-year overall survival between groups (58% vs 65%; $P = .25$). Early morbidity, including hematologic, skin, gastrointestinal, and genitourinary toxicity, was significantly worse with the addition of chemotherapy (48%) versus radiation alone (39%; $P = .03$). Late morbidity did not differ between concurrent therapy and radiation alone (42% vs 38%; $P = .39$).

In the long-term update, with a median follow-up of 13 years, the 5-year locoregional failure rate was 57% for radiation alone versus 32% for chemoradiation ($P<.001$), with this difference maintained out to 10 years.[7] The 5-year cancer-specific survival was 58% for radiation alone versus 70% for concurrent therapy ($P = .004$). As in the initial report, there was no difference in overall survival between groups at 5 years (53% vs 58%; $P = .12$). One outcome not reported in the initial publication was the colostomy-free survival rate, which reflects both the disease-free rate as well as lack of significant late morbidity from treatment that may prompt colostomy in the absence of tumor recurrence. The 5-year colostomy-free survival was increased significantly in patients receiving concurrent therapy (47%) versus radiation alone (37%; $P = .004$). In addition, examination of late morbidity found no difference between arms in rates of ulcers and radionecrosis (23% chemoradiation vs 18%

Table 1
Summary of phase III randomized trials of anal carcinoma with most recent published outcomes

Trial	Number of Patients	Median Follow-up	Comparison Arms	Locoregional Control	Colostomy-Free Survival	Overall Survival
ACT I[7]	585	13 y	RT alone RT+5-FU/MMC	43% 68%[a] at 5 y	37% 47%[a] at 5 y	53% 58% at 5 y
EORTC 22861[8]	110	3.5 y	RT alone RT+5-FU/MMC	50% 68%[a] at 5 y	40% 72%[a] at 5 y	56% 56% at 5 y
RTOG 8704[9]	310	3 y	RT+5-FU RT+5-FU/MMC	66% 84%[a] at 4 y	59% 71%[a] at 4 y	67% 76% at 4 y
RTOG 9811[11]	682	NR (>2.5 y)	RT+5-FU/MMC Induction 5-FU/Cis → RT+5-FU/Cis	80% 74% at 5 y	72% 65% at 5 y	78%[a] 71% at 5 y
ACT II[12]	940	5 y	RT+5-FU/MMC RT+5-FU/Cis	NR	68% 67% at 5 y	79% 77% at 5 y
ACCORD-03[14]	307	4.2 y	Induction 5-FU/Cis → RT+5-FU/Cis RT+5-FU/Cis	80% 81% at 5 y	76% 75% at 5 y	74% 71% at 5 y

Abbreviations: 5-FU, 5-fluorouracil; Cis, cisplatin; MMC, mitomycin C; NR, not reported; RT, radiotherapy.
[a] $P<.05$.

radiation), anorectal morbidity (81% chemoradiation vs 76% radiation), or skin toxicity (59% chemoradiation vs 51% radiation). In summary, the results of the ACT I trial demonstrate that combined modality chemoradiotherapy results in decreased locoregional recurrence, improved colostomy-free survival, and improved anal cancer–specific survival. The lack of impact on overall survival is likely owing to patients having surgical salvage options.

European Organization for the Research and Treatment of Cancer 22861

The European Organization for the Research and Treatment of Cancer (EORTC) trial 22861 had a similar design to ACT I with randomization between (1) radiation therapy alone or (2) combined chemoradiation.[8] From 1987 to 1994, 110 patients were randomized. Inclusion criteria included T3 or T4 primary or any T stage with node-positive disease. Radiation therapy was given as 45 Gy in 25 fractions using a 3- or 4-field technique. After completion of this initial radiation course, patients were reassessed 6 weeks later. For patient with stable or progressive disease, surgery was advised. A differential radiation boost dose was administered to the remaining responders, with patients experiencing a complete response receiving 15 Gy and partial responders receiving 20 Gy. In the chemoradiation arm, chemotherapy consisted of 5-FU (750 mg/m^2/d) on weeks 1 and 5 of radiation and MMC (15 mg/m^2 bolus) on day 1.

Patients receiving chemoradiation had increased clinical complete response rates at the initial assessment (80% for chemoradiotherapy vs 54% for radiotherapy alone). Five-year locoregional control was improved significantly with the addition of chemotherapy to radiation (68% vs 50%; $P = .02$), as was 5-year colostomy-free survival (72% vs 40%; $P = .02$). Similar to the ACT I results, there was no difference between groups in overall survival, with a 5-year combined rate of 56%. The investigators also did not observe significant differences in late toxicity between arms, although there was a trend toward worse late anal ulceration in the chemoradiation treated group.

Taken together, the results of the EORTC 22861 and ACT I trials confirm the superiority of combined modality therapy (chemotherapy with 5-FU and MMC plus pelvic radiation) over radiation alone in the treatment of anal cancer. The clinical phase III trials that follow sought to determine whether alterations in the concurrent 5-FU and MMC chemotherapy regimen could provide similar and/or improved clinical outcomes while limiting the significant acute treatment morbidity.

ROLES OF MITOMYCIN-C, ADJUVANT CHEMOTHERAPY, AND RADIATION BOOST
Radiation Therapy Oncology Group 8704

The US Intergroup (Radiation Therapy Oncology Group [RTOG] 8704/Eastern Cooperative Oncology Group [ECOG] 1289) trial tested whether the addition of MMC to concurrent infusional 5-FU and radiation therapy was necessary to achieve optimal clinical outcomes, because the MMC component of therapy resulted in significant hematologic toxicity.[9] Between 1988 and 1991, 310 patients were randomized to (1) standard chemoradiation with 5-FU and MMC or (2) chemoradiation with 5-FU alone. Any tumor (T) or nodal (N) stage was allowed to enroll, with 85% of patients having T2 to T4 disease and 17% clinically node positive. Radiation was delivered as 45 Gy in 25 fractions with shrinking AP-PA fields after 30.6 Gy; a subsequent radiation boost of 5.4 Gy was permitted to residual primary tumor or involved nodes. Four to 6 weeks later, biopsy of the primary site was performed. If residual disease was observed, an additional 9 Gy was administered to the primary or to palpable inguinal adenopathy along with 5-FU and cisplatin. Initial chemotherapy was given as continuous infusion 5-FU 1000 mg/m^2/d on days 1 to 4 and 29 to 32 of radiation. In arm 2, 5-FU administration was identical with MMC administered as a 10 mg/m^2 bolus on days 1 and 29 of radiation. As mentioned, for patients requiring additional salvage chemoradiation treatment after the 4- to 6-week assessment, chemotherapy consisted of 5-FU and cisplatin 100 mg/m^2 on day 2 of additional radiation, or alternatively MMC, if decreased kidney function was noted.

For both arms, more than 94% of patients received their planned chemotherapy courses. Postinduction biopsy of the primary site was negative in 92% of patients receiving 5-FU and MMC, and in 86% receiving 5-FU alone (P = .135). Initial tumor size also impacted postinduction responses with tumors less than 5 cm having 93% negative biopsies and tumors 5 cm or greater having 83% negative biopsies (P = .02). The 4-year colostomy rates were significantly higher with 5-FU alone (22%) versus 5-FU and MMC (9%; P = .002), and the 4-year colostomy-free survival was inferior (59% vs 71% with MMC; P = .014). Disease-free survival at 4 years was also significantly worse with the omission of MMC (51% vs 73%; P = .0003). There was no difference in overall survival rates between arms. Although the addition of MMC produced better clinical outcomes in terms of reduced disease recurrence and colostomy, this was at the expense of greater acute side effects. Grade 4 acute toxicity was significantly worse with the addition of MMC (23% vs 7%), as was grade 5 toxicity from sepsis (2.7% vs 0.7%). The results of RTOG 8704 indicate that the addition of 5-FU alone to radiation therapy is inferior to combination chemotherapy with 5-FU and MMC for the combined modality treatment of anal cancer. Subsequent phase III studies investigated whether replacing MMC with cisplatin with or without the addition of induction or maintenance chemotherapy would maintain or perhaps improve the effectiveness produced by standard 5-FU and MMC while reducing acute toxicity.

Radiation Therapy Oncology Group 9811

The RTOG initiated a large phase III trial (RTOG 9811) to assess the benefit of induction chemotherapy and the replacement of MMC by cisplatin. In this study, patients were randomized to (1) standard 5-FU and MMC concurrent with radiation or (2) an experimental arm of induction 5-FU and cisplatin followed by chemoradiation with 5-FU and cisplatin.[10] From 1998 to 2005, 682 patients were enrolled among the 2 arms. Inclusion criteria included T2 to T4 primaries and any nodal status, with 35% having T3 to T4 primary disease and 26% being node positive. The control arm was treated much as the 5-FU and MMC arm from RTOG 8704 with 5-FU 1000 mg/m^2/d continuous infusion on days 1 to 4 and 29 to 32 and bolus MMC 10 mg/m^2 on days 1 and 29. In the experimental arm, patients received the initial 2 cycles of chemotherapy alone and the final 2 cycles concurrent with radiation. Induction chemotherapy was continuous infusion 5-FU 1000 mg/m^2/d on days 1 to 4, 29 to 32, 57 to 60, and 85 to 88 with bolus cisplatin 75 mg/m^2 on days 1, 29, 57, and 85. For both arms, radiation was administered as 45 Gy in 25 fractions with AP-PA or multiple field techniques. The initial fields encompassed the pelvis, anus, perineum, and inguinal nodes with the superior border at L5 to S1 and inferiorly 2.5 cm below the anus and tumor. After 30.6 Gy, the superior border was reduced to the bottom of the sacroiliac joints and the pelvis was boosted to 45 Gy. For patients with T3 or T4 primaries, positive inguinal nodes, or T2 with residual disease, after 45 Gy, an additional radiation boost of 10 to 14 Gy at 2 Gy per fraction was delivered to the primary site and involved nodes. Unlike the prior randomized trials discussed, there was no planned radiation break between the initial pelvis treatment and tumor boost.

With a median follow-up of 2.5 years, there was no difference between groups in disease-free survival with a 3-year disease-free survival of 67% for the standard MMC arm versus 61% for cisplatin (P = .17). The 3-year overall survival was also not significantly different (84% MMC vs 76% cisplatin; $P = .10$). In contrast, 3-year colostomy rates were significantly worse with cisplatin (10% vs 16%; $P = .02$). There was no difference in acute grade 3 to 4 nonhematologic side effects between the arms (74% for both arms), but acute grade 3 to 4 hematologic toxicity was significantly worse in the MMC arm (61% vs 42%; $P<.001$). Severe late effects were similar between groups (11% vs 10%).

In the long-term update, cisplatin was found to fare worse as a replacement for MMC, with 5-year disease-free survival (68% vs 58%; $P = .006$), overall survival (78% vs 71%; $P = .026$), and colostomy-free survival (72% vs 65%; $P = .05$) all reduced in the cisplatin arm.[11] Differences in locoregional failure (20% vs 26%; $P = .087$) and colostomy rates (12% vs 17%; $P = .074$) did not attain statistical significance. Additionally, the late grade 3 and 4 side effect rates were comparable over time (13% MMC vs 11% cisplatin; $P = .35$). One potential explanation for the outcome differences between the 2 arms is the decreased efficacy of cisplatin in this setting relative to MMC. Another interpretation is based on the inclusion of induction chemotherapy in the experimental arm, which may have delayed definitive treatment with chemoradiation. Because of these results, chemoradiation with concurrent 5-FU and MMC remains the standard of care in the United States.

Anal Cancer Trial II

The UKCCCR ACT II trial evaluated a more direct comparison of the role of cisplatin in place of MMC with pelvic radiation, as well as assessing whether maintenance chemotherapy would improve outcomes beyond chemoradiation alone.[12] Between 2001 and 2008, 940 patients were accrued. T3 and T4 primaries made up 46% of patients and 32% had involved nodes. Patients were randomized in a 2×2 design to 1 of 4 arms: (1) 5-FU and cisplatin with radiation and no maintenance, (2) 5-FU and cisplatin with radiation followed by maintenance 5-FU and cisplatin, (3) 5-FU and MMC with radiation and no maintenance, or (4) 5-FU and MMC with radiation followed by maintenance 5-FU and cisplatin. Concurrent chemotherapy was administered as 5-FU 1000 mg/m^2/d continuous infusion on days 1 to 4 and 29 to 32 with either bolus cisplatin 60 mg/m^2 on days 1 and 29 or MMC 12 mg/m^2 on day 1. Maintenance chemotherapy was given as an additional 2 cycles of 5-FU on days 71 to 74 and 92 to 95 and cisplatin on days 71 and 92. Radiotherapy was prescribed to 50.4 Gy total in 28 fractions using AP-PA fields, with a field reduction at 30.6 Gy. Treatment response was assessed at 3 time points from the start of treatment: 11, 18, and 26 weeks. The final assessment at 26 weeks included digital anorectal examination and computed tomography imaging; routine biopsy was not recommended.

Of the patients assigned to receive maintenance chemotherapy, 80% began treatment, although only 44% completed maintenance without dose reduction or delay. When comparing MMC versus cisplatin, there was no difference in clinical complete response rates by primary site (89.6% vs 90.5%; $P = .64$) at 26 weeks. With a median follow-up of 5 years, there was no difference between groups in progression-free survival by maintenance (74%) versus no maintenance (73%; $P = .7$). There was also no difference in overall survival or colostomy-free survival, regardless of maintenance regimen or concurrent chemotherapy used. Additionally, there was no difference in acute grade 3 or 4 overall side effects between MMC and cisplatin (71% vs 72%), although there were more hematologic events in the MMC arms (26% vs 16%; $P<.001$).

A post hoc analysis examining the timing of clinical assessment after treatment was recently reported.[13] Although the initial publication defined complete clinical response as response at the primary site only, the updated analysis revised this assessment now using both primary and nodal response. Based on this, at the initial 11-week assessment, 64% of patients were found to have a clinical complete response. By the 26-week (final) assessment, 85% demonstrated clinical complete response. Of the patients who did not experience complete responses at the time of initial assessment, 72% went on to achieve a complete response. The authors examined overall survival based on the presence or absence of complete response by assessment time. At the first assessment, patients with complete response had a 5-year overall survival of 85% versus 75% in those without complete response ($P = .38$). By the final assessment at week 26, patients with complete response had a 5-year overall survival of 87% versus 48% in those patients without response ($P<.0001$). This study confirms that delayed assessment of tumor response after treatment allows for further tumor regression and provides better prognostic value over the response observed at earlier time points.

Although the ACT II trial did not observe the same detriments in disease control and colostomy-free survival that were noted with the replacement of MMC by cisplatin in RTOG 9811, there was also not a significant benefit to this regimen. Furthermore, maintenance chemotherapy does not seem to provide a benefit in improving clinical responses or reducing recurrence rates. Based on the results of the ACT II trial, 5-FU and MMC remain the standard treatment regimen for definitive chemoradiation in localized anal cancer. However, cisplatin-based chemotherapy can be considered as an alternative regimen in patients who may not tolerate the hematologic toxicity associated with MMC.

Action Clinique Coordonnées en Cancérologie Digestive-03

The French Action Clinique Coordonnées en Cancérologie Digestive (ACCORD-03) trial was designed to test the benefits of both induction chemotherapy and a radiotherapy boost.[14] Unlike prior randomized trials, MMC was not included in the chemotherapy regimen. Between 1999 and 2005, 307 patients were randomized in a 2×2 design. Inclusion criteria encompassed patients with primary tumors greater than 4 cm or with involved nodes. The 4 arms were (1) induction 5-FU and cisplatin followed by concurrent 5-FU and cisplatin with radiation to 45 Gy plus a standard 15 Gy primary tumor boost, (2) same as arm 1 with the addition of a 20- to 25-Gy high-dose radiation boost, (3) chemoradiation without induction delivered with a standard radiation boost, and (4) chemoradiation with a high-dose radiation boost. Induction chemotherapy consisted of 5-FU 800 $mg/m^2/d$ continuous infusion on days 1 to 4 and 29 to 32 with bolus cisplatin 80 mg/m^2 on days 1 and 29. The same chemotherapy and dosages were administered concurrently with radiation. Radiation was delivered with an AP/PA or 4-field conformal technique treating superiorly to L5 to S1 and inferiorly the perianal region with a 3 cm normal tissue margin below the tumor. The initial radiation treatment was prescribed as 45 Gy in 25 fractions. The radiation boost began 3 weeks after completion of whole pelvis radiation and was delivered with either external beam or iridium-192 brachytherapy. Standard radiation boost arms received 15 Gy, whereas in the high-dose boost arms, patients received radiation dose based on response (25 Gy for a <80% response; 20 Gy for a >80% response).

In the arms receiving induction chemotherapy, 79% to 82% of patients received the planned course of concurrent chemotherapy with radiation, and in the noninduction arms, 94% to 98% of patients received the planned concurrent chemotherapy. After a median follow-up of 50 months, induction chemotherapy did not significantly improve 5-year colostomy-free survival (76.5% induction vs 75% no induction; $P = .37$). Likewise, a high-dose radiotherapy boost was not found to significantly improve 5-year colostomy-free survival, although this value did approach significance (74% standard boost vs 78% high dose boost; $P = .067$). It should also be noted that a

3-week treatment break was given before the start of the radiotherapy boost, which may have impaired the efficacy of the high dose radiation treatment. There were no differences in 5-year overall survival between groups regardless of induction or high-dose boost. Collectively, these results indicate that neither induction chemotherapy nor radiotherapy dose escalation (at least in the setting of a planned radiation treatment gap) improves outcomes over standard chemoradiation alone.

EFFECT OF A TREATMENT GAP

Many of these early randomized trials in anal cancer were designed with a built-in radiation gap after the initial pelvis treatment to allow patients to recover from acute toxicity and provide time to assess response before a radiotherapy boost. The ACT I investigators examined the effect of this treatment break and prolongation of total treatment time on outcomes in patients receiving a radiation boost.[15] They observed that patients who underwent a boost had lower rates of death from anal cancer ($P = .04$), but no reduction in rates of locoregional failure ($P = .66$). The delayed radiation boost did result in greater rates of late radionecrosis (8% boost vs 0% no boost; $P = .03$). These findings questioned the benefit of delivering a radiation boost after a 6-week treatment gap.

This issue was further addressed by a nonrandomized phase II trial from the Eastern Cooperative Oncology Group (ECOG 4292), which assessed high-dose radiotherapy to 59.4 Gy with concurrent 5-FU and cisplatin.[16] The first cohort of 19 patients received 36 Gy followed by a planned 2-week treatment break before completing the remainder of the treatment. A second cohort of 13 patients received the total 59.4 Gy and chemotherapy without a planned break. The planned radiation gap proved to be deleterious, with superior outcomes observed in patients not receiving a break: complete response rates (92% vs 68%), 5-year progression-free survival (85% vs 53%), and 5-year overall survival (84% vs 58%).

To further assess whether overall treatment time adversely affects outcomes, investigators from the RTOG performed an analysis from completed anal cancer trials and observed a significant association between overall treatment duration and colostomy failure, local failure, regional failure, and time-to-failure rates.[17] Given the totality of these results, combined with the superior outcomes in patients from the RTOG 9811 and ACT II trials that were not treated with a planned treatment gap, current trials of anal cancer no longer include a planned break as part of the design.

INTENSITY-MODULATED RADIOTHERAPY IN REDUCING THE ACUTE TOXICITY OF CHEMORADIATION

The difficulty that remains in administering standard chemoradiation with 5-FU and MMC is the significantly high rates of grade 3 and higher acute morbidity. Intensity-modulated radiotherapy (IMRT) is a form of advanced radiation delivery that uses fluctuating radiation beam intensities to target the radiation dose to the tumor while minimizing dose to the surrounding normal organs. One practical advantage is that the use of IMRT in anal cancer may reduce the chemoradiation acute side effect profile and prevent or reduce treatment breaks that may negatively affect outcomes. IMRT may also allow for further radiation dose escalation in high-risk localized disease. **Fig. 1** demonstrates the highly conformal radiation delivery associated with IMRT in a male patient with a large T3, N1a (right inguinal) anal canal squamous cell cancer with notable tumor extension outside of the anal verge.

Although not randomized, RTOG 0529 was a phase II trial investigating the use of IMRT in reducing the acute side effects of standard 5-FU and MMC chemoradiation

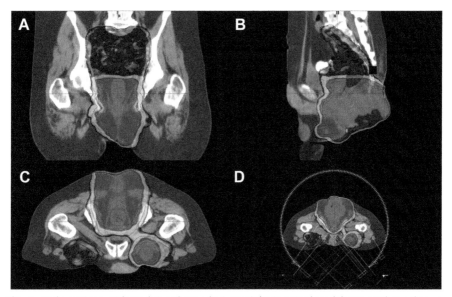

Fig. 1. Male patient with T3 (10 cm) N1a (3.3 cm right inguinal node) M0 anal canal squamous cell carcinoma with notable extension of the primary tumor outside of the anal verge. Patient positioned prone on a bowel displacement device. Representative coronal (*A*), sagittal (*B*), and axial (*C*) images are displayed. Primary tumor, anal canal, and right groin positive node all receive 5400 cGy (180 cGy × 30 fractions; *red color wash*) and elective nodal volume receives 4500 cGy (150 cGy × 30 fractions; blue color wash) with 6 MV photon beam and daily bolus on the external tumor extension. (*D*) This plan utilizes 280° arc therapy to cover the anterior nodal volume(s) and spare entrance dose to anterior organs at risk.

treatment.[18] In comparison with patients treated on the MMC arm of RTOG 9811, IMRT resulted in significantly lower grade 2 and higher hematologic (73% vs 85%; *P* = .032), grade 3 and higher gastrointestinal (21% vs 36%; *P* = .0082), and grade 3 and higher dermatologic (23% vs 49%; *P*<.0001) acute events. The median duration of radiotherapy was 42.5 days using IMRT (range, 32–59), as compared with 49 days (range, 0–102) on the MMC arm of RTOG 9811 (*P*<.0001). Therefore, with modern radiation treatment planning and delivery, the necessity of treatment breaks should become less of an issue, allowing for timely administration of combined modality therapy and the potential of radiation dose escalation.

PROGNOSTIC FACTORS FROM RANDOMIZED TRIALS

Prognostic factors beyond treatment regimen have been examined for several of these trials, either in the primary reports or with secondary analyses (**Table 2**). From the ACT I dataset, multivariable analysis confirmed male sex and palpable inguinal nodes as independent predictors of poor outcomes for locoregional failure, death from anal cancer, and overall survival.[19] Additionally, lower hemoglobin was associated with a higher risk of anal cancer death, whereas advancing age and white blood cell count were associated with poorer overall survival. The authors calculated a prognostic score using these variables and compared this with the ACT II dataset as independent validation. They observed that the prognostic score was a poor predictor of locoregional failure, but had moderate prognostic value for anal cancer death and overall survival in the external dataset. The difference in prognostic value between

Table 2
Patient prognostic factors and associated clinical outcomes from randomized trials

				Prognostic Factor			
Trial	Male	cN+	Size ≥5 cm	Skin Ulceration	Decreased Hemoglobin	Decreased WBC	Age
ACT I[19]	LRF ACD OS	LRF ACD OS			ACD	OS	OS
EORTC[8]		OS LC		OS LC			
RTOG 9811[11,21,23]	DFS OS	DFS OS	DFS OS Colostomy Rate				
ACT II[20]	CFS PFS	CFS PFS	CFS PFS			CFS PFS	

Abbreviations: ACD, anal cancer death; CFS, colostomy-free survival; cN+, clinically node positive; DFS, disease-free survival; LC, local control; LRF, locoregional failure; OS, overall survival; PFS, progression-free survival; WBC, white blood cells.

datasets was interpreted as differences in both the timing of the studies and treatment regimens, particularly with lack of a radiotherapy gap in ACT II.

Secondary analysis of the ACT II data examined predictors of colostomy-free survival.[20] The 5-year colostomy-free survival ranged from 65% to 70% and was not significantly different between treatment arms. For patients with T1 to T2 tumors, the 5-year rate was 79% versus 54% in T3 to T4 patients (P<.001). Similarly, patients with node-negative disease also had a better 5-year colostomy-free rate 72% versus 60% in node-positive patients. When examining patient factors that predicted for poor colostomy-free survival and progression-free survival on multivariable analysis, they determined that male sex (P = .004), lower hemoglobin (P<.001), and primary tumor greater than 5 cm (P<.001) independently influenced outcomes.

As part of their primary report, the EORTC 22861 trial investigators conducted a multivariable analysis to examine prognostic factors in the enrolled patient population.[8] It was observed that nodal involvement (P = .0035), skin ulceration (P = .0033) and absence of chemotherapy (P = .0144) were all significant predictors of local control, with male sex approaching significance (P = .0524). For overall survival, all factors were significant, except for the lack of chemotherapy.

Several secondary analyses of the RTOG 9811 data have also been reported.[21–23] For disease-free survival, poor prognostic factors include male sex (P = .02), clinically node-positive disease (P = .004), and tumor size greater than 5 cm (P = .01).[21] The same factors were determined to be poor predictors for overall survival. With the long-term results published in 2012, treatment with MMC, tumor size greater than 5 cm, and clinically node-positive disease were all predictors of disease-free survival, with male sex approaching significance (P = .06).[11] Likewise, treatment with MMC, male sex, and node-positive status were all predictors of overall survival. Predictors of colostomy included use of cisplatin (P = .03) and tumor size greater than 5 cm (P = .008); node positivity and male gender were not associated with an increased colostomy rate.[23]

When patients were stratified by primary tumor size (2–5 cm vs >5 cm) and node status (N0 node negative vs N+ node positive), 3-year disease-free survival rates were 74% for 5 cm or less and N0, 65% for greater than 5 cm and N0, 48% for 5 cm or less and N+, and 30% for greater than 5 cm and N+.[21] Further categorization into 3 TN staging groups demonstrated significant impact on 5-year disease-free survival, overall survival, locoregional failure, distant metastases, and colostomy failure.[22] The 5-year disease-free survival was 70% for patients with T2 to T3N0, 56% for patients with T4N0 or T2N+, and 36% for patients with T3 to T4N+ disease (*P*<.0001).

From the patients treated in the phase III randomized trials for localized anal cancer, a consistent pattern emerges that those with larger primary tumors, clinically node-positive status, and male sex have poorer outcomes, particularly regarding disease recurrence and colostomy rates. For this reason, the ongoing and proposed trials discussed assess alternative regimens for improving outcomes in these higher at-risk populations or deintensifying treatment in patients with more favorable tumor characteristics.

ONGOING AND FUTURE RANDOMIZED CLINICAL TRIALS

In the United Kingdom, the PLATO (Personalising Anal Cancer Radiotherapy Dose) trial portfolio consists of 3 planned studies (ACT III, ACT IV, and ACT V) to investigate individualized anal cancer treatment regimens based on tumor characteristics.[24] The ACT III trial is designed to evaluate a strategy of selective reduced dose chemoradiotherapy after local excision of T1N0 anal margin tumors. Patients with margins of greater than 1 mm will undergo observation, whereas patients with margins of 1 mm or less will receive pelvic chemoradiation with capecitabine to a lower dose of 41.4 Gy in 23 fractions. Ninety patients are planned for enrollment to this phase II, nonrandomized trial. Patients with clinically staged T1 to T2 up to 4 cm, node-negative anal canal cancers will be eligible for the ACT IV randomized phase II study to evaluate reduced dose chemoradiation to the primary tumor. The deintensified experimental radiation dose arm will deliver 41.4 Gy in 23 fractions, and the standard radiotherapy dose arm will administer 50.4 Gy in 28 fractions. Enrollment is planned at 162 patients with a 2:1 randomization. In accordance with the poor outcomes associated with locally advanced cancers, ACT V will assess radiation dose escalation in patients with greater than 4 cm primary anal tumors or node-positive disease. This phase II/III trial will randomize 677 patients to radiotherapy dose arms of 53.2 Gy, 58.8 Gy, or 61.6 Gy, all in 28 fractions and administered with standard chemotherapy. Only one of the dose-escalated arms (58.8 Gy or 61.6 Gy) will be evaluated for the phase III component. The primary endpoint for each trial is 3-year locoregional failure.

For patients with locally advanced anal cancers, recently completed and developing studies in the United States are evaluating the addition of targeted therapies to standard chemoradiation regimens. Anal cancers strongly express the epidermal growth factor receptor (EGFR).[25] EGFR expression was recently analyzed in 183 pretreatment tumor biopsies of patients treated on RTOG 9811; at a median follow-up of 6 years, EGFR expression was associated with inferior outcomes for all clinical outcomes.[26] Building off of the success of the EGFR inhibitor cetuximab in combination with radiation for squamous cell cancers of the head and neck, the AIDS Malignancy Consortium (AMC) and ECOG completed 2 companion phase II trials (AMC045 and E3205) of radiotherapy with concurrent 5-FU, cisplatin, and cetuximab for anal canal cancer.[27,28] All patients received cetuximab (400 mg/m^2 loading, then 250 mg/m^2 per week IV for 6–8 weeks) with cisplatin (75 mg/m^2 IV every 28 days × 2) and 5-FU (1000 mg/m^2 per day IV infusion on days 1–4 and 29–32) concurrently with radiation (45–54 Gy) starting with the second dose of cetuximab. In E3205, patients also received 2 cycles of cisplatin with 5-FU alone before chemoradiation with cetuximab.

This induction chemotherapy was discontinued after the publication of RTOG 9811. The primary endpoint for both studies was 3-year locoregional failure.

In the AMC045 trial, patients with stage I to III squamous cell cancer of the anal canal with human immunodeficiency virus infection were eligible.[27] The 3-year locoregional failure rate was 42% (95% CI, 28%–56%; 1-sided $P = .9$) by binomial proportional estimate using the prespecified end point (locoregional failure or alive without failure and followed <3 years), and 20% (95% CI, 10%–37%) by Kaplan-Meier estimate in post hoc analysis. Three-year rates of progression-free survival were 72% (95% CI, 56%–84%), and 79% (95% CI, 63%–89%) for overall survival. Grade 4 toxicity occurred in 26%, and 4% had treatment-associated deaths. In the E3205 trial with 61 immunocompetent patients evaluable (28 patients receiving the 2 cycles of induction cisplatin and 5-FU), the 3-year locoregional failure rate was 23% (95% CI, 13%–36%; 1-sided $P = .03$) by binomial proportional estimate using the prespecified end point and 21% (95% CI, 7%–26%) by Kaplan-Meier estimate in post hoc analysis.[28] Three-year rates of progression-free survival were 68% (95% CI, 55%–79%) and 83% (95% CI, 71%–91%) for overall survival. Grade 4 toxicity occurred in 32%, and 5% had treatment-associated deaths. The lack of locoregional control benefit and the significant side effect profile indicate the continued need for more effective and less toxic therapies.

Risk factors associated with the development of anal cancer include immunosuppression from organ transplant, autoimmune disease, and human immunodeficiency virus; however, the vast majority of all cases are attributed to infection by the human papillomavirus.[29,30] As such, great interest exists for the development of immunotherapy as a novel approach to improving clinical outcomes for patients with locally advanced anal cancer. Investigators from Brown University have conducted a phase I/II multicenter human papillomavirus vaccination trial in combination with 5-FU, MMC, and IMRT for locally advanced anal cancer. Four infusions of a listeria-based human papillomavirus-E7 vaccine (ADXS11–001, Advaxis Inc., Princeton, NJ) were administered with standard first-line chemoradiation.[31] Eligibility required tumors greater than 4 cm in size or node-positive disease. Ten patients have been treated, including 6 with large nodal disease. Patients received the first vaccine approximately 2 weeks before chemoradiation, the second vaccine 10 to 28 days after chemoradiation completion, and the third and fourth vaccines at subsequent monthly intervals. All patients have experienced a complete clinical response with an acceptable safety profile. As of March 2017, only 1 patient has experienced a recurrence (systemic), with a median follow-up of 3 years. Based on these encouraging results, the RTOG Foundation is developing a multicenter, randomized trial.

SUMMARY

The management of anal carcinoma has evolved into a multidisciplinary approach involving local excision for very early stage cancers and combined modality sphincter-preserving chemotherapy and radiation for locally advanced disease. Randomized clinical trials have demonstrated a benefit of chemoradiation over radiation therapy alone with improvements in tumor response and disease-free survival. However, subsequent phase III studies have not yielded superior outcomes over the original 5-FU and MMC standard chemoradiation backbone. Refinement in radiation planning and delivery with IMRT has reduced the acute toxicity of treatment, which allows for more patients to complete chemoradiation without significant gaps in delivery, and for further intensification of therapy in the ongoing and future clinical trials in high-risk anal cancer.

REFERENCES

1. Pintor MP, Northover JM, Nicholls RJ. Squamous cell carcinoma of the anus at one hospital from 1948 to 1984. Br J Surg 1989;76(8):806–10.
2. Brown DK, Oglesby AB, Scott DH, et al. Squamous cell carcinoma of the anus: a twenty-five year retrospective. Am Surg 1988;54(6):337–42.
3. Nigro ND, Vaitkevicius VK, Considine B. Combined therapy for cancer of the anal canal: a preliminary report. Dis Colon Rectum 1974;17(3):354–6.
4. Nigro ND, Seydel HG, Considine B, et al. Combined preoperative radiation and chemotherapy for squamous cell carcinoma of the anal canal. Cancer 1983; 51(10):1826–9.
5. Leichman L, Nigro N, Vaitkevicius VK, et al. Cancer of the anal canal. Model for preoperative adjuvant combined modality therapy. Am J Med 1985;78(2):211–5.
6. Northover JMA, Arnott SJ, Cunningham D, et al. Epidermoid anal cancer: results from the UKCCCR randomised trial of radiotherapy alone versus radiotherapy, 5-fluorouracil, and mitomycin. Lancet 1996;348(9034):1049–54.
7. Northover J, Glynne-Jones R, Sebag-Montefiore D, et al. Chemoradiation for the treatment of epidermoid anal cancer: 13-year follow-up of the first randomised UKCCCR Anal Cancer Trial (ACT I). Br J Cancer 2010;102(7):1123–8.
8. Bartelink H, Roelofsen F, Eschwege F, et al. Concomitant radiotherapy and chemotherapy is superior to radiotherapy alone in the treatment of locally advanced anal cancer: results of a phase III randomized trial of the European organization for research and treatment of cancer radiotherapy and gastro. J Clin Oncol 1997;15(5):2040–9.
9. Flam M, John M, Pajak TF, et al. Role of mitomycin in combination with fluorouracil and radiotherapy, and of salvage chemoradiation in the definitive nonsurgical treatment of epidermoid carcinoma of the anal canal: results of a phase III randomized intergroup study. J Clin Oncol 1996;14(9):2527–39.
10. Ajani JA. Fluorouracil, mitomycin, and radiotherapy vs fluorouracil, cisplatin, and radiotherapy for carcinoma of the anal canal. JAMA 2008;299(16):1914.
11. Gunderson LL, Winter KA, Ajani JA, et al. Long-term update of US GI intergroup RTOG 98-11 Phase III trial for anal carcinoma: survival, relapse, and colostomy failure with concurrent chemoradiation involving fluorouracil/mitomycin versus fluorouracil/cisplatin. J Clin Oncol 2012;30(35):4344–51.
12. James RD, Glynne-Jones R, Meadows HM, et al. Mitomycin or cisplatin chemoradiation with or without maintenance chemotherapy for treatment of squamous-cell carcinoma of the anus (ACT II): a randomised, phase 3, open-label, 2×2 factorial trial. Lancet Oncol 2013;14(6):516–24.
13. Glynne-Jones R, Sebag-Montefiore D, Meadows HM, et al. Best time to assess complete clinical response after chemoradiotherapy in squamous cell carcinoma of the anus (ACT II): a post-hoc analysis of randomised controlled phase 3 trial. Lancet Oncol 2017;18(3):347–56.
14. Peiffert D, Tournier-Rangeard L, Gérard JP, et al. Induction chemotherapy and dose intensification of the radiation boost in locally advanced anal canal carcinoma: final analysis of the randomized UNICANCER ACCORD 03 trial. J Clin Oncol 2012;30(16):1941–8.
15. Glynne-Jones R, Sebag-Montefiore D, Adams R, et al. "Mind the gap" - The Impact of variations in the duration of the treatment gap and overall treatment time in the first UK anal cancer trial (ACT I). Int J Radiat Oncol Biol Phys 2011;81(5):1488–94.
16. Chakravarthy AB, Catalano PJ, Martenson JA, et al. Long-term follow-up of a Phase II trial of high-dose radiation with concurrent 5-fluorouracil and cisplatin

in patients with anal cancer (ECOG E4292). Int J Radiat Oncol Biol Phys 2011; 81(4):607–13.

17. Ben-Josef E, Moughan J, Ajani J, et al. Impact of overall treatment time on survival and local control in anal cancer: a pooled data analysis of Radiation Therapy Oncology Group trials 87-04 and 98-11. J Clin Oncol 2010;28(34):5061–6.

18. Kachnic LA, Winter K, Myerson RJ, et al. RTOG 0529: a phase 2 evaluation of dose-painted intensity modulated radiation therapy in combination with 5-fluorouracil and mitomycin-C for the reduction of acute morbidity in carcinoma of the anal canal. Int J Radiat Oncol Biol Phys 2013;86(1):27–33.

19. Glynne-Jones R, Sebag-Montefiore D, Adams R, et al. Prognostic factors for recurrence and survival in anal cancer: generating hypotheses from the mature outcomes of the first United Kingdom Coordinating Committee on Cancer Research Anal Cancer Trial (ACT I). Cancer 2013;119(4):748–55.

20. Glynne-Jones R, Kadalayil L, Meadows HM, et al. Tumour- and treatment-related colostomy rates following mitomycin C or cisplatin chemoradiation with or without maintenance chemotherapy in squamous cell carcinoma of the anus in the ACT II trial. Ann Oncol 2014;25(8):1616–22.

21. Ajani JA, Winter KA, Gunderson LL, et al. Prognostic factors derived from a prospective database dictate clinical biology of anal cancer: the intergroup trial (RTOG 98-11). Cancer 2010;116(17):4007–13.

22. Gunderson LL, Moughan J, Ajani JA, et al. Anal carcinoma: impact of TN category of disease on survival, disease relapse, and colostomy failure in US gastrointestinal intergroup RTOG 98-11 phase 3 trial. Int J Radiat Oncol Biol Phys 2013;87(4):638–45.

23. Ajani JA, Winter KA, Gunderson LL, et al. US intergroup anal carcinoma trial: tumor diameter predicts for colostomy. J Clin Oncol 2009;27(7):1116–21.

24. Sebag-Montefiore D, Adams R, Bell S, et al. The development of an umbrella trial (PLATO) to address radiation therapy dose questions in the locoregional management of squamous cell carcinoma of the anus. Int J Radiat Oncol Biol Phys 2016;96(2, Supplement):E164–5.

25. Alvarez G, Perry A, Tan BR, et al. Expression of epidermal growth factor receptor in squamous cell carcinomas of the anal canal is independent of gene amplification. Mod Pathol 2006;19(7):942–9.

26. Doll CM, Moughan J, Klimowicz A, et al. Significance of co-expression of epidermal growth factor receptor and Ki67 on clinical outcome in patients with anal cancer treated with chemoradiotherapy: an analysis of NRG Oncology RTOG 9811. Int J Radiat Oncol Biol Phys 2017;97(3):554–62.

27. Garg MK, Zhao F, Sparano JA, et al. Cetuximab plus chemoradiotherapy in immunocompetent patients with anal carcinoma: a Phase II Eastern Cooperative Oncology Group-American College of Radiology Imaging Network Cancer Research Group Trial (E3205). J Clin Oncol 2017;35(7):718–26.

28. Sparano JA, Lee JY, Palefsky J, et al. Cetuximab plus chemoradiotherapy for HIV-associated anal carcinoma: a Phase II AIDS Malignancy Consortium Trial. J Clin Oncol 2017;35(7):727–33.

29. Frisch M, Glimelius B, van den Brule AJ, et al. Sexually transmitted infection as a cause of anal cancer. N Engl J Med 1997;337:1350–8.

30. Morris VK, Rashid A, Rodriguez-Bigas M, et al. Clinicopathologic features associated with human papillomavirus/p16 in patients with metastatic squamous cell carcinoma of the anal canal. Oncologist 2015;20:1247–52.

31. Perez K, Safran H, Leonard K, et al. ADXS11-001 immunotherapy with chemoradiation for anal cancer. Int Anal Neoplasia Soc Presented. Atlanta (GE), March 13, 2015.

Advancing Treatment Approach to the Older Patient with Cancer Through Clinical Trials Participation

Efrat Dotan, MD

KEYWORDS

- Clinical trials • Elderly • Older cancer patients

KEY POINTS

- Treatment of older patients with cancer is challenging because of physiologic changes of aging, multiple comorbidities, functional decline, cognitive dysfunction, and limited social support.
- Older patients with cancer are poorly represented in clinical trials because of many barriers that limit their active accrual. Thus, limited data are available to guide the treatment approach to this patient population.
- Barriers to accrual of older patients to clinical trials include strict eligibility criteria, limited support from the treating physician, and patient-related factors.
- Decisions regarding clinical trial participation should be based on functional age rather than chronologic age. Older fit patients who are eligible for clinical trials should be encouraged to enroll.
- Elderly specific clinical trials, and studies evaluating a less fit patient population, are the gold standard for obtaining evidence that can guide oncologic treatment decisions in the clinic.

CANCER IN OLDER ADULTS

With the aging of the population there continues to be a steady increase in the number of older adults routinely seen in oncology clinics, and the challenges associated with the care for this patient population are encountered daily by oncologists worldwide. According to the US Census Bureau by 2050 the number of individuals older than age 65 is projected to surpass 80 million, representing about 20% of the population.[1] Age is known to be a risk factor for many cancers, it is estimated that 60% of the

Disclosure Statement: The author has received research and grant support from Oncomed, Bayer, and Pfizer (22862401).
Department of Medical Oncology, Fox Chase Cancer Center, 333 Cottman Avenue, Philadelphia, PA 19111, USA
E-mail address: Efrat.Dotan@fccc.edu

incidence of cancer and 70% of mortality from cancer occurs in patients that are older than the age of 65 (**Fig. 1, Table 1**).[2,3] Life expectancy carries a significant weight when evaluating and treating older patients with cancer. With improvement in many areas of medicine, life expectancy continues to rise, with projection of an average of 20 years of living for 65-year-old individuals by 2050.[1] This results in a higher portion of older individuals that are seen in practices who are candidates for surgery, and other anticancer therapies. Patients older than the age of 65 accounts for the group that carries the highest personal health care spending in the United States, with continued increase in spending as individuals age.[4]

Surgeons and medical oncologists who are treating older patients with cancer are becoming more comfortable with delivering complex therapies to these individuals. This was demonstrated by Vijayvergia and colleagues[5] who reported an increase in the number of older patients and patients with multiple comorbidities that receive multiagent therapy for metastatic colon cancer over the last two decades. Similarly reports are seen in the literature describing complicated surgical procedures being safely performed on older adults.[6–8] Yet controversy remains with regards to the tolerance of these treatments among older adults, with concerns of increased toxicity in this population. For example, a recent large registry study evaluated the outcomes of older patients with early stage colon cancer who underwent surgical resection. In that study, older age was associated with higher 1-year overall cancer-specific and cardiac-specific mortality.[9] It is clear that age alone could not be used to determine the treatment approach in this patient population because multiple other factors influence the ultimate outcome. The treating physician is challenged daily with predicting

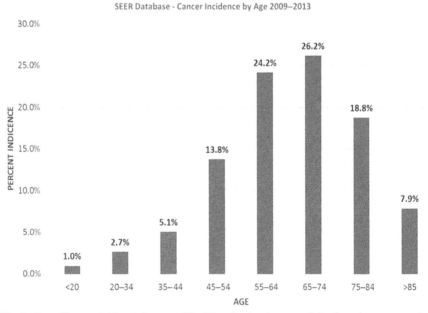

Fig. 1. Surveillance, Epidemiology, and End Results database statistics fact sheet: cancer incidence by age. (*Adapted from* Howlader N, Noone AM, Krapcho M. et al. SEER Cancer Statistics Review, 1975–2013. Bethesda (MD): National Cancer Institute; 2016. Available at: http://seer.cancer.gov/csr/1975_2013/. Based on November 2015 Surveillance, Epidemiology, and End Results data submission, posted to the Surveillance, Epidemiology, and End Results Web site; with permission.)

Table 1
Surveillance, Epidemiology, and End Results database statistics fact sheet: median age at diagnosis

Cancer	Median Age at Diagnosis
All cancers	65
Oral cavity and pharynx	62
Digestive system	68
Respiratory system	70
Breast	62
Female genital system	61
Male genital system	66
Urinary system	69
Lymphoma	65
Myeloma	69
Leukemia	66

From Howlader N, Noone AM, Krapcho M. et al. SEER Cancer Statistics Review, 1975-2013. Bethesda (MD): National Cancer Institute; 2016. Available at: http://seer.cancer.gov/csr/1975_2013/. Based on November 2015 Surveillance, Epidemiology, and End Results data submission, posted to the Surveillance, Epidemiology, and End Results Web site; with permission.

the ability of their older patient to undergo various anticancer therapies, and distinguishing between those who are fit and would benefit from these interventions, and those who are frail and are better served with less aggressive treatment approaches.

Physicians caring for older patients with cancer face multiple challenges. Most importantly, older patients have an altered response to many anticancer therapies compared with their younger counterparts. This is mainly caused by physiologic changes related to the aging process. Decrements in renal and hepatic function, altered gastrointestinal motility, loss of cardiac and marrow reserves, changes in cognition, and decrements in bone and muscle mass may increase the risk for treatment-related toxicity. Furthermore, the high incidence of comorbidities adds additional challenges to the planned therapy. The Centers for Disease Control and Prevention estimates that 80% of older adults have at least one chronic condition and 50% have two or more conditions that affect their care.[10] The presence of multiple comorbidities results in patients receiving additional medications, and often dealing with the challenges of polypharmacy. The reported rate of polypharmacy among older patients with cancer varies in the literature, with one study reporting most patients receiving an average of eight medications.[11,12] Finally, older patients often suffer from decrease in their performance status, and increased need for daily support from family members. Social support directly affects the patient's access to care, and ultimate treatment decisions. All these factors must be assessed before finalizing the treatment decision, and the proposed therapy should be personalized for each patient based on these factors. A comprehensive geriatric assessment (CGA) is the recommended tool for assessing these domains.[13,14] It has been shown to be predictive of disease- and treatment-related outcomes, and unmask underlying disabilities that are not detected with a regular clinical assessment.[15,16] Despite these data, the use of a CGA in routine oncologic practice remains low, and treating physicians rely more on their "eye ball" test rather than objectively collected information. Multiple screening tools have been developed that are easily implemented in an oncology clinic, and alert the physician for the need for a thorough geriatric evaluation.[17,18]

PARTICIPATION OF OLDER PATIENTS WITH CANCER IN CLINICAL TRIALS

In addition to the previously mentioned challenges related to the aging process another pronounced challenge lies in the lack of clear evidence to guide the treatment decisions in this patient population. Clinicians are forced to extrapolate from data derived from studies conducted on younger and healthier patients when deciding on a treatment plan for their older patient with cancer. Older patients with cancer are significantly underrepresented in clinical trials evaluating new cancer therapies. A study by Hutchins and colleagues[19] found that only 25% of patients enrolled on 164 Southwest Oncology Group studies were older than the age of 65, whereas 63% of patients with cancer were older than that age at the same time period. Similar findings were reported by Lewis and colleagues[20] who reviewed the rate of elderly patient participation in National Cancer Institute–supported clinical trials. In this analysis 32% of participants in phase II and III National Cancer Institute–supported studies were older than the age of 65. A more recent analysis evaluated the accrual of older patients with breast cancer to clinical trials run through the Alliance between 1985 to 2012. Similarly, the overall percentage of older patients enrolled on these studies was lower than that seen among the US breast cancer population. The odds of older patients enrolling on adjuvant studies increased over time, yet decreased over time for neoadjuvant and metastatic studies.[21]

The proportion of older patients participating in registration studies that ultimately result in the US Food and Drug Administration approval has also been shown to be low. Talarico and coworkers[22] found only 36% of 28,000 participants in 55 such studies were older than the age of 65, a total of 20% older than the age of 70%, and 9% older than the age of 75. In comparison these subcategories encompass 60%, 46%, and 31% of the overall cancer patient population, respectively. A more recent analysis reviewed 24 new drugs that were approved between 2007 and 2010 for the treatment of cancer and found only 33% of participants in these studies to be older than the age of 65.[23] Regretfully, these data portray lack of progress in this arena and further deepen the gap of knowledge with regards to the treatment approach to this patient population. A recent position paper by the American Society of Clinical Oncology summarized these concerns and urged the oncologic community to take action in improving evidence-based care of the older patient population.[24]

Multiple barriers to enrollment of older patients on oncologic clinical trials have been identified over the years. Overly restrictive eligibility criteria in studies are one of the main reasons for underrepresentation of this patient population in therapeutic studies. A study of 87 clinical trials in patients with non-Hodgkin lymphoma reported 25% of studies excluding patients older than the age of 65, and an additional 54% of studies excluding older adults through selective eligibility criteria aside from age.[25] With stringent eligibility criteria researchers limit the accrual of the "real-life" patients on studies and decrease the ability to learn and produce good evidence that can guide therapy. Multiple societies including the Institute of Medicine have called for the development of eligibility criteria that allow for the broadest participation possible.[24,26]

Another common barrier to clinical trial enrollment lies in the discussion that the patient has with the treating physician. Treating physicians can be a major barrier to enrolling older patients on therapeutic studies out of concern for enhanced toxicities. Javid and colleagues[27,28] found that when studies were available and patients were eligible, these studies were discussed more often with younger than with older patients (78% vs 58%). Conversely, studies have shown that age and comorbidities were not clearly predictive of toxicities on studies.[29] Rather than using chronologic age to determine if a patient is a candidate for a study, biologic and functional age should guide this decision. Clinicians must be educated in appropriate assessment tools that can provide a full evaluation of the patient's overall function, and fitness for clinical trial participation. Those patients who are found to be fit for studies should be encouraged to participate in studies that would enhance the fund of knowledge.

Contrary to the assumption of many physicians, studies have shown that older patients view participation in clinical trials positively, and would be open to this option if given the choice.[30,31] However, there are some patient-related factors that potentially limit participation of this patient population in clinical trials. Older patients fear the loss of autonomy over treatment choice, the loss of decision-making capacity, and the impact of any therapy on quality of life, all of which may occur while on studies. Other barriers include cultural differences in the attitude toward clinical trials, and the perception of the relatives of the benefit of such intervention.[27] Nevertheless, the recommendation from their treating physicians is rated as the highest factor to influence the decision of an older patient.[32] With this in mind, physicians should be educated on having such discussions with an older patient with cancer, and encouraging eligible patients to participate in appropriate clinical trials.

ELDERLY SPECIFIC CLINICAL TRIALS

The need for better evidence to guide the therapy for older patients with cancer has been proclaimed by many national groups.[33] This provides a wide support for elderly specific studies evaluating anticancer therapies, supportive care measures, and assessment tools in this patient population. In addition to evaluating these interventions in fit older patients without any contraindication for therapy, such interventions should also be evaluated in frail patients to clarify the appropriate approach to individuals that cannot tolerate standard of care therapy. Furthermore, trial design and study end points may be different when conducting studies in this patient population. For example, evaluating the "active-life expectancy" (time where the individual remains active, lives independently without disability), and the treatment's effect on physical/cognitive functions is of higher interest in the older patient population in comparison with end points evaluating survival.

Different study designs have been implemented in an older patient population successfully. These studies serve as a model for future elderly specific clinical trials that would advance the field. Randomized controlled trials (RCT) are the gold standard evidence to guide the treatment approach, and those have been conducted in an older population. For example, the MILES study was a phase III RCT evaluating the use of single-agent versus combination chemotherapy in patients 70 years or older with newly diagnosed non–small cell lung cancer.[34] A similar study was CALGB 49907 conducted among older patients with breast cancer evaluating two forms of adjuvant chemotherapy.[35] Another recent study that highlights the ability to conduct elderly specific RCT is the AVEX trial, which enrolled patients older than the age of 70 with newly diagnosed metastatic colorectal cancer evaluating the benefit of the addition of bevacizumab to capecitabine.[36] The FOCUS2 study is an excellent example of an RCT conducted in an unfit older patient population that were not candidates for standard of care therapy.[37] The previous examples outline the feasibility of conducting RCT in elderly patients and unfit patients, and the high utility of the data derived from these studies.

Evaluating every new therapy in an older cohort of patients is not feasible. Therefore, a more attainable goal is to expand the age range of patients eligible for studies, and potentially stratify enrollment into age groups representative of the general population with the cancer target of the trial.[33] This was modeled in the RCT that led to the approval of abiraterone for metastatic prostate cancer, where the median age of patients was 69 (range, 42–95; about 30% of patients older than the age of 75).[38] Supporters of elderly specific studies have also proposed a model of extended trial design with specific attention to the age distribution of the superior arm.[33] In this model, once an RCT is complete the superior arm is examined to ensure it had an age distribution that resembles that of the population with the specific disease. If this was not the case, that arm would then reopen and enroll a sufficient number of older adults. Another alternative is to conduct a phase IV study that would evaluate the new standard in the population of patients that was underrepresented in the registration study. These models are novel, and have not been implemented to date.

Single-arm studies are also a good modality to assess the benefit and toxicities of a certain drug or intervention. This type of study design allows for nontraditional end points that are of high importance in elderly specific studies. These models also inform tolerance to therapy and potential different dosing schedules that better serve the older patient population. An example for such study was the CALGB 9762, which evaluated the relationship between patients' age, paclitaxel pharmacology, and toxicity.[39] Another approach to evaluating the effect of a new treatment modality on an older patient population has been evaluating this population retrospectively following the approval of a new agent. An example for this is the BRITE registry, which collected data regarding tolerance of bevacizumab following its approval. Analysis of older adults who were included in this observational registry allowed us to draw information regarding the tolerance of this agent in the older patient population.[40] As is often the case in oncology, when prospective data are lacking retrospective studies fill the gap to provide additional guidance to the care of patients. Many therapies across different cancers have been studied retrospectively in older adults and these publications provide clinicians with some clinical guidance.[41–44]

ADVANCING KNOWLEDGE ABOUT ASSESSMENT AND SUPPORTIVE CARE OF THE OLDER PATIENT WITH CANCER

Although clinical trials are crucial to advance knowledge and treatment approach to the older patient with cancer, continued evaluation of the optimal process of assessing older patients, and the optimal supportive care measures are of great value. In recent years, landmark studies have validated the importance of CGA in an oncology setting as a predictor of outcomes and toxicities.[45–47] Additional studies have been conducted that define the most robust tool for screening older patients with cancer in a clinical setting, and identifying patients who would benefit from a full geriatric assessment.[17,48] Finally, clinical models have been developed that assist the oncologist in predicting the risk for toxicities associated with chemotherapy in an older cancer population.[49–51] Additionally, the ability to conduct these assessments through a World Wide Web–based patient self-reported assessment has been demonstrated as well.[52] These data provide clear support for the benefit of a CGA in older patients with cancer; additional studies and physician education are needed to define the best way to incorporate these tools into clinical practice.

Because the aging population values quality of life and maintaining their functional status highly, and often over longevity, studies should evaluate supportive care measures that improve these domains. The appropriate dosing for treatment regimens is a commonly debated question among oncologists. Some believe in starting low and slowly intensifying therapy based on tolerance, whereas others believe in starting at standard dosing and dose reducing in the setting of adverse events. Elderly specific studies can help answer these questions. Future studies evaluating various dosing schedules, and the risks associated with them stratified by a profile detected through a geriatric evaluation would be of high value. Evaluation of various supportive care measures including nutritional support, physical therapy, cognitive, and psychological support in the setting of cancer would enhance the care provided to these patients.

SUMMARY

Older patients comprise a large population of patients with cancer, yet they are significantly underrepresented in oncology-based clinical trials. Multiple barriers exist that result in the low accrual of older adults with cancer to studies. Principal investigators, treating physicians, and patients all contribute in different ways to these barriers. Nevertheless, the only way to advance the field and enhance the evidence that guides the care of older adults is through better clinical research that is geared to this patient population. Regulatory agencies and national funding organizations should emphasize the importance of age distribution that mirrors that of the general cancer population in clinical trials. Furthermore, incentives to encourage researchers to obtain elderly specific data would further enhance the applicability of these study results. The oncologic community must bring together different stake holders that focus on enhancing the inclusion of older adults in clinical trials, supporting elderly specific research initiatives, and continued physician education of the importance of this task.

REFERENCES

1. Ortman JM, Velkoff VA, Hogan H. An aging nation: the older population in the US. U.S.D.o.C.E.a.S.A.U.S.C. BUREAU, Editor. US Census Bureau, 2014.
2. Siegel RL, Miller KD, Jemal A. Cancer statistics, 2016. CA Cancer J Clin 2016; 66(1):7–30.
3. Howlader N, Noone AM, Krapcho M, et al. SEER cancer statistics Review, 1975-2013. Bethesda (MD): National Cancer Institute; 2016. Available at: http://seer.cancer.gov/csr/1975_2013/. based on November 2015 SEER data submission, posted to the SEER Web site. Accessed January 12, 2017.
4. Dieleman JL, Baral R, Birger M, et al. US spending on personal health care and public health, 1996-2013. JAMA 2016;316(24):2627–46.
5. Vijayvergia N, Li T, Wong YN, et al. Chemotherapy use and adoption of new agents is affected by age and comorbidities in patients with metastatic colorectal cancer. Cancer 2016;122(20):3191–8.
6. Melis M, Marcon F, Masi A, et al. The safety of a pancreaticoduodenectomy in patients older than 80 years: risk vs. benefits. HPB (Oxford) 2012;14(9):583–8.
7. Niitsu H, Hinoi T, Kawaguchi Y, et al. Laparoscopic surgery for colorectal cancer is safe and has survival outcomes similar to those of open surgery in elderly patients with a poor performance status: subanalysis of a large multicenter case-control study in Japan. J Gastroenterol 2016;51(1):43–54.
8. Miura N, Kohno M, Ito K, et al. Lung cancer surgery in patients aged 80 years or older: an analysis of risk factors, morbidity, and mortality. Gen Thorac Cardiovasc Surg 2015;63(7):401–5.
9. Aquina CT, Mohile SG, Tejani MA, et al. The impact of age on complications, survival, and cause of death following colon cancer surgery. Br J Cancer 2017; 116(3):389–97.
10. Centers for Disease Control and Prevention. Healthy aging: helping people to live long and productive lives and enjoy a good quality of life. Available at: http://stacks.cdc.gov/view/cdc/6114.

11. Maggiore RJ, Gross CP, Hurria A. Polypharmacy in older adults with cancer. Oncologist 2010;15(5):507–22.
12. Riechelmann RP, Moreira F, Smaletz O, et al. Potential for drug interactions in hospitalized cancer patients. Cancer Chemother Pharmacol 2005;56(3):286–90.
13. VanderWalde N, Jagsi R, Dotan E, et al. NCCN guidelines insights: older adult oncology, version 2.2016. J Natl Compr Canc Netw 2016;14(11):1357–70.
14. Extermann M, Aapro M, Bernabei R, et al. Use of comprehensive geriatric assessment in older cancer patients: recommendations from the task force on CGA of the International Society of Geriatric Oncology (SIOG). Crit Rev Oncol Hematol 2005;55(3):241–52.
15. Ramjaun A, Nassif MO, Krotneva S, et al. Improved targeting of cancer care for older patients: a systematic review of the utility of comprehensive geriatric assessment. J Geriatr Oncol 2013;4(3):271–81.
16. Kenis C, Bron D, Libert Y, et al. Relevance of a systematic geriatric screening and assessment in older patients with cancer: results of a prospective multicentric study. Ann Oncol 2013;24(5):1306–12.
17. Soubeyran P, Bellera C, Goyard J, et al. Screening for vulnerability in older cancer patients: the ONCODAGE Prospective Multicenter Cohort Study. PLoS One 2014; 9(12):e115060.
18. Decoster L, Van Puyvelde K, Mohile S, et al. Screening tools for multidimensional health problems warranting a geriatric assessment in older cancer patients: an update on SIOG recommendations dagger. Ann Oncol 2015;26(2):288–300.
19. Hutchins LF, Unger JM, Crowley JJ, et al. Underrepresentation of patients 65 years of age or older in cancer-treatment trials. N Engl J Med 1999;341(27): 2061–7.
20. Lewis JH, Kilgore ML, Goldman DP, et al. Participation of patients 65 years of age or older in cancer clinical trials. J Clin Oncol 2003;21(7):1383–9.
21. Freedman RA, Foster JC, Seisler DK, et al. Accrual of older patients with breast cancer to alliance systemic therapy trials over time: protocol A151527. J Clin Oncol 2016;35(4):421–31.
22. Talarico L, Chen G, Pazdur R. Enrollment of elderly patients in clinical trials for cancer drug registration: a 7-year experience by the US Food and Drug Administration. J Clin Oncol 2004;22(22):4626–31.
23. Scher KS, Hurria A. Under-representation of older adults in cancer registration trials: known problem, little progress. J Clin Oncol 2012;30(17):2036–8.
24. Hurria A, Levit LA, Dale W, et al. Improving the evidence base for treating older adults with cancer: American Society of Clinical Oncology Statement. J Clin Oncol 2015;33(32):3826–33.
25. Bellera C, Praud D, Petit-Monéger A, et al. Barriers to inclusion of older adults in randomised controlled clinical trials on Non-Hodgkin's lymphoma: a systematic review. Cancer Treat Rev 2013;39(7):812–7.
26. Institute of Medicine: A National Cancer Clinical Trials system for the 21st century: reinvigorating the NCI Cooperative Group Program. Washington, DC: National Academies Press; 2015.
27. Javid SH, Unger JM, Gralow JR, et al. A prospective analysis of the influence of older age on physician and patient decision-making when considering enrollment in breast cancer clinical trials (SWOG S0316). Oncologist 2012;17(9):1180–90.
28. Townsley CA, Selby R, Siu LL. Systematic review of barriers to the recruitment of older patients with cancer onto clinical trials. J Clin Oncol 2005;23(13):3112–24.

29. LoConte NK, Smith M, Alberti D, et al. Amongst eligible patients, age and comorbidity do not predict for dose-limiting toxicity from phase I chemotherapy. Cancer Chemother Pharmacol 2010;65(4):775–80.
30. Kemeny MM, Peterson BL, Kornblith AB, et al. Barriers to clinical trial participation by older women with breast cancer. J Clin Oncol 2003;21(12):2268–75.
31. Comis RL, Miller JD, Aldigé CR, et al. Public attitudes toward participation in cancer clinical trials. J Clin Oncol 2003;21(5):830–5.
32. Townsley CA, Chan KK, Pond GR, et al. Understanding the attitudes of the elderly towards enrolment into cancer clinical trials. BMC Cancer 2006;6:34.
33. Hurria A, Dale W, Mooney M, et al. Designing therapeutic clinical trials for older and frail adults with cancer: U13 conference recommendations. J Clin Oncol 2014;32(24):2587–94.
34. Gridelli C, Perrone F, Gallo C, et al. Chemotherapy for elderly patients with advanced non-small-cell lung cancer: the Multicenter Italian Lung Cancer in the Elderly Study (MILES) phase III randomized trial. J Natl Cancer Inst 2003; 95(5):362–72.
35. Muss HB, Berry DA, Cirrincione CT, et al. Adjuvant chemotherapy in older women with early-stage breast cancer. N Engl J Med 2009;360(20):2055–65.
36. Cunningham D, Lang I, Lorusso V, et al. Bevacizumab (bev) in combination with capecitabine (cape) for the first-line treatment of elderly patients with metastatic colorectal cancer (mCRC): results of a randomized international phase III trial (AVEX). J Clin Oncol 2013;30(Suppl 34) [abstract: 337].
37. Seymour MT, Thompson LC, Wasan HS, et al. Chemotherapy options in elderly and frail patients with metastatic colorectal cancer (MRC FOCUS2): an open-label, randomised factorial trial. Lancet 2011;377(9779):1749–59.
38. de Bono JS, Logothetis CJ, Molina A, et al. Abiraterone and increased survival in metastatic prostate cancer. N Engl J Med 2011;364(21):1995–2005.
39. Lichtman SM, Hollis D, Miller AA, et al. Prospective evaluation of the relationship of patient age and paclitaxel clinical pharmacology: Cancer and Leukemia Group B (CALGB 9762). J Clin Oncol 2006;24(12):1846–51.
40. Kozloff MF, Berlin J, Flynn PJ, et al. Clinical outcomes in elderly patients with metastatic colorectal cancer receiving bevacizumab and chemotherapy: results from the BRiTE observational cohort study. Oncology 2010;78(5–6):329–39.
41. Jang S, Zheng C, Tsai HT, et al. Cardiovascular toxicity after antiangiogenic therapy in persons older than 65 years with advanced renal cell carcinoma. Cancer 2016;122(1):124–30.
42. Bouchahahda M, Macarulla T, Spano JP, et al. Cetuximab and irinotecan-based chemotherapy as an active and safe treatment option for elderly patients with extensively pre-treated metastatic colorectal cancer. J Clin Oncol 2007;25(18S) [abstract: 14528].
43. Sorio R, Roemer-Becuwe C, Hilpert F, et al. Safety and efficacy of single-agent bevacizumab-containing therapy in elderly patients with platinum-resistant recurrent ovarian cancer: subgroup analysis of the randomised phase III AURELIA trial. Gynecol Oncol 2017;144(1):65–71.
44. Lubbert M, Suciu S, Hagemeijer A, et al. Decitabine improves progression-free survival in older high-risk MDS patients with multiple autosomal monosomies: results of a subgroup analysis of the randomized phase III study 06011 of the EORTC Leukemia Cooperative Group and German MDS Study Group. Ann Hematol 2016;95(2):191–9.
45. Clough-Gorr KM, Stuck AE, Thwin SS, et al. Older breast cancer survivors: geriatric assessment domains are associated with poor tolerance of treatment

adverse effects and predict mortality over 7 years of follow-up. J Clin Oncol 2010; 28(3):380–6.

46. Decoster L, Kenis C, Van Puyvelde K, et al. The influence of clinical assessment (including age) and geriatric assessment on treatment decisions in older patients with cancer. J Geriatr Oncol 2013;4(3):235–41.

47. Freyer G, Geay JF, Touzet S, et al. Comprehensive geriatric assessment predicts tolerance to chemotherapy and survival in elderly patients with advanced ovarian carcinoma: a GINECO study. Ann Oncol 2005;16(11):1795–800.

48. Luciani A, Ascione G, Bertuzzi C, et al. Detecting disabilities in older patients with cancer: comparison between comprehensive geriatric assessment and vulnerable elders survey-13. J Clin Oncol 2010;28(12):2046–50.

49. Extermann M, Boler I, Reich RR, et al. Predicting the risk of chemotherapy toxicity in older patients: the Chemotherapy Risk Assessment Scale for High-Age Patients (CRASH) score. Cancer 2012;118(13):3377–86.

50. Hurria A, Togawa K, Mohile SG, et al. Predicting chemotherapy toxicity in older adults with cancer: a prospective 500 patient multicenter study. J Clin Oncol 2010;28(15s) [abstract: 9001].

51. Hurria A, Mohile S, Gajra A, et al. Validation of a prediction tool for chemotherapy toxicity in older adults with cancer. J Clin Oncol 2016;34(20):2366–71.

52. Ingram SS, Seo PH, Martell RE, et al. Comprehensive assessment of the elderly cancer patient: the feasibility of self-report methodology. J Clin Oncol 2002;20(3): 770–5.

Randomized Controlled Trials in Hereditary Cancer Syndromes

Chethan Ramamurthy, MD[a], Yana Chertock, MA[b],
Michael J. Hall, MD, MS[b],*

KEYWORDS

- Hereditary cancer syndromes • Clinical trials • HBOC • FAP • Lynch • HNPCC
- Germline mutations

KEY POINTS

- The increase in the recognition of the genetic risk of cancer makes clinical trials in hereditary cancer syndromes important.
- It is challenging to conduct clinical trials in hereditary cancer syndromes because of genetic heterogeneity, established patterns of care, and patient-related factors.
- In hereditary breast and ovarian cancer, randomized controlled trials are few, with most guideline recommendations based on, at best, prospective cohort studies.
- In familial adenomatous polyposis, most randomized controlled trials have focused on chemoprevention, using nonsteroidal antiinflammatory drugs, aspirin, and other agents.
- In Lynch syndrome, there are few randomized controlled trials, with some data on endoscopic surveillance techniques and aspirin for chemoprevention.

INTRODUCTION

Individuals found to have germline mutations in genes that increase the risk of adult-onset cancer constitute a rare but growing population of patients with cancer and at-risk unaffected (ie, no history of cancer) persons. Studies examining germline mutations detected from tumor genomic profiles using next-generation sequencing (NGS) technologies suggest that anywhere from 3% to 15% of patients with cancer may harbor a germline mutation in a hereditary cancer risk gene.[1–4] Although few studies have evaluated this question on a large scale in the average-risk population, these studies paired with mutation prevalence estimates suggest that perhaps 3%

Disclosure: The authors have nothing to disclose.
[a] Department of Medical Oncology, Fox Chase Cancer Center, 333 Cottman Avenue, Philadelphia, PA 19111-9972, USA; [b] Department of Clinical Genetics, Fox Chase Cancer Center, 333 Cottman Avenue, Philadelphia, PA 19111-9972, USA
* Corresponding author.
E-mail address: Michael.Hall@fccc.edu

to 5% of the population carries a germline mutation in a moderate or high penetrance hereditary risk gene that increases cancer risk and affects cancer screening frequency based on current guidelines.[5–7] In the age of increasingly broad (ie, NGS-based multi-gene panel testing and whole-exome/genome sequencing) and inexpensive genetic testing in tumors and in the germline, the relevance of randomized trials that evaluate the efficacy of various medical treatments in individuals with germline mutations in hereditary cancer risk genes must be appreciated.

Individuals with germline mutations in hereditary cancer risk genes are a heterogeneous population that includes patients with active cancer, survivors, and unaffected patients at risk of cancer. With changing approaches to genetic testing and in particular the growing use of multigene hereditary panels, mutation carriers can have a variable degree of family history that accompanies their genetic risk, from highly penetrant families with many cancers to patients who have little to no cancer in their families. Such population heterogeneity can make design and recruitment to randomized controlled trials (RCTs) challenging, because these studies are often focused on disease prevention and screening-related end points, including detection and prevention of new cancers, and prevention of precancerous neoplasia (eg, adenomas in colorectal cancer [CRC]). The outcomes of these trials are often evaluated many years in the future, and thus study retention is difficult. At-risk individuals are often less aware of trials than patients with cancer, whereas oncologists generally have less interaction with at-risk individuals than with patients with cancer.[8] In addition, healthy individuals, even those at high risk, may be less motivated to participate in a study in which frequent follow-up, surveys, and other time burdens are required. However, those more willing to participate may have high perceived risk of cancer coupled with anxiety and cancer worry, and these traits may diminish their willingness to participate in a randomized study, especially if a placebo arm is involved.

Another challenge in hereditary cancer risk assessment is the growing number of genes of moderate to low-moderate penetrance that are now included on commercially available gene panel tests.[9,10] Although the years of 1995 to 2013 provided a fairly stable time of single-gene and oligogene testing in which RCTs could be more easily accrued and conducted in *BRCA1/2*, adenomatous polyposis coli gene (*APC*), Lynch mutation carriers, the past 3 years have seen a proliferation of new genes, many conferring only moderate risks of cancer in carriers. Making matters more complicated, many of these new genes lack randomized data to support effective clinical management for mutation carriers. In this setting, clinical care is often guided by risk magnitude alone, and management of organ-specific risk is based either on expert recommendations or extrapolated clinical trial data from other genes. For example, providers may question the benefit of prophylactic bilateral oophorectomy in a 40-year-old woman found to carry a mutation in a gene called *BRIP1*, which confers a lifetime risk of ovarian cancer 3 to 4 times that of average-risk women ($\sim$4–5%), or the rationale for early and/or increased colonoscopy screening in monoallelic *MUTYH* carriers who harbor $\sim$2-fold increased risk of CRC.[11–14] It seems unlikely that RCTs will be able to keep pace to evaluate screening, prophylaxis, and prevention end points in every new gene discovered and incorporated in a modern gene panel. In the era of inexpensive and power genomic tests, clinicians will increasingly face decisions absent of immediate RCT data specific to the gene mutations found in individual patients, and will rely more heavily on guidelines and recommendations from expert groups and societies.

This article reviews and highlights notable RCTs from the 3 areas of hereditary cancer risk in which most RCTs have been conducted: familial adenomatous polyposis (FAP) and *APC* mutation carriers, hereditary breast ovarian cancer and *BRCA1/2* mutation carriers, and hereditary nonpolyposis CRC (HNPCC; also called Lynch syndrome [LS]) and carriers in the most widely studied and clinically relevant mismatch repair (MMR) genes *MLH1*, *MSH2*, *MSH6*, and *PMS2*. An initial goal in these 3 areas was to focus as much as possible only on those RCTs in which the population of interest was mutation-positive individuals; however, this was nearly impossible, and many more trial participants carry clinical diagnoses of a syndrome than molecular diagnoses of a genetic risk. The lack of confirmatory genetic testing to establish the molecular risk and causative gene means that populations may remain heterogeneous, containing patients with a mix of different germline gene mutations, as well as many who do not have mutations, and thus clinical trial results may be more difficult to interpret.

HEREDITARY BREAST AND OVARIAN CANCER: CLINICAL TRIALS IN SURGICAL ONCOLOGY

The design and conduct of clinical trials in the hereditary breast and ovarian cancer (HBOC) population is a fairly new enterprise and carries many unique opportunities and challenges. Although the high incidence of disease makes the HBOC population ideal for screening and prevention studies, knowledge of the high risk of disease has led to the adoption of several practices into standard of care before demonstration of benefit in gold-standard RCTs. The inclusion criteria and thus composition of participants in HBOC clinical trials have morphed as understanding of the genetic underpinnings of HBOC has matured. Where once familial risk calculators determined eligibility, now gene sequencing is used to ensure a more homogenous population. Like the FAP and LS populations, more advanced screening has shown that the clinical population is molecularly heterogeneous, which means that clinicians must have caution in interpreting older trials in which clinical diagnoses were criteria for participation. As discussed later, these issues have led to most recommendations in screening, chemoprevention, and prophylactic surgery being based on, at best, prospective cohort studies. In addition to these preventive areas of cancer care, there has been the new development of targeted therapeutics based on the presence of certain germline mutations in HBOC as well.

Screening Trials in Hereditary Breast and Ovarian Cancer

The optimal population for screening is one in which the prevalence of a disease is high. To be effective, the screening method also must detect the disease early enough that an intervention can alter the clinical course of the disease. When considering these criteria for screening, the *BRCA1/2* mutation carrier population is ideal for intensified screening given the high prevalence of breast and ovarian cancer, as well as the benefit of detecting these cancers earlier in their clinical course. Newer low-penetrance but high-prevalence hereditary breast, hereditary ovary, and HBOC genes challenge this paradigm, and there is controversy as to how carriers of these genes should be screened.

Mammography and clinical breast examination (CBE) are well-accepted screening methods for women at average risk of breast cancer, showing a survival benefit, although time to initiate screening and screening intervals remain controversial. The United States Preventive Services Task Force recommends biennial mammography screening in women aged 50 to 74 years, whereas the National Comprehensive Cancer Network (NCCN) guidelines recommend annual CBE and mammography beginning at age 40 years for women at average risk.[15] However, the mean ages of breast cancer in *BRCA1* and *BRCA2* carriers are 39.9 years and 42.3 years, respectively, prompting the idea that screening must begin at an earlier age in the *BRCA1/2* carrier population to be effective.[16] Compounding this issue is the poor sensitivity of mammography for detection of breast cancer in young women with dense breasts. A seminal study from the Netherlands in women at high familial risk of breast cancer followed 1198 young women (median age <40 years), including 143 *BRCA1/2* carriers, with mammography and CBE. In the carrier group, the investigators found a ratio of 23.7 for observed/expected cancers, but a sensitivity of only 56% for the screening method used.[17]

This result has led to several clinical trials evaluating earlier age, multimodality imaging (MRI and mammography) screening protocols in women with an increased risk of breast cancer. Note that most of these studies have included patients at increased risk of breast cancer as defined by different risk models, not only *BRCA1/2* carriers. The increased risk is also heterogeneously defined, with some using the BRCAPRO model and others the Gail model to estimate risk, some studies using 15% 10-year risk and others 20% 10-year risk as eligibility. Also, none of these studies obeys a true randomized controlled trial design, with most being prospective cohort studies evaluating a specific screening strategy and the test characteristics of the component imaging techniques. Several large, multicenter, prospective trials were published between 2001 and 2010 showing improved sensitivity for cancer detection with screening strategies using MRI compared with mammography/CBE.[18–25]

Among the studies performed, a few are noteworthy in view of their design, and are summarized in **Table 1**. The Ontario study group is one of the largest to study a cohort restricted to *BRCA1/2* carriers. In 2004, Warner and colleagues[20] published a prospective cohort study in which they screened 236 mutation carriers with a combined screening regimen of CBE, mammography, ultrasonography, and MRI annually for up to 3 years. They showed a sensitivity of 95% for the combined modality screening, 77% for MRI alone, and 45% for mammography and CBE. This finding underscored the poor performance of conventional screening techniques in *BRCA1/2* carriers, and established potential benefit to MRI. A follow-up prospective cohort study published in 2011 by the same group evaluated whether MRI screening reduced the incidence of advanced-stage breast cancer. The investigators followed 1275 women with *BRCA1/2* mutation, 445 of whom were enrolled in an MRI screening trial using a similar combined screening regimen for up to 5 years and 830 in the comparison group for whom a screening regimen was not specified but who were recommended at least annual mammography and CBE. At 6 years, the cumulative incidence of stage II to IV breast cancer was lower for the MRI-screened cohort (1.9%) than for the comparison group (6.6%; $P = .02$), although the incidence of all invasive breast cancer was the same between the groups. Although not a randomized trial, this was one of the few trials in *BRCA1/2* carriers to have a control group for comparison.[26]

Although these and other trials have shown the likely benefit to incorporating MRI into screening strategies of high-risk women and *BRCA1/2* carriers in particular, other recent trials have called into question the utility of other imaging modalities when quality-assured MRI is used. The 2010 EVA trial screened 687 women with increased familial risk with CBE, mammography, ultrasonography, and MRI with median follow-up of 29 months. The cancer yield with MRI alone was better than with mammography plus ultrasonography, and the addition of mammography or ultrasonography to MRI did not significantly improve cancer yield. A subgroup in this study also had 6-month interval mammography and ultrasonography, but this strategy did not lead to increased cancer detection.[27] The Austrian Screening Trial for Familial Breast Cancer, also a prospective cohort study, confirmed that MRI has a higher sensitivity than mammography and ultrasonography, without significant improvement in detection of cancer with the addition of mammography or ultrasonography.[28] However, there remains concern about the sensitivity of MRI for ductal carcinoma in situ, so mammography is still recommended by guidelines such as the NCCN high-risk guidelines. Thus, the available data for screening in *BRCA1/2* carriers come from nonrandomized prospective cohort studies, most of which included women without *BRCA1/2* mutation but who were deemed at high familial risk for breast cancer. The existing data support the incorporation of MRI into breast cancer screening of women with *BRCA1/2* mutation but questions remain as to the impact on breast cancer mortality as well as the specific screening regimen and intervals to be used.

Chemoprevention Trials in Hereditary Breast and Ovarian Cancer

Few studies have investigated the role of chemoprevention in *BRCA1/2* carriers. The only agents with established efficacy in prevention in breast cancer in the general population are antiestrogen therapies, but these are only effective in preventing estrogen receptor–positive breast cancer. However, triple-negative breast cancers are much more common, especially in *BRCA1* carriers, so the role for antiestrogen therapy seems to be more limited in this population. An analysis for germline mutations of 288 patients who developed breast cancer in the National Surgical Adjuvant Breast and Bowel Project (NSABP) P1 Breast Cancer Prevention Trial using tamoxifen revealed 19 patients with pathogenic BRCA1/2 mutations, 8 with BRCA1 mutation and 11 BRCA2 mutation. Based on the number of patients who received tamoxifen in each group, tamoxifen was found to reduce the incidence of breast cancer by 63% in the *BRCA2* group and to not affect breast cancer incidence in healthy *BRCA1* carriers.[29] The study design and the small number of events should influence how these conclusions are interpreted, but these are the only prospective data on the effect of tamoxifen in asymptomatic *BRCA1/2* carriers. Data for tamoxifen secondary prevention in *BRCA1/2* carriers who have had breast cancer come primarily from a case-control study that compared tamoxifen use between *BRCA1/2* carriers with bilateral and unilateral (control) breast cancer. When tamoxifen was used for 2 to 4 years, the risk of contralateral breast cancer was reduced by 75%. They also found a benefit in *BRCA1* carriers, in contrast with the NSABP-P1 study.[30,31]

Surgical Trials in Hereditary Breast and Ovarian Cancer

Knowing the high rates of breast and ovarian cancer in patients with hereditary risk, prophylactic surgeries were offered with only retrospective data to support the practice until the early 2000s. Meijers-Heijboer and colleagues[32] prospectively followed a cohort of 139 women with a pathogenic *BRCA1/2* mutation but no personal history of breast cancer, 76 of whom opted for prophylactic bilateral mastectomy. They found no breast cancers in the mastectomy group but 8 in the control group in nearly 3 years of follow-up, establishing a reduction in risk of breast cancer with prophylactic mastectomy.[32] The PROSE (Prevention and Observation of Surgical Endpoints) study group prospectively followed an even larger cohort of 483 women with *BRCA1/2* mutation and no prior history of breast cancer, 105 whom underwent prophylactic bilateral mastectomy and 378 matched controls who did not. Two (1.9%) women in the mastectomy group and 184 (48.4%) in the control group developed breast cancer, resulting in a greater than 90% reduction in the incidence of breast cancer with bilateral mastectomy.[33] The risk reduction from contralateral mastectomy in a cohort of only *BRCA1/2* carriers with unilateral breast cancer has not been studied prospectively, but is supported by retrospective data.[34]

Bilateral salpingo-oophorectomy (BSO) has also been offered as a prophylactic risk-reduction strategy to women with HBOC, particularly BRCA1/2 carriers. This

Table 1
Select trials in hereditary breast and ovarian cancer

	Design	Population	Size	Intervention	Major Findings
Screening Trials					
Warner et al,[20] 2004	Prospective cohort	BRCA1/2 carriers	236	1–3 annual screening examinations with MRI, mammogram, ultrasonography	Sensitivity for combined screening 95% vs 45% with mammogram + CBE
Warner et al,[26] 2011	Prospective cohort with comparison group	BRCA1/2 carriers	1275 (445 intervention, 830 comparison)	CBE, mammogram, MRI, ultrasonography for 5 y	Cumulative incidence stage II–IV breast cancer at 6 y 1.9% in MRI group vs 6.6% in comparison group (P = .02)
Kuhl et al,[27] 2010	Prospective cohort	Asymptomatic women at increased familial risk (>20%)	687	CBE, mammogram, MRI, ultrasonography read in different combinations	Cancer yield highest with MRI, no improvement with addition of mammogram/ultrasonography
Riedl et al,[28] 2015	Prospective cohort	BRCA1/2 carriers and women at increased familial risk (>20%)	559	CBE, mammogram, MRI, ultrasonography read in different combinations	Sensitivity MRI 90% vs mammography 37.5% vs ultrasonography 37.5% (P<.001); 2 cancers found by mammography alone
Chemoprevention Trials					
King et al,[29] 2001	Retrospective analysis NSABP-P1	BRCA1/2 carriers with breast cancer	228	Tamoxifen	Tamoxifen reduced the risk of primary breast cancer in BRCA2 carriers, but not in BRCA1 carriers
Narod et al,[30] 2000	Case-control study	BRCA1/2 carriers with bilateral and unilateral cancer	—	Tamoxifen	Tamoxifen reduced the risk of contralateral breast cancer in BRCA1 and BRCA2 carriers with history of breast cancer

Surgical Trials

Study	Study design	Population	N	Intervention	Findings
Meijers-Heijboer et al,[32] 2001	Prospective cohort with control	BRCA1/2 carriers	139 (76 mastectomy, 63 control)	Prophylactic mastectomy	Prophylactic bilateral total mastectomy reduced breast cancer incidence at 3 y mean follow-up
Rebbeck et al,[33] 2004	Prospective cohort with matched control	BRCA1/2 carriers	483 (105 mastectomy, 378 control)	Prophylactic mastectomy	Prophylactic mastectomy reduced breast cancer incidence at 6.4 y mean follow-up
Kauff et al,[35] 2002	Prospective cohort with control	BRCA1/2 carriers	170 (98 BSO, 72 control)	Prophylactic oophorectomy	Prophylactic oophorectomy reduced breast BRCA-related gynecologic cancer incidence (HR = 0.25) at 24 mo mean follow-up
Finch et al,[37] 2006	Prospective cohort with control	BRCA1/2 carriers	1828	Prophylactic oophorectomy	Prophylactic oophorectomy reduced risk of BRCA-related gynecologic cancer by 80%
Kauff et al,[38] 2008	Prospective cohort with control	BRCA1 and BRCA2 carriers	1079	Prophylactic oophorectomy	Prophylactic oophorectomy reduced risk of BRCA1-associated gynecologic cancer (HR = 0.11) and BRCA2-associated breast cancer (HR = 0.27)

Treatment Trials

Study	Study design	Population	N	Intervention	Findings
Kaufman et al,[41] 2015	Prospective, nonrandomized phase II trial	Germline BRCA1/2 carriers with platinum-resistant (or platinum-ineligible) ovarian cancer	193 (in ovarian cancer cohort)	Olaparib 400 mg BID	Tumor response rate 31% and 40% stable disease at >8 wk

Abbreviations: BID, twice a day; BSO, bilateral salpingo-oophorectomy; HR, hazard ratio; NSABP, National Surgical Adjuvant Breast and Bowel Project.

strategy was done initially from retrospective data showing a lower incidence of breast and gynecologic cancers with prophylactic BSO in this population, but there were concerns regarding a risk of primary peritoneal cancer after oophorectomy.[35,36] The PROSE study group reported on a matched retrospective cohort of 551 BRCA1/2 carriers, finding a 96% risk reduction in cancers of the coelomic epithelium and 53% risk reduction in breast cancer after Kauff and colleagues[35] conducted the first prospective follow-up study, wherein 170 women were enrolled and 98 chose BSO, whereas the remaining 72 chose surveillance. Their data showed a hazard ratio of 0.15 for BRCA-related gynecologic cancer (including primary peritoneal cancer) and of 0.35 for breast cancer after risk-reducing bilateral salpingo-oopherectomy (RRBSO). A larger study enrolled 1828 BRCA1/2 carriers and found an 80% reduction in risk of BRCA-associated gynecologic cancer with BSO.[37] Another large multicenter prospective study was conducted to separately evaluate the effect of RRBSO between BRCA1 and BRCA2 carriers, given the difference in the receptor phenotype between the respective breast cancers seen in these populations and the differing risks of BRCA-associated gynecologic cancers. The investigators enrolled 1079 women with a pathologic BRCA1 or BRCA2 mutation, and found that, in 3 years of follow-up, there were statistically significant reductions in the risk of BRCA1-associated gynecologic cancer and BRCA2-associated breast cancer, but not in BRCA1-associated breast cancer or BRCA2-associated gynecologic cancer, although there was a suggestion of risk-reducing effect on the last two diseases as well.[38]

Treatment Trials in Hereditary Breast and Ovarian Cancer

The increased understanding of the mechanism of genes implicated in HBOC has led to exciting new developments in targeted therapeutics. BRCA1 and BRCA2 are involved in the DNA repair machinery, specifically in homologous recombination.[39] Poly(ADP-ribose) polymerase (PARP) inhibitors have thus been developed as agents that cause tumor cell death in cells that are homologous-recombination deficient.[40] The PARP inhibitor, olaparib, was the first in class to be approved in the United States and the European Union (EU) for use specifically in germline mutated BRCA ovarian cancer, and this approval was based on results of a phase II single-arm trial that included multiple tumor types.[41] Another PARP inhibitor, rucaparib, has been approved as monotherapy in patients with BRCA1/2 mutant advanced ovarian cancer after 2 lines of prior therapy, but, notably, the mutation can be either somatic or germline. This approval too was based on the results of a nonrandomized, single-arm, phase II trial.[42] However, many more trials, including randomized phase III trials, are underway to investigate the role for PARP inhibitors in the management of BRCA-related HBOC.

RANDOMIZED CONTROLLED TRIALS IN FAMILIAL ADENOMATOUS POLYPOSIS AND CARRIERS OF GERMLINE MUTATIONS IN ADENOMATOUS POLYPOSIS COLI

FAP, previously known as Gardner syndrome, is an uncommon hereditary cancer syndrome with a prevalence of ~1 in 7000 to 1 in 10,000.[43] FAP manifests clinically with development of colorectal adenomatous polyposis in the early to late teens, with risk of CRC approaching 100% before age 50 years. Rarer presentations of FAP include hepatoblastoma in infants and diagnosis after discovery of supernumerary teeth during a routine dental examination. Other manifestations of FAP include upper gastrointestinal (GI) tract polyposis of the stomach and the duodenum and increased relative risks of cancer in these organs, papillary thyroid cancers, and other noncancer manifestations such as desmoid tumors, osteomas, and chronic hypertrophy of the retinal pigment epithelium (CHRPE). Molecularly, FAP is characterized by germline and, most frequently, truncating mutations of the *APC* gene with resultant dysregulation of the WNT signaling pathway.[44] *APC* mutations show a genotype-phenotype correlation, with mutational regions along the *APC* gene identified that correspond with higher risks of dense polyposis, desmoid disease, and CHRPE.[45] In addition, an attenuated version of FAP has also been characterized, and is most commonly found among individuals with mutations nearer the 3' and 5' terminals of the gene.[43]

An important consideration when evaluating the results of trials in patients with FAP conducted in the 1990s and 2000s is that there is unmeasured genetic heterogeneity among participants in these studies. Although patients recruited at the time these trials were conducted had a clinical polyposis syndrome that phenotypically resembled FAP, it is now known that only a portion have a germline *APC* mutation. Others may have biallelic mutations in the *MUTYH* gene, a mutation in *POLE* or *POLD1*, genes also associated with autosomal dominant inheritance of diffuse polyposis, or the *NTHL1* gene.[46]

Chemoprevention of Adenomatous Polyps in Patients with Familial Adenomatous Polyposis

Most randomized clinical trials in patients with FAP have evaluated the benefits of chemoprevention agents in reducing polyp number and size in the lower (colorectum) and upper (duodenum) GI tracts. The agents most tested have been the cyclooxygenase (COX)-1 enzyme inhibitor aspirin and nonsteroidal antiinflammatory drugs (NSAIDs; mainly sulindac), and COX-2 inhibitors (primarily celecoxib) based on ample data in the general population that these agents can reduce the risk of colorectal polyps and CRC.[47,48] At the molecular level, it is inhibition of the COX-1 and COX-2 enzymes and downstream prostaglandin synthesis by aspirinlike drugs and NSAIDs in the colorectal epithelium that seems to be critical in CRC prevention, and has been associated with adenoma initiation, growth, and progression to cancer.[47,48] A list of RCTs in patients with FAP, including chemopreventive agents focused on prevention of lower and upper GI tract polyposis, is provided in **Table 2**.

Chemoprevention of Colorectal Adenomas in Patients with Familial Adenomatous Polyposis

The first RCT to show compelling evidence of chemoprevention in patients with FAP was published by Giardiello and colleagues[49] in 1993. In this study, 22 patients with FAP were randomized to 9 months of twice a day doses of 150 mg of the oral NSAID sulindac (Clinoril) versus placebo. Patients had colonoscopy to evaluate polyp burden every 3 months for 1 year. Statistically significant reductions in number and size of adenomas (both >50% from baseline) were observed for subjects randomized to sulindac. These benefits began to diminish once sulindac was stopped, but polyp number and size did not return fully to baseline levels even at 3 months following discontinuation. No adverse events were attributed to sulindac, and overall compliance with dosing was reported as 85%. A subsequent but smaller trial by Nugent and colleagues[50] in 1993 confirmed these findings in 12 patients with FAP-associated rectal polyposis who had undergone previous subtotal colectomy. Patients were randomized to sulindac 200 mg twice a day versus placebo, and a statistically significant ($P = .01$) improvement in polyp status (a visual assessment of polyposis in the rectum) was reported.

Although infrequent side effects were reported in early prevention trials using NSAIDs, subsequent RCTs investigated the benefits of selective COX-2 inhibitors in polyp prevention in patients with FAP. Steinbach and colleagues[51] in 2000

Table 2
Randomized controlled trials in chemoprevention of familial adenomatous polyposis lower and/or upper gastrointestinal polyposis

RCT	Agents Studied	n	Target Site	Population	Significant Results
Burn et al,[57] 2011	Aspirin 600 mg/resistant starch 30 mg vs placebo (2 × 2 factorial)	133	Lower GI	An age of ≥10 y and ≤21 y and confirmed or a high likelihood of the presence of FAP. FAP status was determined by molecularly confirmed APC mutation or by the determination of having a high probability of carrying the mutation from linked DNA markers or the presence of multiple colonic polyps	Neither intervention significantly reduced polyp count in the rectum or sigmoid colon There was a nonsignificant trend of a reduced number of polyps and the size of the largest polyps in the overall aspirin group vs the nonaspirin group for those treated >1 y. Resistant starch had no clinical effect on adenomas
Giardiello et al,[49] 1993	Sulindac 150 mg BID vs placebo	22	Lower GI	Patients with FAP who either had not undergone colectomy or had undergone subtotal colectomy with ileorectal anastomosis (clinical diagnosis of FAP)	44% decrease in the number of polyps and 35% in size of polyps (P = .001) in sulindac 150 mg arm. No side effects from sulindac were reported
Giardiello et al,[72] 2002	Sulindac 75 mg or sulibdac 150 mg vs placebo	41	Lower GI	Young patients with FAP (8–25 y) genotypically affected with FAP (had genetic testing for APC mutation), phenotypically unaffected (no endoscopically detectable colorectal adenomatous polyps and no history of colonic surgery)	No significant difference in the number or size of polyps between groups
Higuchi et al,[73] 2003	Rofecoxib 25 mg vs placebo Note: rofecoxib (Vioxx) was taken off the market in 2004	21	Lower GI	Patients with clinical diagnosis of FAP. Patients with attenuated FAP were not included	6.8% reduction in polyp number in rofecoxib 25 mg arm vs placebo (P = .004). Significant reduction in the polyp size as well (P<.001)

Study	Treatment	N		Inclusion Criteria	Findings
Lynch et al,[52] 2016	Celecoxib vs celecoxib + DFMO	112	Lower GI	Patients 18–65 y of age with clinical diagnosis of FAP	No significant difference in adenoma count was seen between 2 study arms. Fatigue is the only significant adverse event, worse on celecoxib arm
West et al,[54] 2010	EPA-FFA 2g vs placebo	55	Lower GI	Patients ≥18 y of age with clinical diagnosis of FAP	Treatment with EPA-FFA for 6 mo was associated with 22.4% reduction in polyp number ($P = .012$) and 29.8% decrease in polyp size ($P = .027$) in EPA-FFA arm vs placebo. EPA-FFA was well tolerated with an incidence of AE similar to placebo
van Heumen et al,[61] 2013	Celecoxib 400 mg + UDCA vs celecoxib + placebo	37	Upper GI	The diagnosis FAP was established either clinically, by the presence of >100 colorectal polyps, or genetically, by the presence of APC gene mutations. Eligible patients were between 18 and 70 y of age	Celecoxib-alone treatment reduces duodenal polyp density in patients with FAP, and, unexpectedly, high dose UDCA cotreatment counteracts this effect ($P = .014$); 81% reported 1 or more adverse event
Nugent et al,[50] 1993	Sulindac 200 mg BID vs placebo	24	Upper GI	Patients with FAP and advanced duodenal polyposis (Spigelman stage 3 or 4)	Sulindac was associated with a reduction in epithelial cell proliferation in the duodenum and a trend toward duodenal polyp regression. In the rectum, cell proliferation showed a marked reduction, and significant ($P = .01$) polyp regression was seen
Parc et al,[60] 2012	UDCA vs placebo	71	Upper GI	Patients aged 18–65 y with diagnosis of FAP with proven APC mutation or clinical diagnosis of FAP	UCDA given for 2 y had no effect on the evolution and severity of duodenal adenomas of patients with FAP. No side effects or change in digestive function were observed

(continued on next page)

Table 2
(continued)

RCT	Agents Studied	n	Target Site	Population	Significant Results
Phillips et al,[58] 2002	Celecoxib 100 mg BID vs 400 mg BID vs placebo	83	Upper GI	Clinical diagnosis of FAP. Some of the patients were tested for APC mutation	A reduction was found in duodenal polyposis after 6 mo of treatment with celecoxib 400 mg vs placebo (14.5% vs 1.4%, $P = .436$). Higher reduction for patients with clinically significant disease (>5% covered by polyps) at baseline (31% vs 8%, $P = .049$)
Steinbach et al,[51] 2000	Celecoxib 100 mg or 400 mg vs placebo	77	Lower GI	Patients aged 18–65 y with clinical diagnosis of FAP	Treatment with celecoxib 400 mg was associated with 28% reduction in the number of polyps ($P = .003$), and 30.7% in size of polyps ($P = .001$) Statistically significant reductions were not observed in the celecoxib 100 mg group
Samadder et al,[62] 2016	Sulindac + erlotinib vs placebo	92	Upper GI	Patients aged 18–69 y with proven pathogenic APC mutation or a clinical diagnosis of FAP	The use of sulindac + erlotinib vs placebo resulted in a lower duodenal polyp burden after 6 mo. Author reported frequency of adverse events in 83% of participants; 29% with grade 2 or 3 adverse events

Abbreviations: AE, adverse event; DFMO, difluoromethylornithine; EPA, eicosapentaenoic acid; UDCA, ursodeoxycholic acid.

randomized 77 patients with FAP to placebo versus celecoxib 100 or 400 mg twice a day for 6 months. Relative to placebo, those patients randomized to 400 mg of celecoxib twice daily had a 28% reduction in the mean adenoma number ($P = .003$) and a 31% reduction in the overall adenoma burden (a score equaling the sum of polyp diameters) ($P = .001$). Statistically significant reductions were not observed in the celecoxib 100 mg group. Adverse events were reported in 57% of those randomized to celecoxib 400 twice a day, including diarrhea (19%) and abdominal pain (7%). More recently, an RCT tested celecoxib 400 mg twice a day alone versus the same dose in combination with difluoromethylornithine (DFMO), a treatment of African trypanosomiasis and inhibitor of ornithine decarboxylase, an enzyme predicted to be key in the production of carcinogenic polyamines in colorectal mucosa.[52,53] In total, 112 patients with FAP were randomized to celecoxib alone or celecoxib plus DFMO. The study's primary end point was not met: DFMO plus celecoxib failed to reduce adenoma count more than celecoxib alone. Studies of DFMO in the FAP prevention setting are ongoing. In a second study, West and colleagues[54] in 2010 evaluated another agent in patients with FAP with preexisting polyps, the omega-3 polyunsaturated fatty acid eicosapentaenoic acid (EPA), in an RCT in patients with FAP with retained rectum after colectomy.[55] In total, 55 patients were evaluated (EPA-free fatty acid (FFA), 28; placebo, 27). EPA-FFA for 6 months reduced mean polyp number by 22.4% (95% confidence interval, 5.1%–39.6%; $P = .012$) and reduced polyp size by 29.8% (3.6%–56.1%; $P = .027$). EPA-FFA was well tolerated, with an incidence of adverse events similar to placebo.

RCTs have also evaluated early chemoprevention of FAP-associated polyposis in young patients. In the first study, Giardiello and colleagues[56] in 2004 randomized 41 young subjects with FAP who had not yet manifested polyposis (ages 8–25 years) to 75 mg versus 150 mg of sulindac orally twice a day versus placebo. Disappointingly, the primary outcome was not met: sulindac failed to prevent polyp development, with polyps developing in 43% of patients receiving celecoxib and 55% of those receiving placebo ($P = .54$). Size and number of polyps were also no different between the study arms. More recently, Burn and colleagues[57] in 2011 enrolled adolescents aged 10 to 21 years with FAP in a 2×2 factorial design RCT to study the effects of aspirin (600 mg orally daily) and resistant starch (30g orally day) versus placebo on colorectal polyposis. Of 206 randomized subjects, 133 completed at least 1 follow-up colonoscopy. Neither aspirin nor starch showed a significant benefit in reducing polyp number in this population. However, aspirin did show a trend toward reducing polyp size, with more benefit seen in those treated for more than 1 year.

Chemoprevention of Upper Gastrointestinal Adenomas

With total colectomy in the 20s being the standard of care for managing patients with FAP, several trials have moved to investigate chemoprevention of the rarer, but surgically technically more challenging, upper GI tract (duodenum) polyposis among patients with FAP. An early RCT by Nugent and colleagues[50] in 1993 failed to show a reduction in duodenal polyposis with sulindac 200 mg by mouth twice a day. In 2002, Phillips and colleagues[58] randomized 83 patients with FAP and upper GI polyposis to celecoxib 100 mg twice a day, 400 mg twice a day, or placebo. Patients randomized to celecoxib 400 mg twice daily experienced a 15% statistically nonsignificant overall reduction of involved polyposis. A subgroup analysis of those patients with the most severe polyposis found that this group experienced a statistically significant reduction in polyposis (31% vs 8% on placebo; $P = .049$).

Ursodeoxycholic acid (UDCA) or ursodiol has been under investigation as a chemopreventive agent for many years because of its antiapoptotic properties, especially in the GI tract.[59] Parc and colleagues[60] in 2012 reported on the results of an RCT of UDCA versus placebo in patients with FAP (n = 71) with duodenal polyposis, but this was a negative trial with no differences in posttreatment polyposis burden seen. A second RCT combined celecoxib plus UDCA versus celecoxib plus placebo and evaluated the impact on duodenal polyposis.[61] Surprisingly, UDCA seemed to counteract the benefits of celecoxib, with patients randomized to the dual drug arm (celecoxib plus UDCA) developing worsening polyp density.

In 2016, Samadder and colleagues[62] broke new ground with their *JAMA* publication evaluating erlotinib, a US Food and Drug Administration–approved oral cancer therapy in lung and pancreatic cancers targeted to the epithelial growth factor receptor, in the prevention of FAP-associated upper GI polyposis. In this RCT, patients with FAP with duodenal polyposis received either sulindac plus erlotinib or sulindac plus placebo. The investigators reported a statistically significant reduction in polyp burden and polyp number in patients randomized to the dual intervention (sulindac plus erlotinib). In total, 29% of subjects had grade 2 or 3 adverse events, most commonly rash, which was seen in 87% of those treated with erlotinib. Further studies are warranted, including RCTs that evaluate optimal dosing to mitigate side effects for this novel indication.

Summary of Randomized Controlled Trials in Familial Adenomatous Polyposis

Multiple RCTs have investigated the efficacy of chemopreventive agents in the prevention of upper and lower GI polyposis in patients with FAP. Several agents have shown the ability to decrease polyp burden and polyp size in the colon, rectum, and duodenum, including sulindac and celecoxib. In patients with FAP and upper GI polyposis or lower GI polyposis in a rectal remnant, these agents may be appropriate to help control polyp growth. Nonetheless, the negative trial by Giardello and colleagues[56] in 2004 of sulindac in the setting of primary polyp prevention urges caution among providers about the ability of chemopreventive agents to suppress new polyposis and/or prevent cancers in this disease. More RCTs are needed, and the recent data from Samadder and colleagues[62] from 2016 are an encouraging first step in the use of targeted agents like erlotinib in this disease.

RANDOMIZED CONTROLLED TRIALS IN LYNCH SYNDROME/HEREDITARY NONPOLYPOSIS COLORECTAL CANCER

LS or HNPCC is the among most common hereditary CRC syndromes, with most recent estimates projecting that ~1 in 280 individuals in the population is a carrier of a germline mutation in one of the 4 clinically relevant MMR proteins MLH1, MSH2, MSH6, and PMS2.[63] MMR deficiency is characterized by an increased rate of mutation in daughter cells following DNA replication, with the most vulnerable region of the genome being areas of DNA base pair repeats called microsatellites, which tend to shorten or lengthen during DNA replication, a process that is detectable by tumor-based testing.[64] Like the germline *APC* mutations of FAP, LS is inherited in an autosomal dominant fashion. Thus, a second somatic hit is required for MMR deficiency to manifest in a daughter cell and lead to cancer.[63] Overall, germline mutations in *PMS2* and *MSH6* seem to be more common in the general population relative to *MLH1* and *MSH2*,[6] but seem to cause a more attenuated LS phenotype with overall lower lifetime risks of CRC and endometrial cancer and later onset disease.[63] Cancer risks in LS include CRC, endometrial cancer, stomach cancer, ovarian cancer, and several other rarer cancers, with risks ranging from 20% to 80% lifetime risk for

CRC depending on the gene affected.[63] Screening and management guidelines from the NCCN are an excellent resource for interested providers.[14]

Overall, the authors found the number of RCTs conducted in patients with LS to be limited. A summary of the studies discussed here is provided in **Table 3**.

Randomized Clinical Trials Associated with Colorectal Cancer Screening in Lynch Syndrome

Although several prospective trials are evaluating new endoscopic techniques, only 2 RCTs have assessed new forms of CRC screening in LS/HNPCC and 1 RCT has studied colonic preparation regimens before colonoscopy. In 2008, Stoffel and colleagues[65] reported the results of an RCT that examined the value of chromoendoscopy (intervention) compared with standard endoscopy alone. This technique uses narrow-band light plus a special dye to visualize precancerous lesions at a smaller and earlier stage[66] and in theory could offer an advantage for cancer prevention in high-risk persons. Chromoendoscopy is among several advanced colorectal imaging techniques, including narrow-band imaging and autofluorescence endoscopy, that have shown potential advantage in high-risk populations like the LS population.[66] In the Stoffel and colleagues[65] trial, 54 patients with clinically and molecularly diagnosed LS were randomized to standard colonoscopy or standard colonoscopy plus chromoendoscopy. The study failed to meet its primary outcome (improved detection of adenomas). A second study of chromoendoscopy, by Rahmi and colleagues[67] in 2015, randomized 78 patients with genetically proven LS to standard colonoscopy versus standard colonoscopy plus pancolonic chromoendoscopy. Contrary to the findings of Stoffel and colleagues,[65] this study showed a significant benefit in improved detection of adenomas (total detected was higher in the intervention arm) and in the proportion of patients with at least 1 adenoma detected. Nonetheless, national guidelines for LS management do not endorse chromoendoscopy for all patients with LS.[14] Related to colonoscopy, an RCT conducted by van Vugt van Pinxteren and colleagues[68] in 2012 evaluated the efficacy of precolonoscopy prep (enema) by polyethylene glycol electrolyte (PEG) versus sodium phosphate (NaP). Results favored PEG for quality of preparation in the cecum (42% vs 22% excellent) and in the ascending colon (11% vs 2% excellent). However, disappointingly, only 27.2% of patients had an excellent result after preparation with either formulation, and patients preferred the inferior performing regimen (NaP).

Randomized Clinical Trials of Chemoprevention in Lynch Syndrome

Only 1 RCT of chemoprevention in LS has been reported, but its results are highly noteworthy and await recapitulation in another trial. In a study by Burn and colleagues[69,70] in 2008, known as Cancer Prevention Programme 2, 746 individuals with molecular and genetic diagnoses of LS were randomized to 2 interventions in a 2 × 2 factorial design: 600 mg of acetylsalicylic acid per day versus placebo and 30 mg/d of resistant starch versus placebo. Although the primary outcome (reduction in incidence of intestinal neoplasm) in the intention-to-treat population was not met, a subgroup analysis of patients who were able to sustain use of aspirin for 25 months or more showed a significant reduction in the incidence of CRC (63% reduction in incidence of CRC; $P = .008$) and non-CRC LS cancers at 4 years. Like chromoendoscopy, the NCCN Guidelines Committee has not fully endorsed the use of 600 mg of aspirin for all LS mutation carriers until additional studies confirm these results.[14]

Table 3
Randomized controlled trials in Lynch syndrome

RCT	Agents Studied	n	Target Site	Population	Significant Results
Clinical Studies					
Burn et al,[69] 2008	Aspirin 600 mg, resistant starch (Novelose) 30 g vs placebo (2 × 2 factorial)	746	Lower GI polyp prevention	Adults with LS (clinical diagnosis and genetic diagnosis)	Neither aspirin 600 mg nor resistant starch 30 mg alone or in combination, given for up to 4 y has any detectable effect on the incidence of intestinal neoplasms among adults with LS
Burn et al,[70] 2011	Aspirin 600 mg, resistant starch (Novelose) 30 g vs placebo (2 × 2 factorial)	861	Lower GI polyp prevention	Adults with LS (clinical diagnosis and genetic diagnosis)	600 mg aspirin per day for a mean of 25 mo reduced incidence of colorectal cancer with the effect becoming apparent after 3–4 y from the start of aspirin intervention
Rahmi et al,[67] 2015	Colonoscopy vs colonoscopy + pancolonic chromoscopy	78	Lower GI polyp detection	Asymptomatic adults aged ≥30 y with LS (genetic diagnosis: germline mutation in one of the *MMR* genes)	Standard colonoscopy followed by pancolonic chromocolonoscopy doubled both the total number of adenomas detected and the proportion of patients with at least 1 adenoma detected compared with standard colonoscopy alone ($P<.001$)

Study	Intervention	N	Outcome	Population	Results
Van Vugt van Pinxteren et al,[68] 2012	PEG solution vs NaP	116	Lower GI prep adequacy for scope	LS gene carriers	Excellent clean colon only in 27.6% of the participants, regardless of the bowel cleansing. Significant difference in an excellent clean cecum was found in favor for PEG preparation (42% vs 22%). In the ascending colon the quality of bowel cleansing was significantly poorer in the NaP group (11% vs 2%). Patients with Lynch tolerated NaP better and preferred this formula for future bowel preparation. Nausea and feeling cold were side effects of both the PEG and NaP groups
Stoffel et al,[65] 2008	Colonoscopy vs colonoscopy + chromoendoscopy	54	Lower GI polyp detection	Adults aged ≥18 y with LS (clinical diagnosis and genetic diagnosis)	Chromoendoscopy did not detect more missing adenomas than intensive standard white-light colonoscopy examinations
Biomarker Studies					
Lu et al,[71] 2013	OCP vs Depo-Provera (Depo-MPA)	51	Endometrial proliferation	Women aged 25–50 y with a known mutation in MLH1, MSH2, or MSH6, or personal history of an LS-associated cancer. No prior hysterectomy, pelvic radiation, chemotherapy	Both OCP and Depo-MPA induced a dramatic decrease in endometrial proliferation as measured by Ki-67. Depo-MPA mean before 51.8%; mean after 13.1% ($P<.001$); and OCP mean before 48.3%, mean after 3.1% ($P<.001$)

Abbreviations: OCP, oral contraceptive pill; PEG, polyethylene glycol electrolyte.

Randomized Biomarker Studies in Lynch Syndrome

Although the primary focus of this article is clinical studies with primary cancer end points, one biomarker trial in LS is important to note. In 2013, Lu and colleagues[71] reported the results of an RCT of 51 women aged 25 to 50 years with a molecular diagnosis of LS or a history or an LS-associated cancer. A pre-post design was used, so although subjects were randomized, they served as their own controls for analyses. The study compared the benefits of oral contraceptive pills (OCPs) versus Depo-medroxyprogesterone acetate (MPA) (Depo-Provera) on biomarkers of endometrial proliferation in high-risk individuals. Both OCPs and Depo-Provera decreased Ki-67 by a significant degree (Depo-MPA 51.8% to 13.1%, $P<.001$; OCPs 48.3% to 3.1%, $P<.001$). Although not definitive, this finding suggests a potential chemoprevention benefit in women with LS with an intact uterus.

Summary of Randomized Controlled Trials in Lynch Syndrome/Hereditary Nonpolyposis Colorectal Cancer

A paucity of RCTs have been conducted in LS/HNPCC. At present, clinical guidelines are primarily based on expert recommendations and accumulated evidence from prospective cohort studies among individuals with clinical and/or molecular diagnoses of LS. To date, RCTs have shown promise for chromoendoscopy when paired with traditional colonoscopy for CRC screening, but larger trials are needed to establish benefit. One important RCT has shown substantial protective benefit from daily aspirin use in LS; a follow-up trial examining other dosing levels is currently accruing.

REFERENCES

1. Schrader KA, Cheng DT, Joseph V, et al. Germline variants in targeted tumor sequencing using matched normal DNA. JAMA Oncol 2016;2(1):104–11.
2. Hall MJ, Daly MB, Ross EA, et al. Germline variants in cancer risk genes detected by NGS-based comprehensive tumor genomic profiling (CGP). J Clin Oncol 2015;33(15):11084.
3. Raymond CM, Stoffel EM, Innis JW, et al. Inherited gastrointestinal cancer diagnoses in a tumor-normal sequencing project. Paper presented at: Collaborative Group of the Americas Annual Meeting. Baltimore (MD), October 11-12, 2015.
4. Ellingson MS, Hart SN, Kalari KR, et al. Exome sequencing reveals frequent deleterious germline variants in cancer susceptibility genes in women with invasive breast cancer undergoing neoadjuvant chemotherapy. Breast Cancer Res Treat 2015;153(2):435–43.
5. Johnston JJ, Rubinstein WS, Facio FM, et al. Secondary variants in individuals undergoing exome sequencing: screening of 572 individuals identifies high-penetrance mutations in cancer-susceptibility genes. Am J Hum Genet 2012; 91(1):97–108.
6. Win AK, Jenkins MA, Dowty JG, et al. Prevalence and penetrance of major genes and polygenes for colorectal cancer. Cancer Epidemiol Biomarkers Prev 2016; 26(3):404–12.
7. Maxwell KN, Domchek SM, Nathanson KL, et al. Population frequency of germline BRCA1/2 mutations. J Clin Oncol 2016;34(34):4183–5.
8. Hall MJ, Egleston B, Miller SM, et al. Barriers to participation in cancer prevention clinical trials. Acta Oncol 2010;49(6):757–66.
9. Lynce F, Isaacs C. How far do we go with genetic evaluation? Gene, panel, and tumor testing. Am Soc Clin Oncol Educ Book 2016;35:e72–8.

10. Slavin TP, Niell-Swiller M, Solomon I, et al. Corrigendum: clinical application of multigene panels: challenges of next-generation counseling and cancer risk management. Front Oncol 2015;5:271.

11. Ramus SJ, Song H, Dicks E, et al. Germline mutations in the BRIP1, BARD1, PALB2, and NBN genes in women with ovarian cancer. J Natl Cancer Inst 2015;107(11) [pii:djv214].

12. Balmaña J, Domchek SM. BRIP1 as an ovarian cancer susceptibility gene: ready for the clinic? J Natl Cancer Inst 2015;107(11) [pii:djv262].

13. Win AK, Dowty JG, Cleary SP, et al. Risk of colorectal cancer for carriers of mutations in MUTYH, with and without a family history of cancer. Gastroenterology 2014;146(5):1208–11.e1-5.

14. NCCN guidelines colorectal prevention. 2017. Available at: https://www.nccn.org/store/login/login.aspx?ReturnURL=https://www.nccn.org/professionals/physician_gls/pdf/colon.pdf. Accessed January 13, 2017.

15. Bevers TB, Anderson BO, Bonaccio E, et al. NCCN clinical practice guidelines in oncology: breast cancer screening and diagnosis. J Natl Compr Canc Netw 2009;7(10):1060–96.

16. Rebbeck TR, Mitra N, Wan F, et al. Association of type and location of BRCA1 and BRCA2 mutations with risk of breast and ovarian cancer. JAMA 2015;313(13): 1347–61.

17. Brekelmans C, Seynaeve C, Bartels C, et al. Effectiveness of breast cancer surveillance in BRCA1/2 gene mutation carriers and women with high familial risk. J Clin Oncol 2001;19(4):924–30.

18. Warner E, Plewes D, Shumak R, et al. Comparison of breast magnetic resonance imaging, mammography, and ultrasound for surveillance of women at high risk for hereditary breast cancer. J Clin Oncol 2001;19(15):3524–31.

19. Kriege M, Brekelmans CT, Boetes C, et al. Efficacy of MRI and mammography for breast-cancer screening in women with a familial or genetic predisposition. N Engl J Med 2004;351(5):427–37.

20. Warner E, Plewes DB, Hill KA, et al. Surveillance of BRCA1 and BRCA2 mutation carriers with magnetic resonance imaging, ultrasound, mammography, and clinical breast examination. JAMA 2004;292(11):1317–25.

21. MARIBS Study Group. Screening with magnetic resonance imaging and mammography of a UK population at high familial risk of breast cancer: a prospective multicentre cohort study (MARIBS). Lancet 2005;365(9473):1769–78.

22. Kuhl CK, Schrading S, Leutner CC, et al. Mammography, breast ultrasound, and magnetic resonance imaging for surveillance of women at high familial risk for breast cancer. J Clin Oncol 2005;23(33):8469–76.

23. Hagen AI, Kvistad KA, Maehle L, et al. Sensitivity of MRI versus conventional screening in the diagnosis of BRCA-associated breast cancer in a national prospective series. Breast 2007;16(4):367–74.

24. Sardanelli F, Podo F, D'Agnolo G, et al. Multicenter comparative multimodality surveillance of women at genetic-familial high risk for breast cancer (HIBCRIT study): interim results 1. Radiology 2007;242(3):698–715.

25. Rijnsburger AJ, Obdeijn I-M, Kaas R, et al. BRCA1-associated breast cancers present differently from BRCA2-associated and familial cases: long-term follow-up of the Dutch MRISC Screening Study. J Clin Oncol 2010;28(36):5265–73.

26. Warner E, Hill K, Causer P, et al. Prospective study of breast cancer incidence in women with a BRCA1 or BRCA2 mutation under surveillance with and without magnetic resonance imaging. J Clin Oncol 2011;29(13):1664–9.

27. Kuhl C, Weigel S, Schrading S, et al. Prospective multicenter cohort study to refine management recommendations for women at elevated familial risk of breast cancer: the EVA trial. J Clin Oncol 2010;28(9):1450–7.

28. Riedl CC, Luft N, Bernhart C, et al. Triple-modality screening trial for familial breast cancer underlines the importance of magnetic resonance imaging and questions the role of mammography and ultrasound regardless of patient mutation status, age, and breast density. J Clin Oncol 2015;33(10):1128–35.

29. King M-C, Wieand S, Hale K, et al. Tamoxifen and breast cancer incidence among women with inherited mutations in BRCA1 and BRCA2: National Surgical Adjuvant Breast and Bowel Project (NSABP-P1) Breast Cancer Prevention Trial. JAMA 2001;286(18):2251–6.

30. Narod SA, Brunet J-S, Ghadirian P, et al. Tamoxifen and risk of contralateral breast cancer in BRCA1 and BRCA2 mutation carriers: a case-control study. Lancet 2000;356(9245):1876–81.

31. Gronwald J, Tung N, Foulkes WD, et al. Tamoxifen and contralateral breast cancer in BRCA1 and BRCA2 carriers: an update. Int J Cancer 2006;118(9):2281–4.

32. Meijers-Heijboer H, van Geel B, van Putten WL, et al. Breast cancer after prophylactic bilateral mastectomy in women with a BRCA1 or BRCA2 mutation. N Engl J Med 2001;345(3):159–64.

33. Rebbeck TR, Friebel T, Lynch HT, et al. Bilateral prophylactic mastectomy reduces breast cancer risk in BRCA1 and BRCA2 mutation carriers: the PROSE Study Group. J Clin Oncol 2004;22(6):1055–62.

34. Van Sprundel T, Schmidt M, Rookus M, et al. Risk reduction of contralateral breast cancer and survival after contralateral prophylactic mastectomy in BRCA1 or BRCA2 mutation carriers. Br J Cancer 2005;93(3):287–92.

35. Kauff ND, Satagopan JM, Robson ME, et al. Risk-reducing salpingo-oophorectomy in women with a BRCA1 or BRCA2 mutation. N Engl J Med 2002;346(21):1609–15.

36. Rebbeck TR, Lynch HT, Neuhausen SL, et al. Prophylactic oophorectomy in carriers of BRCA1 or BRCA2 mutations. N Engl J Med 2002;346(21):1616–22.

37. Finch A, Beiner M, Lubinski J, et al. Salpingo-oophorectomy and the risk of ovarian, fallopian tube, and peritoneal cancers in women with a BRCA1 or BRCA2 Mutation. JAMA 2006;296(2):185–92.

38. Kauff ND, Domchek SM, Friebel TM, et al. Risk-reducing salpingo-oophorectomy for the prevention of BRCA1-and BRCA2-associated breast and gynecologic cancer: a multicenter, prospective study. J Clin Oncol 2008;26(8):1331–7.

39. Farmer H, McCabe N, Lord CJ, et al. Targeting the DNA repair defect in BRCA mutant cells as a therapeutic strategy. Nature 2005;434(7035):917–21.

40. Konecny G, Kristeleit R. PARP inhibitors for BRCA1/2-mutated and sporadic ovarian cancer: current practice and future directions. Br J Cancer 2016; 115(10):1157–73.

41. Kaufman B, Shapira-Frommer R, Schmutzler RK, et al. Olaparib monotherapy in patients with advanced cancer and a germline BRCA1/2 mutation. J Clin Oncol 2015;33(3):244–50.

42. Kristeleit R, Swisher E, Oza A, et al. 2700 Final results of ARIEL2 (Part 1): A phase 2 trial to prospectively identify ovarian cancer (OC) responders to rucaparib using tumor genetic analysis. Eur J Cancer 2015;51:S531.

43. Jasperson KW, Patel SG, Ahnen DJ. APC-Associated Polyposis Conditions. In: Pagon RA, Adam MP, Ardinger HH, et al, editors. GeneReviews® [Internet]. Seattle (WA): University of Washington, Seattle; 1993-2017.

44. Clevers H, Nusse R. Wnt/beta-catenin signaling and disease. Cell 2012;149(6): 1192–205.
45. Nielsen M, Bik E, Hes FJ, et al. Genotype-phenotype correlations in 19 Dutch cases with APC gene deletions and a literature review. Eur J Hum Genet 2007; 15(10):1034–42.
46. Valle L. Recent discoveries in the genetics of familial colorectal cancer and polyposis. Clin Gastroenterol Hepatol 2017;15(6):809–19.
47. Drew DA, Cao Y, Chan AT. Aspirin and colorectal cancer: the promise of precision chemoprevention. Nat Rev Cancer 2016;16(3):173–86.
48. Hawk ET, Umar A, Viner JL. Colorectal cancer chemoprevention – an overview of the science. Gastroenterology 2004;126(5):1423–47.
49. Giardiello FM, Hamilton SR, Krush AJ, et al. Treatment of colonic and rectal adenomas with sulindac in familial adenomatous polyposis. N Engl J Med 1993; 328(18):1313–6.
50. Nugent KP, Farmer KC, Spigelman AD, et al. Randomized controlled trial of the effect of sulindac on duodenal and rectal polyposis and cell proliferation in patients with familial adenomatous polyposis. Br J Surg 1993;80(12):1618–9.
51. Steinbach G, Lynch PM, Phillips RK, et al. The effect of celecoxib, a cyclooxygenase-2 inhibitor, in familial adenomatous polyposis. N Engl J Med 2000;342(26):1946–52.
52. Lynch PM, Burke CA, Phillips R, et al. An international randomized trial of celecoxib versus celecoxib plus difluoromethylornithine in patients with familial adenomatous polyposis. Gut 2016;65(2):286–95.
53. Meyskens FL, Gerner EW. Development of difluoromethylornithine (DFMO) as a chemoprevention agent. Clin Cancer Res 1999;5(5):945–51.
54. West NJ, Clark SK, Phillips RK, et al. Eicosapentaenoic acid reduces rectal polyp number and size in familial adenomatous polyposis. Gut 2010;59(7):918–25.
55. Kim B, Giardiello FM. Chemoprevention in familial adenomatous polyposis. Best Pract Res Clin Gastroenterol 2011;25(4–5):607–22.
56. Giardiello FM, Casero RA Jr, Hamilton SR, et al. Prostanoids, ornithine decarboxylase, and polyamines in primary chemoprevention of familial adenomatous polyposis. Gastroenterology 2004;126(2):425–31.
57. Burn JD, Bishop TD, Chapman PD. A randomized placebo-controlled prevention trial of aspirin and/or resistant starch in young people with familial adenomatous polyposis. Cancer Prev Res 2011;4(5):655–65.
58. Phillips RKS, Wallace MH, Lynch PM, et al. A randomised, double blind, placebo controlled study of celecoxib, a selective cyclooxygenase 2 inhibitor, on duodenal polyposis in familial adenomatous polyposis. Gut 2002;50(6):857–60.
59. Serfaty L, Bissonnette M, Poupon R. Ursodeoxycholic acid and chemoprevention of colorectal cancer. Gastroenterol Clin Biol 2010;34(10):516–22.
60. Parc Y, Desaint B, Flejou JF, et al. The effect of ursodesoxycholic acid on duodenal adenomas in familial adenomatous polyposis: a prospective randomized placebo-control trial. Colorectal Dis 2012;14(7):854–60.
61. van Heumen BW, Roelofs HM, Vink-Borger ME, et al. Ursodeoxycholic acid counteracts celecoxib in reduction of duodenal polyps in patients with familial adenomatous polyposis: a multicentre, randomized controlled trial. Orphanet J Rare Dis 2013;8:118.
62. Samadder NJ, Neklason DW, Boucher KM, et al. Effect of sulindac and erlotinib vs placebo on duodenal neoplasia in familial adenomatous polyposis: a randomized clinical trial. JAMA 2016;315(12):1266–75.

63. Kohlmann W, Gruber SB. GeneReviews. Lynch syndrome. 2014. Available at: https://www.ncbi.nlm.nih.gov/books/NBK1211/. Accessed January 13, 2017.

64. Boland CR, Goel A. Microsatellite instability in colorectal cancer. Gastroenterology 2010;138(6):2073–87.e3.

65. Stoffel EM, Turgeon DK, Stockwell DH, et al. Missed adenomas during colonoscopic surveillance in individuals with Lynch syndrome (hereditary nonpolyposis colorectal cancer). Cancer Prev Res (Phila) 2008;1(6):470–5.

66. Haanstra JF, Kleibeuker JH, Koornstra JJ. Role of new endoscopic techniques in Lynch syndrome. Fam Cancer 2013;12(2):267–72.

67. Rahmi G, Lecomte T, Malka D, et al. Impact of chromoscopy on adenoma detection in patients with Lynch syndrome: a prospective, multicenter, blinded, tandem colonoscopy study. Am J Gastroenterol 2015;110(2):288–98.

68. van Vugt van Pinxteren MW, van Kouwen MC, van Oijen MG, et al. A prospective study of bowel preparation for colonoscopy with polyethylene glycol-electrolyte solution versus sodium phosphate in Lynch syndrome: a randomized trial. Fam Cancer 2012;11(3):337–41.

69. Burn J, Bishop DT, Mecklin JP, et al. Effect of aspirin or resistant starch on colorectal neoplasia in the Lynch syndrome. N Engl J Med 2008;359(24):2567–78.

70. Burn J, Gerdes AM, Macrae F, et al. Long-term effect of aspirin on cancer risk in carriers of hereditary colorectal cancer: an analysis from the CAPP2 randomised controlled trial. Lancet 2011;378(9809):2081–7.

71. Lu KH, Loose DS, Yates MS, et al. Prospective multicenter randomized intermediate biomarker study of oral contraceptive versus depo-provera for prevention of endometrial cancer in women with Lynch syndrome. Cancer Prev Res 2013;6(8): 774–81.

72. Giardiello FM, Yang VW, Hylind LM, et al. Primary chemoprevention of familial adenomatous polyposis with sulindac. N Engl J Med 2002;346(14):1054–9.

73. Higuchi T, Iwama T, Yoshinaga K, et al. A randomized, double-blind, placebo-controlled trial of the effects of rofecoxib, a selective cyclooxygenase-2 inhibitor, on rectal polyps in familial adenomatous polyposis patients. Clin Cancer Res. 2003;9(13):4756–60.

Randomized Controlled Trials in Neuroendocrine Tumors

John C. McAuliffe, MD, PhD[a], Edward M. Wolin, MD[b],*

KEYWORDS

- Neuroendocrine tumor • Somatostatin • Clinical trial • Carcinoid

KEY POINTS

- Neuroendocrine tumors are a diverse group of tumors with variable clinical presentation and biological behavior, making evaluation, diagnosis, and treatment planning difficult in the absence of an experienced multidisciplinary team.
- Treatment is predicated on accurate staging and biologic work-up; namely, the differentiation, grade, and presence of somatostatin receptors.
- Somatostatin analogues, mammalian target of rapamycin inhibitors, receptor tyrosine kinase inhibitors, antiangiogenics, targeted radiopeptides, immune therapy, and cytotoxic chemotherapy have shown efficacy in the treatment of neuroendocrine tumors.
- Multidisciplinary evaluation and treatment are recommended to give patients with neuroendocrine tumors the best chance at a durable survival with optimal quality of life.

INTRODUCTION

Carcinoid tumor was identified more than 100 years ago. The term carcinoid described a carcinomalike tumor with an indolent course. These tumors arise from the resident endocrine cells with the gastrointestinal (GI) tract and lung as the predominant sites of occurrence, and are designated endocrine tumors because of their endocrine and paracrine function and the resemblance to endocrine cells elsewhere, as in the pancreas. Submucosal endocrine cells can be found in multiple organs, including pancreas, lungs, thymus, upper respiratory tract, ovary, uterine cervix, bladder, prostate, kidney, and biliary tree, but the great preponderance are in the GI tract.

Well-differentiated neuroendocrine malignancies are referred to as tumor, neoplasia, carcinoid, or neuroendocrine tumor, whereas poorly differentiated tumors

Disclosures: The authors have nothing to disclose.
[a] Department of Surgery, Montefiore-Einstein Center for Cancer Care, 1521 Jarrett Place, Suite 207, Bronx, NY 10461, USA; [b] Neuroendocrine Tumor Program, Division of Medical Oncology, Department of Medicine, Montefiore-Einstein Center for Cancer Care, 1695 Eastchester Road, 2nd Floor, Bronx, NY 10461, USA
* Corresponding author.
E-mail address: ewolin@montefiore.org

represent small cell carcinoma. At present, neuroendocrine tumors are divided into grade 1 and grade 2 based on their proliferative rate and are also discriminated by their differentiation (**Table 1**). This pathologic reporting is paramount in a multidisciplinary discussion regarding management of neuroendocrine tumors.

Localized tumors rarely produce symptoms unless obstructive. Many of these tumors are found incidentally during endoscopic evaluation or cross-sectional imaging and are already metastatic. Up to 35% of these tumors release vasoactive peptides such as serotonin, histamine, or tachykinins, causing clinical syndromes, including carcinoid syndrome.[1] Typical manifestations of functional neuroendocrine tumors are episodic flushing, wheezing, diarrhea, glycemic instability, hypertension, weight change, cosmetic change, and heart disease.[2] Discussion of these syndromes is beyond the scope of this article, but astute physicians must assess for symptoms to appropriately evaluate patients with neuroendocrine tumors.

The prevailing axiom in the management of neuroendocrine tumor is that treatment should be influenced by the distribution and bulk of tumor, the biology of the tumor, and the severity and manner of the associated symptoms. Once determined to treat, physicians target the systems that propel the metastatic machinery of neuroendocrine tumor: DNA repair, somatostatin receptor signaling, receptor tyrosine kinase signaling, and mammalian target of rapamycin (mTOR) signaling. There are no curative interventions for metastatic neuroendocrine tumor. Therefore, managing the patient's expectations of observation or therapeutic intervention remains a critical aspect of cancer care in this disease. This article provides a review of the important randomized controlled trials that have shaped the management of neuroendocrine tumor over the last 2.5 decades (**Table 2**).

CYTOTOXIC CHEMOTHERAPY

In 1992, a multi-institutional study conducted by the Eastern Cooperative Oncology Group (ECOG) was published presenting the outcomes of the randomized controlled trial studying the effect of streptozocin plus fluorouracil, streptozocin plus doxorubicin, or chlorozotocin alone in the treatment of advanced pancreatic neuroendocrine tumor.[3] Previous reports supported the use of these agents in the treatment of neuroendocrine tumor and provided the rationale for this randomized control trial. Patients were randomly assigned after stratification according to the ECOG performance score to 1 of the 3 arms. After failure of therapy, patients were randomly assigned to receive alternative arms of therapy. An intention-to-treat analysis was performed on the outcome measures to determine efficacy. One-hundred and twenty-five patients were enrolled between 1978 and 1985. However, only 105 patients received therapy.

Table 1			
Classification of neuroendocrine tumors			
Grade	**GI and Pancreatic**	**Lung and Thymic Tumors**	**Differentiation**
Low (G1)	<2 mitoses/10 HPF and/or <3% Ki-67 index	<2 mitoses/10 HPF and no necrosis	Well
Intermediate (G2)	2–20 mitoses/10 HPF and/or 3%–20% Ki-67 index	2–10 mitoses/10 HPF and/or foci of necrosis	Well
High (G3)	>20 mitoses/10 HPF and/or >20% Ki-67 index	>10 mitoses/10 HPF	Poor

Abbreviation: HPF, high-power field.

Table 2
Published important randomized trials for neuroendocrine tumors

Study	Study Group	Disease	Intervention	Control	Outcome of Primary End Point	Limitation	Significance
Moertel et al,[3] 1992		Advanced/metastatic NET	Streptozocin plus doxorubicin; chlorozotocin	Streptozocin plus 5-FU	Tumor response 69% vs 45% and 30%; OS 2.2 vs 1.4 and 1.5 y	Mixed histologies; treatment not well tolerated	Streptozocin plus doxorubicin standard of care for advanced NET
Jacobsen et al,[7] 1995		Metastatic NET with carcinoid symptoms	Octreotide SC	Placebo	Flushing, diarrhea, quality of life improved	Few patients	Confirmed octreotide SC can benefit symptoms of carcinoid syndrome
Rubin et al,[9] 1999		Advanced/metastatic NET with carcinoid symptoms	Octreotide LAR	Octreotide SC	Control of symptoms equivalent	New tumor response assessment	Octreotide LAR as good as octreotide SC; octreotide LAR standard for control of carcinoid symptoms
Arnold et al,[8] 2005		Metastatic GI and pancreatic NET	Octreotide SC plus interferon α	Octreotide SC	Treatment failure equivalent at 50%; survival 51 vs 35 mo ($P = .55$)	Not powered for survival	Combination therapy not superior; somatostatin blockade alone is the standard
Rinke et al,[13] 2009	PROMID	Advanced/metastatic well-differentiated NET	Octreotide LAR	Placebo	Time to tumor progression 14.3 vs 6.0 mo	Crossover allowed and OS no different. Low-grade tumors have low hepatic metastasis volume	Octreotide LAR standard of therapy for both functional and nonfunctional advanced NETs

(continued on next page)

Table 2
(continued)

Study	Study Group	Disease	Intervention	Control	Outcome of Primary End Point	Limitation	Significance
Pavel et al,[21] 2011	RADIANT-2	Advanced/metastatic well-differentiated, grade 1 or 2 NET with carcinoid symptoms	Everolimus plus octreotide LAR	Octreotide LAR	Median PFS 16.4 vs 11.3 mo (P = .026)	Imbalanced randomization in favor of placebo. Not powered adequately for predefined statistical benchmarks. P value not significant	Everolimus (mTOR blockade) seems to be an active agent in NET
Yao et al,[22] 2011	RADIANT-3	Advanced/metastatic well-differentiated, grade 1 or 2 pancreatic NET	Everolimus	Placebo	Median PFS 11 vs 4.6 mo (P<.001)	Crossover allowed and no change in OS; symptoms of carcinoid not evaluated; only pancreatic NET included	Everolimus is a standard regimen for advanced/ metastatic, progressive, pancreatic NET
Raymond et al,[24] 2011		Advanced/metastatic, well-differentiated, progressive pancreatic NET	Sunitinib	Placebo	Median PFS 11.4 vs 5.5 mo (P<.01)	Study interrupted at interim analysis because of serious events in placebo arm	Sunitinib is an active agent in progressive, well-differentiated pancreatic NETs
Caplin et al,[15] 2014	CLARINET	Advanced/metastatic well-differentiated, grade 1 or 2, nonfunctioning, somatostatin receptor–positive GI or pancreatic NET	Lanreotide	Placebo	PFS not reached vs 18 mo	OS same because of crossover; tumor stable at inclusion rather than progressive; nonfunctioning tumors	Lanreotide has efficacy in well-differentiated, grade 1 and 2 NETs and is well tolerated

Study	Population	Treatment	Control	Outcome	Comments	Conclusion
Wolin et al,[16] 2015	Advanced/metastatic GI NETs with poorly controlled carcinoid symptoms	Pasireotide LAR	Octreotide LAR	Symptoms control 20.9% vs 26.7% (P = .53)	PFS post hoc analysis; pasireotide causes nausea and hyperglycemia	Octreotide LAR remains the standard for advanced/metastatic NET with carcinoid symptoms
RADIANT-4 Yao et al,[23] 2016	Advanced/metastatic, nonfunctional, well-differentiated, grade 1 or 2 GI or pulmonary NET	Everolimus	Placebo	Median PFS 11 vs 3.9 mo (P<.01)	45% of patients treated with everolimus censored at analysis	Everolimus has activity in a variety of NETs and is a standard regimen for progressive NET
Vinik et al,[12] 2016 ELECT	Advanced/metastatic NETs with carcinoid symptoms	Lanreotide	Placebo	Use of rescue octreotide for carcinoid symptoms 33.7% vs 48.5% (P = .017)	Patients treated with placebo were not receiving long-acting octreotide analogues	Lanreotide controls symptoms of carcinoid
Kulke et al,[17] 2017	Metastatic, well-differentiated NET with refractory carcinoid symptoms	Telotristat ethyl	Placebo	BM frequency improvement 44% and 42% vs 20% (OR = 3.49)	Different somatostatin analogues used at baseline	Telotristat ethyl may benefit those with refractory symptoms of carcinoid and represents a second-line therapy
NETTER-1 Strosberg et al,[18] 2017	Advanced/metastatic midgut somatostatin receptor–positive, well-differentiated, grade 1 or 2 NET	177 Lu-Dotatate	Octreotide LAR	PFS 65.2% vs 10.8% at 20 mo	Inclusion of patients required somatostatin receptor positivity by scintigraphy	177 Lu-Dotatate has efficacy in progressive, refractory, somatostatin receptor–positive NET

Abbreviations: BM, bowel movement; 5-FU, 5-fluorouracil; LAR, long-acting release; NET, neuroendocrine tumor; OS, overall survival; PFS, progression-free survival; SC, subcutaneous.

Three patients did not have evaluation of their response, which left 102 patients for analysis. Patients randomized to the 3 arms were well balanced for age, time from diagnosis, ECOG performance status, and endocrine abnormality. Importantly, functional and nonfunctional tumors were included in this study.

Patients treated with doxorubicin and streptozocin had a statistically greater rate of regression compared with the other 2 arms. The median duration of response for the doxorubicin plus streptozocin arm was 18 months compared with 14 months for fluorouracil plus streptozocin, and 17 months for the chlorozotocin arm ($P = .005$). Eleven patients had durable regression in the doxorubicin plus streptozocin group, providing 2 or more years of disease control. The median overall survival for the patients treated with doxorubicin plus streptozocin was 2.2 years, as opposed to 1.5 years for the other treatment arms ($P = .001$). Toxicity was evaluated in this trial. Patients treated with streptozocin had significant toxicities compromising quality of life and compliance. Despite this, the trial provided evidence for standard therapy for streptozocin plus doxorubicin for fit patients diagnosed with advanced pancreatic neuroendocrine tumor.

An anticipated trial is ongoing evaluating alternative cytotoxic chemotherapeutics for pancreatic neuroendocrine tumors. ECOG has sponsored a study evaluating temozolomide with or without capecitabine (CAPTEM) for advanced pancreatic neuroendocrine tumors (clinicaltrials.gov NCT01824875). The rationale is supported by preclinical studies showing synergistic induction of apoptosis in neuroendocrine cell lines. Likewise, multiple clinical studies suggest this combination's efficacy.[4] Stable disease with temozolomide combinations can be as high as 68%. One such study showed that, in patients with metastatic, well-differentiated pancreatic neuroendocrine tumor, CAPTEM was an active agent.[5] This study's primary outcome was objective response rate. Thirty patients received treatment and 70% had a radiographic response with a median progression-free survival of 18 months. Congruent results are anticipated from the ongoing phase II clinical trial, which will provide mounting evidence for a change in the standard first-line cytotoxic chemotherapeutic regimen for metastatic pancreatic neuroendocrine tumors.

SOMATOSTATIN ANALOGUE THERAPIES

Somatostatin was first discovered in hypothalamic tissue in the 1970s and has paninhibitory effects on GI peptides. However, its clinical use is limited by a short half-life. In the 1980s, analogues of somatostatin, namely octreotide, were brought into clinical use. Studies were not randomized but showed efficacy in relieving symptoms and decreasing tumor marker levels.[6] These early studies provided the rationale for randomized controlled trials, which began to appear in the late 1990s. Somatostatin required dosing subcutaneously every 8 hours and was used at that time principally for acromegaly and carcinoid syndrome. A small randomized study proved its utility in this regard.[7] Eleven consecutive patients with midgut metastatic neuroendocrine tumor or pancreatic neuroendocrine tumor were randomized to octreotide or placebo. Patients were followed for 8 weeks. Mean 5-Hydroxyindoleacetic acid (5-HIAA) levels and symptoms were improved significantly with octreotide compared with placebo ($P<.05$). In addition, patients treated with octreotide reported an improved quality of life ($P<.05$). However, this study did not evaluate for response to therapy by tumor burden. Although this was a small study, it confirmed the mounting evidence of the efficacy of octreotide treatment in this disease.

An alternative to subcutaneous octreotide, interferon-alfa was reported to result in stabilization or tumor shrinkage of neuroendocrine tumors. It was unknown whether interferon-alfa was better than or equivalent to octreotide. Therefore, a randomized controlled trial was performed accruing patients between 1995 and 1998 with metastatic midgut and pancreatic neuroendocrine tumors.[8] At the time of recruitment, octreotide Long-Acting Release (LAR) was not available. Patients were treated with subcutaneous octreotide thrice daily or subcutaneous octreotide thrice daily plus interferon-alfa thrice weekly. Patients were stratified based on symptoms, age, location of the primary tumor, prior chemotherapy, and prior octreotide therapy. Tumor progression was the primary outcome of this study. Secondary outcomes of the study were biochemical response adverse events, and quality of life. Of the 125 patients registered for the study, 105 patients were evaluable (51 monotherapy, 54 combination). Importantly, 11 of the 54 patients discontinued combination therapy because of side effects compared with 2 of 51 receiving monotherapy. The patients treated with both octreotide and interferon-alfa had a lower global quality of life than patients treated with octreotide alone ($P = .039$). Symptomatic biochemical responses were essentially the same between treatment arms. Treatment response was likewise equivalent in the 2 arms. The median follow-up times were 32 months and 54 months for monotherapy and combination therapy, respectively. The median survival time was 35 months for those treated with monotherapy versus 51 months for those treated with combination ($P = .55$). Patients responding to either treatment had improved survival overall compared with those who did not respond to treatment ($P = .006$). In light of the decreased quality of life of the combination arm and the nonsuperior response, combination octreotide and interferon-alfa is not recommended in the treatment of midgut and pancreatic neuroendocrine tumors.

Administration of octreotide was challenging. It required subcutaneous dosing every 8 hours, limiting its feasibility. A series of long-acting formulations were developed through the 1990s to improve this shortcoming of therapy.

Octreotide acetate, also known as octreotide LAR, consists of microspheres of poly-DL-lactide-co-glycolide glucose containing octreotide. The pharmacokinetics of this formulation allowed once-a-month dosing. The goal of this formulation was to improve patient compliance and quality of life while providing similar efficacy to subcutaneous octreotide. This treatment was studied in a multicenter randomized control trial published in 1999[9] comparing the efficacy of 10 mg, 20 mg, and 30 mg of octreotide LAR (Sandostatin) versus subcutaneous octreotide every 8 hours in the control of carcinoid symptoms. Efficacy was defined by the degree and duration of suppression of carcinoid symptoms as indicated by the use of subcutaneous rescue therapy. In addition, 24-hour urinary 5-HIAA was sampled. Safety assessments were likewise performed. Ninety-three patients constituted the intention-to-treat analysis, with 79 patients returning for at least a 20-week follow-up. Once at steady state, octreotide LAR had equivalent efficacy compared with subcutaneous octreotide. The efficacy of the 20-mg octreotide LAR dosage was superior with regard to symptomatic control at steady state compared with the 10-mg dose. In addition, the 20-mg dose had equivalent efficacy compared with the 30-mg dose. Therefore, the recommended dose was 20 mg of octreotide LAR to replace subcutaneous octreotide as standard of care for carcinoid symptoms.

Lanreotide is another long-acting somatostatin analogue and its efficacy in the management of carcinoid symptoms for GI neuroendocrine tumors was studied and published in 1999.[10] This trial was a phase 2 study conducted at 7 European sites. Eligible patients were diagnosed with malignant GI neuroendocrine tumor with symptoms related to hormone production (48 with carcinoid, 6 with gastrinoma, 1 with VIPoma). Intradermal injections were given every 2 weeks for a 6-month period and symptoms, biochemical markers, echocardiography, quality of life, and tumor size were evaluated. Fifty-five patients were included in the study. Twelve (22%) patients discontinued lanreotide during the study, with a mean duration of treatment of 20.7 weeks. Symptomatic or biochemical improvement was achieved in most patients. Four patients had progression in tumor size, whereas the remainder had stable disease with only 2 patients having tumor regression. Quality of life was also improved with lanreotide.

Shortly after publication of this study, results of a randomized control trial were published evaluating lanreotide versus subcutaneous octreotide in patients with carcinoid syndrome.[11] Somatostatin analogue–naive patients were eligible for the trial if they had diarrhea or flushing. This prospective, open, comparative study with crossover design was performed for 35 patients at 15 different centers. Quality of life, clinical symptoms, and tumor markers were analyzed. Patients were also asked which treatments they would rather have: octreotide or lanreotide. After randomization, the treatment groups were well matched. The intensity of flushes and diarrhea as well as the mean stools per day were not statistically different between the 2 groups. The mean number of flushes per day was less in the lanreotide-treated patients ($P = .05$). There was no statistically significant difference in the quality of life. To summarize, subcutaneous octreotide and lanreotide were essentially equivalent in this study. However, most patients preferred the simplified mode of lanreotide administration, suggesting lanreotide as a more feasible therapy for long-term control of carcinoid symptoms. Another randomized trial evaluating the efficacy and safety of lanreotide in the control of carcinoid syndrome was published recently (ELECT).[12] A total of 115 patients were enrolled to receive lanreotide versus placebo in a randomized, double-blind, phase III trial. Patients were able to use short-acting octreotide for a rescue medication for control of carcinoid symptoms. The need for short-acting octreotide rescue was 14.8% less for those treated with lanreotide ($P = .017$). The odds for treatment success were significantly greater with lanreotide compared with placebo (odds ratio [OR], 2.4; $P = .036$).

The first randomized controlled study assessing the efficacy of octreotide LAR as an antiproliferative agent was performed by the PROMID study group and published in 2009.[13] Patients with locally inoperable or metastatic midgut well-differentiated neuroendocrine tumor were randomized to receive octreotide LAR 30 mg versus placebo. The primary end point was time to tumor progression. Treatment-naive patients were stratified and randomized based on tumor functionality, presence of distant metastasis, Ki-67, and age. Ninety patients were registered between 2001 and 2008. At the interim analysis, 26 patients had progression or tumor-related death in the octreotide LAR group compared with 40 in the placebo group. Median time to tumor progression was 14.3 months in the octreotide LAR group compared with 6 months in the placebo group ($P<.001$). Symptomatic response as well as biochemical response was seen more frequently in those treated with octreotide LAR. Both treatment groups had equivalent quality of life and treatment with octreotide LAR was tolerated with no treatment-related deaths. A follow-up study was performed recently assessing long-term survival from this PROMID study.[14] An important aspect of the PROMID study was the potential for crossover at the time of progression. Of the 43 patients randomized to the placebo arm, 38 crossed over and received octreotide LAR at progression. The study was not powered to detect a survival benefit of octreotide LAR. However, tumor burden was a predictor of long-term survival, and progression-free survival is an appropriate outcome measure for studying neuroendocrine tumor.

The largest and most important randomized controlled trial evaluating the antiproliferative effects of a somatostatin analogue was called CLARINET.[15] Lanreotide was used for the treatment of neuroendocrine tumors of the GI tract and pancreas. This study was a double-blind, placebo controlled, multinational study. Eligible patients were those with somatostatin receptor positive, locally advanced or metastatic sporadic, nonfunctioning neuroendocrine tumors, well-differentiated or moderately differentiated, with a Ki-67 less than 10% and mitotic index of less than 2 mitoses per 10 high-power fields. Patients were excluded if they had received previous interferon, octreotide, chemoembolization, chemotherapy, or a radionucleotide. Patients were given deep subcutaneous injections of either 120 mg of lanreotide or placebo every 28 days in a 96-week period. The primary end point of the study was progression-free survival. Secondary end points included overall survival, time to tumor progression, quality of life, chromogranin A level, and safety. End points were analyzed on an intention-to-treat population basis. A total of 204 patients were registered between 2006 and 2013. The median progression-free survival was not reached in those patients treated with lanreotide, versus 18 months in those who received placebo ($P<.001$). At 24 months, the estimated progression-free survival was 65.1% in the lanreotide group and 33% in the placebo group. Overall survival did not differ significantly between the 2 groups, likely related to the ability to cross over and receive lanreotide after progression on the placebo arm. Forty-two percent of those treated with lanreotide had an improvement in the chromogranin A levels compared with 5% in the placebo arm. Safety of treatment was no different between the 2 groups. Lanreotide provided a prolonged progression-free survival for those with gut and pancreatic neuroendocrine tumors. With definitive proof of efficacy, the subcutaneous administration of lanreotide is the approved treatment of metastatic neuroendocrine tumors that are somatostatin receptor positive.

Another somatostatin analogue, called pasireotide (SOM230), has better specificity and affinity for somatostatin receptors 1 to 3 and 5. A randomized control trial was conducted testing the efficacy and safety of pasireotide LAR versus octreotide LAR.[16] The primary end point was symptom control. A secondary end point was progression-free survival. Patients who had inadequately controlled carcinoid symptoms were randomized to receive pasireotide LAR versus octreotide LAR. Patients were required to have histologically confirmed metastatic carcinoid of the digestive system and inadequately controlled symptoms as well as measurable disease on cross-sectional imaging. Patients were stratified based on symptoms. Patients received either 16 mg of pasireotide LAR every 28 days or 40 mg of octreotide LAR every 28 days. Patients on the octreotide arm were allowed to cross over if not responding to treatment. Patients were allowed to have rescue subcutaneous injections of pasireotide or octreotide if needed to control symptoms. One-hundred and ten patients were enrolled between 2008 and 2012. In an intention-to-treat analysis, patients receiving pasireotide LAR or octreotide LAR had equivalent symptom control at 6 months ($P = .53$), and 60.8% of patients treated with pasireotide LAR achieved stable disease compared with 42.3% in those treated with octreotide LAR. However, this result did not approach statistical significance ($P = .57$). Median progression-free survival for those treated with pasireotide LAR was 11.8 months, whereas the median progression-free survival was 6.8 months for those treated with octreotide LAR ($P = .45$). However, treatment was not as well tolerated for those receiving pasireotide LAR. Typical adverse events included hyperglycemia, fatigue, and nausea, with a treatment discontinuation rate of 17% for those receiving pasireotide LAR. The treatment discontinuation rate for those receiving octreotide LAR was 7%. Drug-related serious adverse events occurred more frequently in the pasireotide LAR group (17% compared with 3.5%). This study showed that pasireotide LAR and high-dose octreotide LAR have similar symptom control and suggested improvement in progression-free survival for the pasireotide LAR group. However, because of adverse events, pasireotide is not standard first-line therapy in the treatment of neuroendocrine tumors at this time and requires further study.

Somatostatin analogues are the initial treatment of carcinoid symptoms. However, patients may develop recurrent symptoms despite maximal somatostatin receptor blockade. For these patients, treatments are limited. The pathophysiology of carcinoid syndrome is attributed to the overproduction of serotonin. The rate-limiting enzyme in its synthesis is tryptophan hydroxylase. Inhibition of this enzyme with telotristat ethyl was studied to evaluate the improvement of carcinoid symptoms for those refractory to somatostatin analogue therapy.[17] This international study recruited 135 patients from 2013 to 2015 and randomized patients to placebo versus 2 different doses of telotristat ethyl. Patients treated with telotristat ethyl realized improvements in bowel movement frequency 44% of the time compared with 20% for those treated with placebo (OR, 3.49; confidence interval, 1.33–9.16). Likewise, urine 5-HIAA levels were significantly decreased for those treated with telotristat ethyl compared with placebo. Importantly, telotristat ethyl seemed to be safe and well tolerated. This phase 3 study provides evidence that patients refractory to somatostatin receptor blockade may find relief of carcinoid symptoms with telotristat ethyl.

A long-awaited randomized controlled trial has recently studied somatostatin receptors on neuroendocrine tumors. The NETTER-1 trial investigators studied the efficacy of lutitium^{177} (^{177}Lu)-DOTATATE for midgut neuroendocrine tumors.[18] Octreotate is radiolabeled with ^{177}Lu, which is a beta and gamma emitting radionucleotide with a particle range of 2 mm and a half-life of 160 hours. Previous reports showed up to a 28% remission rate and a median progression-free survival of approximately 33 months for those with advance neuroendocrine tumors. Patients with well-differentiated, somatostatin receptor–positive, metastatic midgut neuroendocrine tumors were treated with ^{177}Lu-DOTATATE plus octreotide LAR or octreotide LAR alone. The primary end point was progression-free survival with secondary end points including response rate, overall survival, safety, and side effect profile. Patients treated with ^{177}Lu-DOTATATE received infusions every 8 weeks for a total of 4 infusions. Between 2012 and 2016, a total of 229 patients were recruited and underwent randomization, whereas 221 patients received the treatment. The groups were well balanced with regard to grade and somatostatin radiotracer uptake. The 20-month progression-free survival was 65.2% for those treated with ^{177}Lu-DOTATATE compared with 10.8% in the control group. The median progression-free survival had not been reached for the ^{177}Lu-DOTATATE group, as opposed to 8.4 months in the control group ($P<.001$). The estimated risk of death was 60% lower in patients treated with ^{177}Lu-DOTATATE. Seventy-seven percent of patients received all 4 infusions of ^{177}Lu-DOTATATE, suggesting it was well tolerated. The most common adverse events among patients treated with ^{177}Lu-DOTATATE were nausea (59%) and vomiting (47%), attributed mostly to the required administration of amino acid infusions with the ^{177}Lu-DOTATATE. Only 1 patient had cytopenia following administration of ^{177}Lu-DOTATATE. Despite treating patients with refractory disease, progressing through octreotide therapy, this study validates the extraordinary efficacy of radiolabeled somatostatin receptor targeting. This study represents a landmark in the treatment of neuroendocrine tumors.

SMALL MOLECULE INHIBITORS OF MAMMALIAN TARGET OF RAPAMYCIN AND RECEPTOR TYROSINE KINASES

mTOR has been implicated in multiple steps in the tumor progression of neuroendocrine tumors, as reviewed elsewhere.[19,20] Everolimus is an oral inhibitor of mTOR that showed activity in phase II trials. The RADIANT study groups issued 3 sequential randomized control trials evaluating the efficacy of everolimus in the treatment of advanced neuroendocrine tumor.

The first, RADIANT-2, evaluated the antitumor activity in patients with advanced or metastatic, low-grade or intermediate-grade, progressive neuroendocrine tumors.[21] Patients were treated with 10 mg of everolimus or placebo combined with octreotide LAR. The treatment was continued until disease progression or until withdrawal of treatment because of adverse events. The primary end point was progression-free survival. Secondary end points included objective response rate, overall survival, and changes in baseline 5-HIAA and chromogranin A concentrations, along with safety. The primary sites of cancer included the small intestine, lung, colon, pancreas, and liver, with most metastatic lesions within the liver. Most patients were previously treated with a somatostatin analogue. Most patients were diagnosed with a well-differentiated tumor. The treatment arms were imbalanced, favoring the placebo arm with regard to the primary tumor site being lung, a worse performance status, and previous use of chemotherapy. Two-hundred and eleven patients were randomized to receive everolimus, whereas 204 received placebo. At a median follow-up of 28 months, the median duration of treatment was 37 weeks in both arms. Dose reductions or interruptions of therapy were required in 65% of those treated with everolimus and 35% treated with placebo. Despite this, the median progression-free survival was 16.4 months for those treated with everolimus and octreotide LAR versus 11.3 months for placebo and octreotide LAR ($P = .026$). Importantly, the statistical strategy prespecified a $P \leq .0246$. Therefore, this difference in progression-free survival was deemed insignificant. However, combined everolimus and octreotide LAR was associated with a 23% reduction in estimated risk for progression. Of patients who could be assessed, 75% in the everolimus plus octreotide LAR group versus 45% in the placebo plus octreotide LAR group experienced tumor shrinkage. Moreover, 84% of patients had stable disease in the everolimus plus octreotide LAR group compared with 81% in the placebo arm. Likewise, patients treated with both everolimus and octreotide LAR had higher degrees of reduction in chromogranin A and 5-HIAA compared with combined placebo and octreotide LAR. Most common adverse events were stomatitis, rash, fatigue, and diarrhea, but most of these were grade 1 or 2. This study was a landmark event. Patients with progressive neuroendocrine tumor despite somatostatin analogue therapy have limited systemic options with diminutive benefit. Results from this study suggested everolimus to be an active agent in this disease. However, this required validation.

In the same year, the RADIANT-3 study was published.[22] This study's focus was solely on low-grade or intermediate-grade pancreatic neuroendocrine tumors. At that point in history, streptozocin was the only approved cytotoxic therapy for pancreatic neuroendocrine tumors. Importantly, treatments were not combined with octreotide LAR. Patients were randomized to receive 10 mg of everolimus daily versus placebo. Treatment continued until progression was evident or adverse events occurred. Patients were recruited between 2007 and 2009 and a total of 410 patients were accrued worldwide. After randomization, the treatment groups were well balanced. At a median follow-up of 17 months, the median duration of treatment with everolimus was 8.8 months compared with 3.7 months for placebo. The median progression-free survival was 11 months in the everolimus group compared with 4.6 months in the placebo group ($P < .001$). This difference represented a 65% reduction in the estimated risk of progression favoring everolimus. A decrease in the size of the target lesion was seen in 64% of patients treated with everolimus as opposed to 21% those treated with placebo. On progression, patients in the placebo arm could cross over to receive everolimus. The overall survival was no different between the 2 groups despite not reaching a median overall survival, the study. Importantly, most patients received prior treatments. Therefore, this study represents a landmark in the treatment of progressive neuroendocrine tumors and provides another well-tolerated therapeutic tool for those with the disease.

Baseline characteristics in the treatment arms of the RADIANT-2 study were implicated for not achieving a statistically significant improvement in progression-free survival for everolimus. Therefore, a repeat randomized controlled trial was performed (RADIANT-4) and recently published.[23] This international multicenter study recruited patients with advanced or metastatic, nonfunctional, well-differentiated neuroendocrine tumors of the lung or GI tract. Those with pancreatic neuroendocrine tumors were excluded as well as those with carcinoid syndrome. Patients were not treated with octreotide LAR, but with everolimus or placebo. The primary end point was progression-free survival with the secondary end point of overall survival. All analyses were performed on an intention-to-treat basis. Three-hundred and two patients were recruited between 2012 and 2013. The treatment arms were well balanced, with 205 patients receiving everolimus and 97 receiving placebo. The median progression-free survival was 11 months in those treated with everolimus versus 3.9 months in those receiving placebo, with a 52% reduction in estimated risk of disease progression or death for those treated with everolimus ($P<.001$). The estimated progression-free survival at 12 months was 44% in those treated with everolimus versus 28% in those receiving placebo, suggesting a durable benefit for those treated with everolimus. A decrease in the target lesion was seen in 64% of those treated with everolimus compared with 26% of those treated with placebo. Results from this trial confirm that everolimus is an active agent in refractory, progressive neuroendocrine tumors.

Streptozocin alone or in combination with doxorubicin were the only chemotherapeutic agents accepted for the use of pancreatic neuroendocrine tumors in 2011. Between the late 1990s and 2010, small molecule inhibitors targeting receptor tyrosine kinases were finding utility in the treatment of cancers. One such drug, sunitinib (Sutent), was found to inhibit platelet-derived growth factor receptor, vascular endothelial growth factor receptor, and c-kit, all of which are implicated in tumor progression. Phase I and II trials suggested that sunitinib had antitumor activity in pancreatic neuroendocrine tumors. This finding provided the rationale for a randomized controlled trial that resulted in 2011.[24] Patients with well-differentiated advanced or metastatic pancreatic endocrine tumors were recruited between 2007 and 2009. The primary end point of this study was progression-free survival, with secondary end points being overall survival, the objective response rate, the time to tumor response, duration of response, safety, and patient-reported outcomes. Patients received either 37.5 mg of sunitinib daily or placebo. A total of 171 patients were accrued. The trial was discontinued early because of a greater number of deaths and serious adverse events in the placebo group along with improvement of progression-free survival favoring sunitinib. Sunitinib was well tolerated. In an intention-to-treat analysis, the progression-free survival was 11.4 months for those treated with sunitinib compared with 5.5 months for those treated with placebo ($P<.001$). Progression-free survival at 6 months was 71.3% in the sunitinib group versus 43.2% in the placebo group. The hazard ratio for death was 0.41 in favor of sunitinib ($P = .02$). However, the median overall survival could not be estimated for either study group because of the number of censored events. No objective responses were observed in those treated with placebo. However, 9.3% of patients had an objective response when treated with sunitinib. Common adverse events in those treated with sunitinib were diarrhea, nausea, asthenia, vomiting, and fatigue in about 30% of patients. This study represented another landmark in the treatment of advanced or metastatic neuroendocrine tumors. This study confirmed that neuroendocrine tumors are sensitive to receptor tyrosine kinase inhibition. In an updated analysis published recently, the efficacy of sunitinib was confirmed in the treatment of neuroendocrine tumors with a progression-free survival of 12.6 months versus 5.8 months for those treated with placebo.[25] Median overall survival was 38.6 months for those treated with sunitinib and 29.1 months for those treated with placebo ($P = .094$). Importantly, 69% of patients who were assigned to the placebo arm crossed over to the sunitinib arm, which is the likely reason that overall survival was not statistically different.

SUMMARY

Contemporary evaluation and management continue to improve for neuroendocrine tumors as a consequence of an ever-evolving understanding of the pathophysiology of this disease. As shown by the publication date of each of the discussed studies, knowledge is in its infancy. However, the medical community has made progress and will continue to learn, as shown by multiple clinical investigations pending completion (**Table 3**). This disease process is a prototypical example of the utility of the multidisciplinary care of patients. For patients who are not surgical candidates, level 1 evidence shows that multiple rational systemic therapies and radionucleotides provide benefit for those with neuroendocrine tumors.

Table 3
Pending randomized trials of interest

Sponsor or Lead Institution	Title of Study	Status
Hutchison Medipharma Limited	Phase III Study of Sulfatinib in Treating Advanced Extrapancreatic Neuroendocrine Tumors	Recruiting
Ipsen	SPINET	Recruiting
Abramson Cancer Center of the University of Pennsylvania	Randomized Embolization Trial for Neuroendocrine Tumor Metastases to the Liver	Recruiting
GERCOR	TERAVECT	Recruiting
ECOG-ACRIN Cancer Research Group	Cisplatin and Etoposide or Temozolomide and Capecitabine in Treating Patients with Neuroendocrine Carcinoma of the GI Tract or Pancreas that is Metastatic or Cannot Be Removed by Surgery	Recruiting
Federation Francophone de Cancerologie Digestive	REMINET	Recruiting
University of California, San Francisco	Combination Chemotherapy and Bevacizumab in Treating Patients with Advanced Neuroendocrine Tumors	Active, not recruiting

Abbreviations: ACRIN, American College of Radiology Imaging Network; ECOG, Eastern Cooperative Oncology Group; GERCOR, Groupe Cooperateur Multidisciplinaire en Oncologie; REMINET, Study Evaluating Lanreotide as Maintenance Therapy in Patients With Non-Resectable Duodeno-Pancreatic Neuroendocrine Tumors; SPINET, Efficacy and Safety of Lanreotide Autogel/Depot 120 mg Versus Placebo in Subjects with Lung Neuroendocrine Tumors; TERAVECT, Metabolic Radiotherapy After Complete Resection of Liver Metastases in Patient with Digestive Neuroendocrine Tumor.

REFERENCES

1. Rorstad O. Prognostic indicators for carcinoid neuroendocrine tumors of the gastrointestinal tract. J Surg Oncol 2005;89(3):151–60.
2. Modlin IM, Kidd M, Latich I, et al. Current status of gastrointestinal carcinoids. Gastroenterology 2005;128(6):1717–51.
3. Moertel CG, Lefkopoulo M, Lipsitz S, et al. Streptozocin-doxorubicin, streptozocin-fluorouracil or chlorozotocin in the treatment of advanced islet-cell carcinoma. N Engl J Med 1992;326(8):519–23.
4. Koumarianou A, Kaltsas G, Kulke MH, et al. Temozolomide in advanced neuroendocrine neoplasms: pharmacological and clinical aspects. Neuroendocrinology 2015;101(4):274–88.
5. Strosberg JR, Fine RL, Choi J, et al. First-line chemotherapy with capecitabine and temozolomide in patients with metastatic pancreatic endocrine carcinomas. Cancer 2011;117(2):268–75.
6. Kvols LK, Moertel CG, O'Connell MJ, et al. Treatment of the malignant carcinoid syndrome. N Engl J Med 1986;315(11):663–6.
7. Jacobsen MB, Hanssen LE. Clinical effects of octreotide compared to placebo in patients with gastrointestinal neuroendocrine tumours. Report on a double-blind, randomized trial. J Intern Med 1995;237(3):269–75.
8. Arnold R, Rinke A, Klose K-J, et al. Octreotide versus octreotide plus interferon-alpha in endocrine gastroenteropancreatic tumors: a randomized trial. Clin Gastroenterol Hepatol 2005;3(8):761–71.
9. Rubin J, Ajani J, Schirmer W, et al. Octreotide acetate long-acting formulation versus open-label subcutaneous octreotide acetate in malignant carcinoid syndrome. J Clin Oncol 1999;17(2):600–6.
10. Wymenga AN, Eriksson B, Salmela PI, et al. Efficacy and safety of prolonged-release lanreotide in patients with gastrointestinal neuroendocrine tumors and hormone-related symptoms. J Clin Oncol 1999;17(4):1111.
11. O'Toole D, Ducreux M, Bommelaer G, et al. Treatment of carcinoid syndrome: a prospective crossover evaluation of lanreotide versus octreotide in terms of efficacy, patient acceptability, and tolerance. Cancer 2000;88(4):770–6.
12. Vinik AI, Wolin EM, Liyanage N, et al, ELECT Study Group*. Evaluation of lanreotide depot/autogel efficacy and safety as a carcinoid syndrome treatment (ELECT): a randomized, double-blind, placebo-controlled trial. Endocr Pract 2016;22(9):1068–80.
13. Rinke A, Muller H-H, Schade-Brittinger C, et al. Placebo-controlled, double-blind, prospective, randomized study on the effect of octreotide LAR in the control of tumor growth in patients with metastatic neuroendocrine midgut tumors: a report from the PROMID study group. J Clin Oncol 2009;27(28):4656–63.
14. Rinke A, Wittenberg M, Schade-Brittinger C, et al. Placebo-controlled, double-blind, prospective, randomized study on the effect of octreotide LAR in the control of tumor growth in patients with metastatic neuroendocrine midgut tumors (PROMID): results of long-term survival. Neuroendocrinology 2017;104(1):26–32.
15. Caplin ME, Pavel M, Ćwikła JB, et al. Lanreotide in metastatic enteropancreatic neuroendocrine tumors. N Engl J Med 2014;371(3):224–33.
16. Wolin E, Jarzab B, Eriksson B, et al. Phase III study of pasireotide long-acting release in patients with metastatic neuroendocrine tumors and carcinoid symptoms refractory to available somatostatin analogues. Drug Des Devel Ther 2015;9:5075.

17. Kulke MH, Hörsch D, Caplin ME, et al. Telotristat ethyl, a tryptophan hydroxylase inhibitor for the treatment of carcinoid syndrome. J Clin Oncol 2017;35(1):14–23.
18. Strosberg J, El-Haddad G, Wolin E, et al. Phase 3 trial of (177)Lu-Dotatate for midgut neuroendocrine tumors. N Engl J Med 2017;376(2):125–35.
19. Meric-Bernstam F, Gonzalez-Angulo AM. Targeting the mTOR signaling network for cancer therapy. J Clin Oncol 2009;27(13):2278–87.
20. Bjornsti M-A, Houghton PJ. The tor pathway: a target for cancer therapy. Nat Rev Cancer 2004;4(5):335–48.
21. Pavel ME, Hainsworth JD, Baudin E, et al. Everolimus plus octreotide long-acting repeatable for the treatment of advanced neuroendocrine tumours associated with carcinoid syndrome (RADIANT-2): a randomised, placebo-controlled, phase 3 study. Lancet 2011;378(9808):2005–12.
22. Yao JC, Shah MH, Ito T, et al. Everolimus for advanced pancreatic neuroendocrine tumors. N Engl J Med 2011;364(6):514–23.
23. Yao JC, Fazio N, Singh S, et al. Everolimus for the treatment of advanced, nonfunctional neuroendocrine tumours of the lung or gastrointestinal tract (RADIANT-4): a randomised, placebo-controlled, phase 3 study. Lancet 2016; 387(10022):968–77.
24. Raymond E, Dahan L, Raoul J-L, et al. Sunitinib malate for the treatment of pancreatic neuroendocrine tumors. N Engl J Med 2011;364(6):501–13.
25. Faivre S, Niccoli P, Castellano D, et al. Sunitinib in pancreatic neuroendocrine tumors: updated progression-free survival and final overall survival from a phase III randomized study. Ann Oncol 2017;28(2):339–43.

Randomized Clinical Trials in Pancreatic Cancer

Neha Goel, MD, Sanjay S. Reddy, MD*

KEYWORDS

- Randomized trials • Pancreatic cancer • Chemotherapy • Chemoradiation
- Randomized control trails

KEY POINTS

- To gain a thorough understanding of the evolution of pancreatic cancer management.
- To discuss the most recent level 1a evidence for management of pancreatic cancer.
- To discuss the future of pancreatic cancer management and ongoing clinical trials.

REVIEW OF OLDER ADJUVANT TRIALS
Adjuvant Chemotherapy

The CONKO-001 (Charite Onkologie 001) trial was designed to compare adjuvant intravenous gemcitabine with observation alone in patients undergoing complete curative resection for pancreatic cancer.[1] Three-hundred and sixty-eight patients without prior chemotherapy or radiation were randomized to 6 cycles of standard-dose gemcitabine or observation, following complete resection. More than 80% of patients had an R0 resection. During median follow-up of 53 months, 133 patients (74%) in the gemcitabine group and 161 patients (92%) in the control group developed recurrent disease. Median disease-free survival was 13.4 months in the gemcitabine group and 6.9 months in the control group (P<.001). Estimated disease-free survival at 3 and 5 years was 23.5% and 16.5% in the gemcitabine group, and 7.5% and 5.5% in the control group, respectively. Subgroup analyses showed that the effect of gemcitabine on disease-free survival was significant in patients with either R0 or R1 resection. There was no difference in overall survival between the gemcitabine group and the control group (median, 22.1 months and 20.2 months, respectively; P = .06). However, there were differences in estimated 3-year and 5-year survival. In the gemcitabine group, the estimated survivals were 34% at 3 years and 22.5% at 5 years compared with the control group, in which estimated survivals were 20.5% at 3 years and 11.5% at 5 years. This study has been criticized for its high local failure rate (92% in

Department of Surgical Oncology, Fox Chase Cancer Center, 333 Cottman Avenue, Philadelphia, PA 19111, USA
* Corresponding author.
E-mail address: sanjay.reddy@fccc.edu

Surg Oncol Clin N Am 26 (2017) 767–790
http://dx.doi.org/10.1016/j.soc.2017.05.005
1055-3207/17/© 2017 Elsevier Inc. All rights reserved.
surgonc.theclinics.com

observation arm). Nevertheless, this study further strengthened the efficacy of gemcitabine-based chemotherapy for patients in the adjuvant setting.

Long-term outcomes analyzing whether the previously reported improvement in disease-free survival with adjuvant gemcitabine therapy translated into improved overall survival were published in *JAMA* in 2013. With a median follow-up of 136 months, long-term follow-up of the CONKO-001 study showed a significant improvement in overall survival that favors gemcitabine (median survival, 22.8 months vs 20.2 months; $P = .01$). The median disease-free survival was 13.4 months in the treatment group compared with 6.7 months in the observation group ($P<.001$). Gemcitabine compared with observation alone yielded improved survival rates at 5 years of 20.7% for the gemcitabine arm versus 10.4% for the observation-alone arm, and at 10 years the survival rates were 12.2% for the gemcitabine arm versus 7.7% for the observation-alone arm. Thus, among patients with macroscopic complete removal of pancreatic cancer, the use of adjuvant gemcitabine for 6 months compared with observation alone resulted in increased overall survival as well as disease-free survival. These findings provide strong support for the use of gemcitabine in this setting.[2]

Adjuvant Chemoradiation

The Gastrointestinal Tumor Study Group (GITSG) trial published in 1985 was one of the first phase III trials exploring the role of adjuvant therapy in pancreas adenocarcinoma. The GITSG trial reported that the median survival of patients undergoing pancreatoduodenectomy could be prolonged almost 2-fold with adjuvant chemoradiation.[3] Patients were randomly assigned to either observation or radiation therapy (RT) combined with an intermittent bolus of 5-fluorouracil (5-FU) postresection. A standard split course of 4000 cGy was used. 5-FU, 500 mg/m^2 daily for 3 days, was given concurrently with each 2000-cGy segment of RT. The 5-FU regimen was then continued weekly for 2 years. In addition to a prolonged median survival, chemoradiation also resulted in a 2-year actuarial survival of 42%, compared with 15% in the control group. Criticisms of this study include having a small patient population and inadequate quality assurance of RT. Furthermore, although patients in this study derived a survival benefit with adjuvant treatment, it is unclear whether the benefit was from the systemic chemotherapy or the chemoradiation or both. Although the GITSG study has been used by some as a basis for 5-FU–based chemoradiation in the adjuvant setting, other studies have challenged the value of chemoradiation.[4]

The European Organisation for Research and Treatment of Cancer (EORTC) 40891 trial was a large multicenter phase III study of patients with resected pancreatic head cancer and periampullary tumors performed to investigate the results of the GITSG trial from 1985, and reported their 5-year and 10-year follow-up. Two-hundred and eighty patients with resected cancers of the pancreatic head or periampullary region were randomized to surgery alone or surgery and chemoradiation (5-FU and 40 Gy). Subgroup analysis of 114 patients with pancreatic head cancers revealed a trend toward improved overall survival for those who received adjuvant therapy compared with the surgery-only arm (median, 17.1 months vs 12.6 months), but this difference was not statistically significant ($P = .99$). Long-term results in the patients with pancreatic head cancer over a greater than 10-year follow-up period reported median survivals of 1.3 and 1 year, which were not statistically significant. Overall, unlike the previous, much smaller 43-patient GITSG trial, EORTC-40891 did not support the benefit of 5-FU-based chemoradiation.[5]

The European Study Group of Pancreatic Cancer (ESPAC)-1 trial further investigated the impact of chemoradiation and suggested that chemotherapy alone provided a survival benefit in the adjuvant setting. ESPAC-1 enrolled 541 patients who were randomized to one of 4 arms: observation, chemotherapy with bolus 5-FU and leucovorin, radiation (20 Gy) plus bolus 5-FU during the first 3 days of split-course external beam RT (EBRT), or radiation followed by 6 months of chemotherapy with bolus 5-FU and leucovorin. The study analyzed the survival outcomes using a 2 × 2 factorial design, pooling survival data based on randomization to chemotherapy (yes or no) or chemoradiation (yes or no). Median follow-up of the 227 patients (42%) still alive was 10 months (range, 0–62). Results showed no benefit for adjuvant chemoradiotherapy (median survival, 15.5 months in 175 patients with chemoradiotherapy vs 16.1 months in 178 patients without; $P = .24$). There was evidence of a survival benefit for adjuvant chemotherapy (median survival, 19.7 months in 238 patients with chemotherapy vs 14.0 months in 235 patients without; $P = .0005$). The investigators concluded that this study showed no survival benefit for adjuvant chemoradiotherapy but revealed a potential benefit for adjuvant chemotherapy.[6]

Final results of this study published in 2004 showed an estimated 5-year survival rate of 10% among patients assigned to receive chemoradiotherapy and 20% among patients who did not receive chemoradiotherapy ($P = .05$). The 5-year survival rate was 21% among patients who received chemotherapy and 8% among patients who did not receive chemotherapy ($P = .009$). This study further supported the previously described significant survival benefit of chemotherapy, and deleterious effect of chemoradiation, in the adjuvant setting.[7]

The ESPAC-1 trial has been criticized for lack of standardized trial methodology, the large number of patients who did not receive the intended therapy (31% to receive chemotherapy and 19% to receive chemoradiation did not receive it), and its high local recurrence rate >60%.[4] Despite the various limitations of the study, ESPAC-1 led to a trend away from chemoradiation in Europe and beyond in favor of systemic chemotherapy alone as the main adjuvant treatment choice for resected pancreas adenocarcinoma. Regardless, ESPAC-1 remains the first randomized controlled trial (RCT) to show a statistically significant benefit of adjuvant systemic therapy alone in resected pancreas cancer.[6]

At approximately the same time as the CONKO-001 study was being conducted in Germany and Austria, investigators in North America conducted the Radiation Therapy Oncology Group (RTOG) 9704 study. RTOG 9704 was a phase III trial to determine whether the addition of gemcitabine to adjuvant 5-FU chemoradiation improved survival in patients with resected pancreatic adenocarcinoma. RTOG 9704 was a phase III study that evaluated postoperative adjuvant treatment of resected pancreatic adenocarcinoma using either gemcitabine or 5-FU for 3 weeks before and 12 weeks after 5-FU–based chemoradiation for both groups.[8] This trial, which used daily fractionated radiotherapy, included prospective quality assurance of all patients, including central review of preoperative computed tomography imaging and radiation fields. For patients with tumors of the pancreas head (representing 388 of the 451 patients enrolled in the trial), there was a non–statistically significant increase in overall survival in the gemcitabine arm compared with the 5-FU arm (median and 3-year survival of 20.5 months vs 16.9 months; $P = .05$).[8]

The 5-year analysis of RTOG 9704 showed that there was no difference in overall survival between the two groups, although patients with tumors in the head of the pancreas showed a trend toward improved overall survival with gemcitabine ($P = .08$) on multivariate analysis.[9] Although not statistically significant, the investigators concluded that the addition of gemcitabine given before and after chemoradiation was associated with a survival benefit in the adjuvant setting. The major criticisms of this trial included the lack of a radiation-only arm and that at least 50% of patients had an unknown or positive margin.[4] A follow-up study by Abrams and colleagues[10] on the RTOG 9704 in 2010 noted that, on multivariate analysis for patients with pancreatic head tumors, adherence to RT per protocol and gemcitabine treatment were both correlated with improved median survival (P = .016 and P = .043, respectively). Therefore, the investigators further concluded that it was a failure to adhere to specified RT guidelines during the trial that was associated with reduced survival (**Table 1**).

RECENT ERA OF ADJUVANT THERAPY
Adjuvant Chemotherapy

In more recent years, the ESPAC investigators began to build on results from their ESPAC-1 trial. The ESPAC-3(v1) trial was developed as an initial 3-arm study randomizing patients with resected pancreas adenocarcinoma to adjuvant 5-FU and leucovorin versus gemcitabine versus observation. Chemoradiation was not evaluated in this study. As the ESPAC-1 trial results were finalized showing a benefit to adjuvant 5-FU, the observation arm for ESPAC-3(v1) was removed, and ESPAC-3 (v2) accrued a total of 1088 patients from 2000 to 2007. The ESPAC-3 (NCT00058201) trial randomly assigned 1088 patients who had undergone complete macroscopic resection to either 6 months of 5-FU and leucovorin or 6 months of gemcitabine. The primary end point of the study was 2-year overall survival. The final analysis was performed after a median follow-up of 34.2 months and revealed equivalency between the 2 different chemotherapy agents with a median survival of 23.0 months for patients treated with 5-FU plus leucovorin and 23.6 months for those patients treated with gemcitabine (P = .39). The study also reported that 14% of patients treated with 5-FU plus leucovorin developed serious (>grade 3) treatment-related adverse events compared with only 7.5% of patients treated with gemcitabine (P<.001). Based on these results, the ESPAC-3 trial argued that adjuvant gemcitabine should be the

Table 1
Overall survival data from older prospective, randomized trials of adjuvant therapy in resected pancreas cancer

Trial	N	Randomization	Overall Survival (mo)	P	Classification
CONKO-001	368	Chemotherapy (gemcitabine) vs observation	22.1 vs 20.1 Long follow-up: 22.8 vs 20.2	.06 .01	1a
GITSG	43	Observation or radiation/ bolus 5-FU	20 vs 11	Not reported	1a
ESPAC-1	541	Chemoradiation (5-FU, 20 Gy) vs no chemoradiation	15.5 vs 16.1	.24	1a
		Chemotherapy vs observation	19.7 vs 14.0	.0005	
EORTC 40,891	114	Chemoradiation (5-FU 1 40 Gy EBRT) vs observation	17.1 vs 12.6	.99	1a
RTOG 9704	451	Gemcitabine and 5-FU 1 50.4 Gy EBRT vs 5-FU 1 50.4 Gy EBRT	20.5 vs 16.9	.05	1a

standard of care based on similar survival to, and less toxicity than, adjuvant 5-FU/leucovorin.[11] Nevertheless, this study also supported the use of 5-FU/leucovorin when gemcitabine cannot be safely continued or administered, such as in patients with a history of gemcitabine-related pneumonitis, hemolytic uremic syndrome, or idiopathic pulmonary fibrosis in which there is a high risk of gemcitabine-related pneumonitis.[11]

In March of 2017, the results of the ESPAC-4 phase III, multicenter, randomized trial in which gemcitabine combined with capecitabine was compared with gemcitabine monotherapy for the adjuvant setting were published. Patients were randomly, within 12 weeks of surgery, to receive 6 cycles of either gemcitabine alone administered once a week for 3 of every 4 weeks (1 cycle) or oral capecitabine administered for 21 days followed by 7 days' rest (1 cycle). The primary end point was overall survival, measured as the time from randomization until death from any cause, and assessed in the intention-to-treat population. Of 732 patients enrolled, 730 were included in the final analysis. Of these, 366 were randomly assigned to receive gemcitabine and 364 to gemcitabine plus capecitabine. The median overall survival for patients in the gemcitabine plus capecitabine group was 28.0 months compared with 25.5 months in the gemcitabine group ($P = .032$). Six-hundred and eight grade 3 to 4 adverse events were reported by 226 of 359 patients in the gemcitabine plus capecitabine group compared with 481 grade 3 to 4 adverse events in 196 of 366 patients in the gemcitabine group. This study concluded that the adjuvant combination of gemcitabine and capecitabine should be the new standard of care following resection for pancreatic ductal adenocarcinoma.[12]

In July 2016 the results of the Japan Adjuvant Study Group of Pancreatic Cancer (JASPAC)-01 trial suggested that S-1, an oral fluoropyrimidine designed with the aim of improving antitumor activity and reducing the toxicity of 5-FU, seems to be not only noninferior to gemcitabine but also superior to gemcitabine in the adjuvant setting for the Japanese patient subpopulation. This study investigated the noninferiority of S-1 to gemcitabine as adjuvant chemotherapy for pancreatic cancer in terms of overall survival. Three-hundred and eighty-five patients with resected pancreas adenocarcinoma from 2007 to 2010 were randomized to 6 cycles of intravenous gemcitabine or 4 cycles of oral S-1. The study was a noninferiority study with 80% power with the primary end point of overall survival. Median overall survival was greater for S-1 at 46.5 months compared with gemcitabine at 25.5 months. Three-year and 5-year survival rates were 59.7% and 44.1%, respectively, for S-1, and 38.8% and 24.4%, respectively, for gemcitabine. S-1 was generally well tolerated, and the treatment of patients randomized to receive gemcitabine was more likely to be discontinued, relative to the treatment of patients randomized to receive S-1 ($P = .005$). Although the results are impressive, it is unclear whether the survival benefit with adjuvant S-1 will translate to a broader population. Specifically, white people receiving S-1 have been known to develop more severe gastrointestinal toxicities compared with Asian people, possibly because of metabolic and pharmacogenomic differences between the populations. Therefore, lower doses of S-1 may be required if S-1 is introduced to a broader patient population, which could affect the overall efficacy of the drug in the adjuvant setting.[13]

Adjuvant Chemoradiation

The role of adjuvant chemoradiation therapy (CRT) in resectable pancreatic cancer is still debated. The EORTC-40013-22012/FFCD-9203/GERCOR randomized phase II intergroup study explores the feasibility and tolerability of a gemcitabine-based CRT regimen after R0 resection of pancreatic head cancer. Within 8 weeks after surgery, patients were randomly assigned to receive either 4 cycles of gemcitabine (control arm) or gemcitabine for 2 cycles followed by weekly gemcitabine with concurrent radiation (50.4 Gy; CRT arm). The primary objective was to exclude a less than 60% treatment completion and a greater than 40% rate of grade 4 hematologic or gastrointestinal toxicity in the CRT arm with type I and II errors of 10%. Secondary end points were late toxicity, disease-free survival, and overall survival. Between September 2004 and January 2007, 90 patients were randomly assigned. No differences were seen in overall survival (24.4 months vs 24.3 months) or disease-free survival (10.9 months vs 11.8 months) between the groups, but, with only 45 patients in each arm, no P values were reported. The investigators concluded that adjuvant gemcitabine-based CRT is feasible, well tolerated, and not deleterious. Adding this treatment to full-dose adjuvant gemcitabine after resection of pancreatic cancer should be evaluated in a phase III trial.[14]

In addition, the multicenter, open-label, randomized, phase III CapRI trial evaluated adjuvant chemoradiation with 5-FU, cisplatin, and interferon alfa-2b (IFN α-2b) followed by 5-FU chemotherapy compared with 5-FU alone. Between 2004 and 2007, 132 R0/R1 resected patients received FU, cisplatin, and IFN α-2b plus radiotherapy followed by 2 cycles of FU (arm A, n = 64) or 6 cycles of FU monotherapy (arm B, n = 68). One-hundred and ten patients (arm A, n = 53; arm B, n = 57) received at least 1 dose of the study medication, and these patients composed the per-protocol (PP) population. Biomarkers were analyzed longitudinally for their predictive value. Median survival for all randomly assigned patients was 26.5 months in arm A and 28.5 months in arm B. Median survival for the PP population was 32.1 months in arm A and 28.5 months in arm B ($P = .49$). Eighty-five percent of patients in arm A and 16% of patients in arm B experienced grade 3 or 4 toxicity. The quality of life was temporarily negatively affected in arm A. This study concluded that the 5-FU, cisplatin, and IFN α-2b plus radiotherapy regimen did not improve the survival compared with 5-FU monotherapy.[15]

Adjuvant Targeted Therapy

The CONKO-005 (DRKS00000247) phase III randomized trial has completed recruitment and is currently in the follow-up phase. This study evaluated gemcitabine plus erlotinib compared with gemcitabine alone in patients with R0 resected pancreas cancer. The primary end point of the study was relapse-free survival based on 436 patients. Two-hundred and nineteen patients were randomized to gemcitabine/erlotinib and 217 to gemcitabine. Preliminary results presented at American Society of Clinical Oncology (ASCO) in 2015 revealed that this combination regimen did not significantly improve overall survival or disease-free survival, compared with gemcitabine monotherapy. Median disease-free survival for gemcitabine/erlotinib was 11.6 months versus 11.6 months for gemcitabine alone. Median overall survival for gemcitabine/erlotinib was24.6 months compared with 26.5 months for gemcitabine alone. Based on the data discussed earlier, no definite standard has been established in the adjuvant treatment of pancreatic cancer at this time.[16]

Adjuvant Immunotherapy

An area of increasing research in the adjuvant setting for pancreas adenocarcinoma has been the development of the use of vaccinations and immunotherapy. A vaccine composed of long synthetic mutant ras peptides designed mainly to elicit T-helper responses was developed for KRAS mutated pancreatic adenocarcinomas. A small phase I/II trial of 23 patients treated with a KRAS vaccine in the adjuvant setting showed an immune response to the vaccine in 85% of patients with a median survival of 28 months. The 5-year survival was 22% for all patients and 29% for responders.

The 10-year survival was 20% (4 out of 20) versus 0% (0 out of 87) in a cohort of non-vaccinated patients treated in the same period. The present observation of long-term immune response together with 10-year survival following surgical resection indicates that KRAS vaccination may consolidate the effect of surgery and represent an adjuvant treatment option for the future.[17]

Another target besides KRAS has been telomerase. A recent phase III randomized trial of 1062 patients with locally advanced or metastatic pancreatic cancer treated with gemcitabine and capecitabine with or without the telomerase vaccination (GV1001) found that there was no significant overall survival benefit with the addition of GV1001 to chemotherapy, compared with chemotherapy alone.[18]

Allogeneic granulocyte-macrophage colony-stimulating factor (GM-CSF)–secreting pancreatic tumor vaccines have also been studied. Investigators at the Johns Hopkins University developed an allogeneic whole-cell GM-CSF vaccine (GVAX). A phase I trial studying adjuvant GVAX revealed that 3 of 14 patients treated with the vaccine and chemoradiation developed specific immunity. Mean disease-free survival for this vaccine study was 13 months, although 3 patients were still disease free at 25 to 30 months. The investigators concluded that this vaccine approach seems to induce dose-dependent systemic antitumor immunity as measured by increased postvaccination delayed-type hypersensitivity responses against autologous tumors.[19] A follow-up single-arm phase II trial of approximately 60 patients treated with GVAX in the adjuvant setting found that there was no improvement in survival compared with a contemporary patient cohort treated without the vaccine at the same institution.[20]

Overall, no vaccines or immunotherapies have shown significant improvements in overall survival in phase III clinical trials of patients with resected pancreas adenocarcinoma. However, new agents are continually being developed and studied. Using the concept of hyperacute rejection, a vaccine (algenpantucel-L) has been developed using genetically modified pancreas cancer cells with a mouse gene leading to foreign protein expression of alpha (1,3)-galactosyl (αGal). Preexisting anti-αGal antibodies then trigger a significant immune response leading to cell destruction of any tumor cells in patients undergoing treatment with this form of immunotherapy.[21,22] A phase II study evaluating the role of this form of algenpantucel-L immunotherapy in addition to therapy with gemcitabine with 5-FU–based chemoradiation in the adjuvant setting showed an impressive 1-year disease-free survival of 63% and overall survival of 86%, which is encouraging based on historical controls.[23]

Ongoing Adjuvant Trials

Ongoing clinical trials in the adjuvant setting include RTOG 0848 (NCT01013649), which is assessing gemcitabine with or without subsequent chemoradiation; a phase II study comparing FOLFIRINOX with albumin-bound paclitaxel (NCT02243007); the Advanced Pancreatic Adenocarcinoma Clinical Trial study (NCT01964430), comparing albumin-bound paclitaxel with gemcitabine; and the Immunotherapy for Pancreatic Resectable cancer Study trial, which is comparing gemcitabine (with or without chemoradiation) with and without algenpantucel-L immunotherapy (NCT01072981). A phase III trial of chemotherapy and chemoradiotherapy with or without algenpantucel-L immunotherapy in 722 subjects with surgically resected pancreatic cancer recently completed recruitment in May 2016 with pending results (**Table 2**) (NCT01072981).

NEOADJUVANT THERAPY IN BORDERLINE RESECTABLE DISEASE

Patients with borderline resectable disease should be considered for neoadjuvant therapy, followed by restaging and resection in patients without disease progression.

Table 2
Overall survival data from recent prospective, randomized trials of adjuvant therapy in resected pancreas cancer

Trial	N	Randomization	Overall Survival (mo)	P	Classification
ESPAC-3	1088	5-FU and leucovorin or gemcitabine	23 vs 23.6	.39	1a
ESPAC-4	732	Gemcitabine/capecitabine or gemcitabine	28.0 vs 25.5	.032	1a
JASPAC-01	385	Gemcitabine or S-1	25.2 vs 46.5	.005	1b
EORTC-40013-22012/ FFCD-9203/ GERCOR	90	Gemcitabine or gemcitabine/50.4 Gy	24.4 vs 24.3	Not reported	1b
CapRI trial	132	Chemoradiation with 5-FU, cisplatin, and IFN α-2b followed by 5-FU chemotherapy or 5-FU alone	26.5 vs 28.5	.49	1b

The use of neoadjuvant therapy in the setting of borderline resectable disease has been highly debated and is supported mainly by trials at the phase I and phase II levels. Nevertheless, according to the 2016 National Comprehensive Cancer Network (NCCN) guidelines, up-front resection in patients with borderline resectable disease is no longer recommended because it is becoming clear that patients with borderline resectable pancreatic cancer, especially those at high risk for R1 resections, need a different management strategy. More recent approaches to perioperative treatment have focused on neoadjuvant therapy for patients with borderline resectable disease with the goal of improving overall survival. The theoretic benefits of neoadjuvant therapy include a higher chance of patients completing chemotherapy and/or radiation in the preoperative setting given they are not debilitated after surgery. In addition, there is the potential benefit of downsizing tumors or shrinking them away from vasculature, allowing an R0 resection. Neoadjuvant chemotherapy also has the potential to select for those patients with more stable disease or disease that is responsive to therapy. There is the potential benefit of treating micrometastases at an earlier stage. Surgery following neoadjuvant treatment seems to be safe.[24,25]

Several trials have shown that preoperative treatment of borderline resectable pancreatic adenocarcinoma can be effective and well tolerated. E1200, a randomized phase I/II trial of neoadjuvant therapy in borderline resectable disease, eventually allowed 5 of 21 patients to be resected posttherapy. This trial was designed to assess toxicities and surgical resection rates in 2 neoadjuvant gemcitabine–based chemoradiation regimens in patients with borderline resectable pancreatic cancer. Arm A patients (n = 10) received gemcitabine weekly for 6 weeks, with radiation followed by surgical resection. Arm B patients (n = 11) received preoperative gemcitabine, cisplatin, and 5-FU, followed by radiation with a continuous infusion of 5-FU for 6 weeks. Three patients in arm A and 2 patients in arm B were resected.[26]

A recent multi-institutional phase II trial found that full-dose gemcitabine, oxaliplatin, and radiation given preoperatively to patients with resectable (n = 23), borderline resectable (n = 39), or unresectable disease (n = 6) resulted in a high percentage of R0 resections. Forty-three patients underwent resection (63%), and complete (R0) resection was achieved in 36 of those 43 patients (84%). The median overall survival was18.2 months for all patients, 27.1 months for those who underwent resection, and 10.9 months for those who did not undergo resection.[27]

A multicenter nonrandomized phase II trial evaluating neoadjuvant/adjuvant gemcitabine and erlotinib (American College of Surgeons Oncology Group [ACOSOG] Z5041; NCT003733746) has completed recruitment and may provide additional valuable results regarding the delivery of systemic therapy in the neoadjuvant setting. This study has proved the feasibility of multicenter participation in a neoadjuvant study. A phase III trial of 310 patients exploring the role of neoadjuvant gemcitabine with oxaliplatin in addition to adjuvant gemcitabine compared with adjuvant gemcitabine alone in resectable pancreatic cancer with the primary end point of progression-free survival (NEOPAC [Neoadjuvant Gemcitabine/Oxaliplatin Plus Adjuvant Gemcitabine in Resectable Pancreatic Cancer]; NCT01521702) is projected to be completed by December 2015. Several phase II clinical trials are currently underway to determine the R0 resection rate following neoadjuvant chemotherapy in patients with borderline resectable or unresectable locally advanced disease (NCT00557492). In addition, the Alliance A021101 trial (NCT01821612) is a single-arm pilot study evaluating the safety and efficacy of FOLFIRINOX before capecitabine-based chemoradiation and surgery in this population (**Table 3**).

NEOADJUVANT THERAPY IN RESECTABLE DISEASE

The standard approach to therapy in patients with resectable disease has been (and remains) adjuvant therapy, with median survivals in the range of 20.1 to 23.6 months under the most optimal phase III trials.[1,6–8] Neoadjuvant chemotherapy in resectable patients has yet to be fully defined with regard to value because results from prior phase II studies have been limited and mostly are based on single-institution experiences. Although most studies investigating the neoadjuvant experience in patients with resectable pancreatic cancer are retrospective, several small phase II studies have been published.[25]

In a randomized phase II trial of 50 patients evaluating the safety and efficacy of gemcitabine-based chemotherapy regimens as neoadjuvant therapy for patients

Table 3				
Neoadjuvant therapy in borderline resectable pancreatic cancer				
Trial	**N**	**Treatment**	**Significance**	**Classification**
Kim et al,[27] 2013	68	Full-dose gemcitabine, oxaliplatin, and radiation given preoperatively to patients with resectable (n = 23), borderline resectable (n = 39), or unresectable disease (n = 6)	Preoperative therapy with full-dose gemcitabine, oxaliplatin, and RT was feasible and resulted in a high percentage of R0 resections	IIa
E1200	21	Gemcitabine/XRT (arm A) vs gemcitabine, cisplatin, 5-FU, followed by XRT with a continuous infusion 5-FU (arm B)	3 out of 10 (A) and 2 out of 11 (B) were resectable. Both regimens were tolerable, and resectability was comparable with previous studies	Ia

Abbreviation: XRT, Radiation.

with resectable pancreatic cancer, 9 patients (38%) in the gemcitabine-only arm and 18 patients (70%) in the gemcitabine and cisplatin arm were able to undergo resection compared with those in the gemcitabine-only arm.[28]

A single 28-patient phase II prospective trial evaluating neoadjuvant gemcitabine and cisplatin for resectable head of pancreas adenocarcinoma showed feasibility with favorable overall and disease-free survival. Patients received 4 biweekly cycles of gemcitabine and cisplatin, and were then restaged before surgery. Twenty-six patients (93%) had resectable cancer on restaging, and the R0 resection rate was 80%. On intention-to-treat analysis, the actuarial overall survival was 26.5 months, which did not change after exclusion of the patient without invasive cancer (n = 27). Those with resected ductal adenocarcinoma had a median overall survival of 19.1 months. Twenty patients developed disease recurrence, resulting in an actuarial recurrence-free survival of 9.2 months on an intention-to-treat analysis, which did not change after excluding the patient without proof of invasive cancer. Patients with resected ductal adenocarcinoma had a median recurrence-free survival of 9 months. The investigators concluded that neoadjuvant chemotherapy with gemcitabine and cisplatin is well tolerated and does not impair the resectability of pancreatic cancer.[29]

Another phase II trial studied the outcomes of patients who received preoperative gemcitabine-based chemoradiation and resection for stage I/II pancreatic adenocarcinoma.[30] Preoperative radiation and gemcitabine was administered to 86 patients with resectable disease, and patients were restaged 4 to 6 weeks following completion. Those without progression of disease were taken to surgery for a pancreatoduodenectomy. Although all patients were able to complete neoadjuvant therapy, at the time of restaging, only 73 patients (85%) were able to undergo surgery, and at the time of surgery 9 patients were had extrapancreatic disease. Median overall survival was 22.7 months with a 27% 5-year survival. The investigators concluded that preoperative gemcitabine-based chemoradiation followed by restaging and evaluation for surgery separated the study population into 2 different subsets: those patients likely to benefit from resection (n = 64) and those in whom surgery would be unlikely to provide clinical benefit (n = 22).[30]

Similar results were observed in another phase II trial involving preoperative gemcitabine/cisplatin followed by gemcitabine-based chemoradiation.[31] Of the 90 patients enrolled in this study, 79 patients (88%) were able to complete neoadjuvant therapy, and 52 patients (66%) underwent surgery. The median overall survival of all 90 patients was 17.4 months. Median survival for the 79 patients who completed chemotherapy-chemoradiation was 18.7 months, with a median survival of 31 months for the 52 patients who underwent resection and 10.5 months for the 27 patients who did not undergo resection of their primary tumors ($P<.001$). Preoperative gemcitabine/cisplatin followed by gemcitabine-based chemoradiation did not improve survival beyond that achieved with preoperative gemcitabine-based chemoradiation alone. The longer preoperative interval was not associated with local tumor progression.[31]

A recent randomized phase II trial, which was terminated early because of slow accrual, compared gemcitabine/cisplatin neoadjuvant chemoradiation with up-front surgery. Both arms received adjuvant chemotherapy.[32] With only 66 patients eligible for analysis, no significant differences were seen in the R0 resection rate, which was 52% in patients who had neoadjuvant chemoradiation and 48% in up-front surgery group. The (y)pN0 rate was 39% in the neoadjuvant chemoradiation arm and 30% in the up-front surgery arm. Overall survival was not statistically significant at 25 months in the neoadjuvant chemoradiation arm versus 18.9 months in the up-front surgery arm. Nevertheless, all results favored the neoadjuvant arm and no safety issues were noted.[32]

At this time, the NCCN does not recommend neoadjuvant therapy for clearly resectable patients without high-risk features, except in a clinical trial. Ongoing trials include the phase III NEOPA trial, which is comparing neoadjuvant gemcitabine CRT with upfront surgery in patients with clearly resectable pancreatic cancer. The primary end point is overall survival (ClinicalTrials.gov, NCT01900327).[33] A phase II trial with R0 resection as the primary end point is also ongoing (**Table 4**) (ClinicalTrials.gov, NCT01389440).[34,35]

CHEMOTHERAPY IN LOCALLY ADVANCED OR METASTATIC DISEASE

The BAYPAN study was a multicenter, placebo-controlled, double-blind, randomized phase III trial comparing gemcitabine/sorafenib and gemcitabine/placebo in the

Table 4
Neoadjuvant therapy in resectable pancreatic cancer

Trial	N	Treatment	Significance	Classification
Palmer et al,[28] 2007	50	Gemcitabine or gemcitabine/cisplatin	27 (54%) underwent pancreatic resection, 9 (38%) in the gemcitabine arm and 18 (70%) in the combination arm, with no increase in surgical complications	Ib
Heinrich et al,[29] 2008	28	Gemcitabine and cisplatin	26 patients (93%) had resectable cancer on restaging, and the R0 resection rate was 80%	IIa
Evans et al,[30] 2008	86	Gemcitabine-based chemoradiation	Preoperative gemcitabine-based chemoradiation followed by restaging and evaluation for surgery separated the study population into 2 different subsets: those patients likely to benefit from resection (n = 64) and those in whom surgery would be unlikely to provide clinical benefit (n = 22)	IIa
Varadhachary et al,[31] 2008	90	Gemcitabine/cisplatin followed by gemcitabine-based chemoradiation	Preoperative gemcitabine/cisplatin followed by gemcitabine-based chemoradiation did not improve survival beyond that achieved with preoperative gemcitabine-based chemoradiation alone	IIa
Golcher et al,[32] 2015	66	Gemcitabine/cisplatin neoadjuvant chemoradiation or up-front surgery	Overall survival was not statistically significant at 25 mo in the neoadjuvant chemoradiation arm vs 18.9 mo in the up-front surgery arm. Nevertheless, all results favored the neoadjuvant arm and no safety issues were noted	Ib

treatment of chemotherapy-naive patients with advanced or metastatic disease. Between December 2006 and September 2009, 104 patients were enrolled on the study (52 patients in each arm) and 102 patients were treated. The median and 6-month progression-free survival were 5.7 months and 48% for gemcitabine/placebo and 3.8 months and 33% for gemcitabine/sorafenib (P = .902). The median overall survivals were 9.2 and 8 months, respectively (P = .231). The investigators concluded that the addition of sorafenib to gemcitabine does not improve progression-free survival.[36]

Gemcitabine plus Albumin-bound Paclitaxel

Albumin-bound paclitaxel is a nanoparticle form of paclitaxel. In a publication of a phase I/II trial, 67 patients with advanced pancreatic cancer received gemcitabine plus albumin-bound paclitaxel. At the maximum tolerated dose, the partial response rate was 48%, with an additional 20% of patients showing stable disease for greater than 16 weeks. The median overall survival at this dose was 12.2 months.[37]

Based on these results, the large, open-label, international, randomized phase III Metastatic Pancreatic Adenocarcinoma Clinical Trial (MPACT) trial was initiated in 861 patients with metastatic pancreatic cancer and no prior chemotherapy.[38] Patients were randomized to receive gemcitabine plus albumin-bound paclitaxel or gemcitabine alone. The trial met its primary end point of overall survival (8.7 months vs 6.6 months; P<.0001).[38] The addition of albumin-bound paclitaxel also improved other end points, including 1-year survival, 2-year survival, response rate, and progression-free survival. Overall survival was associated with a decrease in cancer antigen (CA) 19-9 (P = .001).[39] Tumor response was validated with PET imaging.[40] The most common grade 3 or higher adverse events attributable to albumin-bound paclitaxel were neutropenia, fatigue, and neuropathy. Updated results of the MPACT trial show that long-term survival is possible with gemcitabine plus albumin-bound paclitaxel. Three percent of patients from that arm were alive at 42 months, whereas no patients were alive from the control arm at that time.[41] This combination of gemcitabine plus albumin-bound paclitaxel is a preferred treatment option for patients with metastatic disease and good performance status.

Gemcitabine plus Erlotinib and Other Targeted Therapeutics

Although early phase II trial results of gemcitabine combined with new targeted drugs such as bevacizumab [42] and cetuximab[43] were encouraging, results of phase III studies of combinations of gemcitabine with a biologic agent have indicated that only gemcitabine plus erlotinib is associated with a statistically significant increase in survival compared with gemcitabine alone. This finding was described in the phase III, double-blind, placebo-controlled National Cancer Institute of Canada Clinical Trials Group (NCIC-CTG) trial, in which 569 patients were randomized to receive standard gemcitabine plus erlotinib or gemcitabine plus placebo. Patients in the erlotinib arm showed statistically significant improvements in overall survival (P = .038) and progression-free survival (P = .004) compared with patients receiving gemcitabine alone. Median survival was 6.24 months and 1-year survival was 23%, compared with 5.91 months and 17% in the control arm.[44]

Adding to the previous study that reported that gemcitabine plus erlotinib shows a small but significant improvement in overall survival versus gemcitabine alone, a double-blind, phase III trial was developed of 607 patients with metastatic pancreatic adenocarcinoma studying gemcitabine, erlotinib, and bevacizumab compared with gemcitabine, erlotinib, and placebo. A total of 301 patients were randomly assigned to the placebo group and 306 to the bevacizumab group. Median overall survival was 7.1 and 6.0 months in the bevacizumab and placebo arms, respectively (hazard ratio [HR], 0.89; 95% confidence interval [CI], 0.74–1.07; P = .2087); this difference was not statistically significant. Adding bevacizumab to gemcitabine-erlotinib significantly improved progression-free survival (HR, 0.73; 95% CI, 0.61–0.86; P = .0002). Treatment with bevacizumab plus gemcitabine-erlotinib was well tolerated and safe.[45]

Another phase III trial of 745 patients evaluating the addition of cetuximab to standard gemcitabine therapy revealed no significant difference in median survival between the gemcitabine plus cetuximab arm and the gemcitabine-alone arm (6.3 months vs 5.9 months; P = .23).[46]

Given the initial encouraging results of gemcitabine plus bevacizumab with a 21% response rate and a median survival of 8.8 months in a multicenter phase II trial in patients with metastatic pancreatic cancer, the Cancer and Leukemia Group B (CALGB) conducted a double-blind, placebo-controlled, randomized phase III trial of gemcitabine/bevacizumab versus gemcitabine/placebo in patients with advanced pancreatic cancer.[42] Five-hundred and thirty-five patients were treated and the median overall survival was 5.8 months for gemcitabine/bevacizumab and 5.9 months for gemcitabine/placebo (P = .95). Median progression-free survival was 3.8 and 2.9 months for gemcitabine/bevacizumab and gemcitabine/placebo, respectively (P = .07). Overall response rates were 13% and 10% for gemcitabine/bevacizumab and gemcitabine/placebo, respectively. The investigators concluded that the addition of bevacizumab to gemcitabine does not improve survival in patients with advanced pancreatic cancer.[42]

Targeted therapies in addition to erlotinib have been assessed in combination with gemcitabine but none have been shown to significantly improve outcomes. For example, axitinib, a potent selective inhibitor of vascular endothelial growth factor (VEGF) receptors, was studied in a randomized phase II trial studying gemcitabine alone or with axitinib in advanced pancreatic cancer. Results suggested increased overall survival in axitinib-treated patients. From these results, Kindler and colleagues[47] assessed the effect of treatment with gemcitabine plus axitinib on overall survival in a phase III trial. Six-hundred and thirty-two patients were enrolled and assigned to 2 treatment groups. Three-hundred and sixteen patients were in the gemcitabine/axitinib group compared with 316 patients in the gemcitabine/placebo group. An interim analysis in January 2009 revealed that the addition of axitinib to gemcitabine does not improve overall survival in advanced pancreatic cancer.[46]

Other phase II/III trials of gemcitabine plus ziv-aflibercept,[48] a VEGF inhibitor; rigosertib,[49] a Ras mimetic and small-molecule inhibitor of multiple signaling pathways; ganitumab,[50] an insulinlike growth factor 1 receptor monoclonal antibody; and sunitinib,[51] an angiogenesis inhibitor showed no improved overall survival, compared with gemcitabine alone, in patients with metastatic pancreatic cancer.

Poly (ADP-ribose) polymerase (PARP) inhibitors are another avenue of research for cancers associated with breast cancer antigen gene (BRCA)1/2 mutations. In a phase II trial assessing the efficacy and safety of olaparib, an oral PARP, the tumor response rate for patients with metastatic pancreatic cancer and a germline BRCA1/2 mutation (n = 23) was 21.7%.[52] The PARP inhibitor rucaparib is being assessed in the ongoing RUCAPANC trial, targeting patients with a BRCA1/2 mutation.[53] Preliminary data from this phase II trial presented at ASCO in 2016 revealed that 19 patients with a BRCA1/2 mutation and relapsed disease showed an objective response rate of 11% with rucaparib, a PARP inhibitor, in patients with pancreatic cancer and a known deleterious germline or somatic BRCA mutation.[53] The phase III randomized POLO trial

(NCT02184195), in which the effectiveness of maintenance olaparib monotherapy following cisplatin, carboplatin, or oxaliplatin is being assessed, is currently in progress.[54]

Gemcitabine plus Cisplatin

Data regarding the survival impact of combining gemcitabine with a platinum agent are conflicting and results of RCTs have not provided support for the use of gemcitabine plus cisplatin in the treatment of patients with advanced pancreatic cancer. Three phase III trials evaluating the combination of gemcitabine with cisplatin versus gemcitabine alone in patients with advanced pancreatic cancer failed to show a significant survival benefit for combination therapy compared with gemcitabine monotherapy.[55–57]

Gemcitabine plus Capecitabine

Several randomized trials have investigated the combination of gemcitabine with capecitabine, a fluoropyrimidine, in patients with advanced pancreatic cancer. A randomized study of 533 patients with advanced disease found that progression-free survival and objective response rates were significantly improved in patients receiving gemcitabine plus capecitabine compared with gemcitabine alone. There was also a trend toward an improvement in overall survival in the combination arm; however, it did not reach statistical significance.[58] Results from another, smaller phase III trial evaluating gemcitabine and capecitabine did not show an overall survival advantage, although a post-hoc analysis showed overall survival to be significantly increased in the subgroup of patients with good performance status.[59]

Gemcitabine and Other Fluoropyrimidine-based Therapies

FU-based, irinotecan–based, and gemcitabine-based regimens are the standard of care as first-line treatment of patients with metastatic pancreatic cancer. Whether a sequential approach alternating irinotecan, FU, and gemcitabine may be effective and tolerable in patients with metastatic pancreatic cancer is unknown. In a phase II randomized trial, the effects of the FIRGEM regimen (irinotecan delivered before and after infusion of 5-FU/leucovorin [FOLFIRI.3], alternating with fixed-dose-rate gemcitabine) were assessed in 98 patients with metastatic pancreatic cancer.[60] Patients were randomized to receive the FIRGEM regimen or fixed-dose-rate gemcitabine monotherapy. The primary objective of a 45% progression-free survival rate at 6 months was reached, and progression-free survival was a median of 5 months in those randomized to receive the FIRGEM regimen, whereas those randomized to receive only gemcitabine had a median progression-free survival of 3.4 months. Study investigators deemed FIRGEM to be effective and feasible in the metastatic setting.[60]

A recent randomized trial from Asia showed that gemcitabine combined with the oral fluoropyrimidine S-1 may improve response and survival in patients with locally advanced pancreatic cancer, although trial results are inconsistent regarding whether outcomes are improved compared with gemcitabine monotherapy.[61]

FOLFIRINOX

Results from the randomized phase III PRODIGE trial evaluating FOLFIRINOX versus gemcitabine in patients with metastatic pancreatic cancer and good performance status showed dramatic improvements in both median progression-free survival (6.4 months vs 3.3 months; P<.001) and median overall survival (11.1 months vs 6.8 months; P<.001), in favor of the group receiving FOLFIRINOX.[62] However, the eligibility criteria for this trial were stringent, limiting ability to generalize to real-world settings. For example, patients with abnormal bilirubin levels were excluded from participating. There are also some concerns about the toxicity of the FOLFIRINOX regimen. In the PRODIGE trial, some of the grade 3 to 4 toxicity rates that were significantly greater in the FOLFIRINOX group than in the gemcitabine group were 45.7% for neutropenia, 12.7% for diarrhea, 9.1% for thrombocytopenia, and 9.0% for sensory neuropathy.[63] Despite the high levels of toxicity, no toxic deaths have been reported.[62,63] Furthermore, the PRODIGE trial determined that, despite this toxicity, fewer patients in the FOLFIRINOX group than in the gemcitabine group experienced a degradation in their quality of life at 6 months (31% vs 66%, P<.01).[63]

The efficacy and toxicity of a modified FOLFIRINOX regimen in which the initial dosings of bolus 5-FU and irinotecan were each reduced by 25% were assessed in a phase II single-arm prospective trial of 75 patients.[64] In patients with metastatic disease, the efficacy of the modified regimen was comparable with that of the standard regimen, with a median overall survival of 10.2 months. In patients with locally advanced disease, the median overall survival was 26.6 months. Patients who received the modified regimen experienced significantly less neutropenia, fatigue, and vomiting, relative to patients who received the standard FOLFIRINOX regimen.

Capecitabine and Continuous-infusion 5-Fluorouracil

Capecitabine monotherapy and continuous-infusion 5-FU is also considered a first-line treatment option for patients with locally advanced unresectable or metastatic disease. The capecitabine recommendation is supported by a randomized phase III trial from the Arbeitsgemeinschaft Internistische Onkologie (AIO) group in which overall survival was similar in patients with advanced pancreatic cancer receiving capecitabine plus erlotinib followed by gemcitabine monotherapy or gemcitabine plus erlotinib followed by capecitabine monotherapy.[65] Two-hundred and eighty-one treatment-naive patients were randomly assigned to either the capecitabine plus erlotinib arm (A) or the gemcitabine plus erlotinib arm (B). Interim analysis of toxicity evaluated data from the first 127 randomized patients. Grade 3 to 4 hematological toxicity was less than 10% in both the arms. Major grade 3 to 4 toxicities in arms A and B were diarrhea (9% vs 7%), skin rash (4% vs 12%), and hand-foot syndrome (7% vs 0%). No treatment-related death was observed. This interim safety analysis suggests that treatment with erlotinib 150 mg/d is feasible in combination with capecitabine or gemcitabine.[65]

Possible Role of Maintenance Therapy in Advanced Disease

Given the success of more effective regimens in patients with advanced disease, clinicians are now determining how best to manage the treatment-free interval before disease progression. Options include stopping treatment, eliminating the most toxic agents, and switching to an alternative agent for maintenance therapy. A recent randomized phase II trial (PACT-12) had interesting results, suggesting that maintenance therapy with sunitinib after a full course of first-line treatment may have a benefit in some patients with metastatic disease.[66] In this trial, 55 patients with pathologic diagnosis of metastatic pancreatic adenocarcinoma, performance status greater than 50%, and no progression after 6 months of chemotherapy (mostly gemcitabine combinations) were randomized to observation (arm A) or sunitinib until progression or a maximum of 6 months (arm B). The primary outcome measure was the probability of being progression free at 6 months from randomization. Median overall survival was 9.2 months in the observation group versus 10.6 months in the sunitinib group ($P = .11$). A criticism of this study is the small sample size. However, the 1-year and 2-year survival rates were 36% and 7% in the observation arm compared with 41% and 23% in the sunitinib arm, suggesting that a subset of patients may derive significant benefit. Overall, results of the PACT-12 trial suggest that there may be a role for antiangiogenic agents after more effective first-line treatments.[66]

Second-line Systemic Therapy in the Advanced Setting

Final results of the 160-patient phase III CONKO-003 trial initially presented in 2008 were published in 2014. This study assessed the efficacy of a second-line regimen of oxaliplatin and folinic acid–modulated FU (OFF) in patients with advanced pancreatic cancer who experienced progression while receiving gemcitabine monotherapy. The median overall survival in the OFF arm was 5.9 months and was 3.3 months in the 5-FU/leucovorin arm, for a significant improvement in the HR ($P = .01$).[67]

However, results from the open-label phase III PANCREOX trial show that the addition of oxaliplatin to 5-FU/leucovorin in second-line treatment may be detrimental.[68] In this trial, 108 patients with advanced pancreatic cancer who progressed on gemcitabine-based treatment were randomized to receive second-line FOLFOX or infusional 5-FU/leucovorin. No difference was seen in median progression-free survival (3.1 vs 2.9 months; $P = .99$), but median overall survival was worse in those in the FOLFOX arm (6.1 vs 9.9 months; $P = .02$). Furthermore, the addition of oxaliplatin resulted in increased toxicity, with rates of grade 3 to 4 adverse events of 63% in the FOLFOX arm and of 11% in the 5-FU/leucovorin arm.[68]

In the recent NAPOLI-1 phase III randomized trial, the effects of nanoliposomal irinotecan were examined in patients with metastatic pancreatic cancer who previously received gemcitabine-based therapy. Four-hundred and seventeen patients were randomized to receive the nanoliposomal irinotecan monotherapy, 5-FU/leucovorin, or both. Median progression-free survival was 3.1 months versus 1.5 months, which was statistically significantly greater for patients who received nanoliposomal irinotecan with 5-FU/leucovorin compared with patients who did not receive irinotecan ($P<.001$). Updated analyses showed that median overall survival was 6.2 months versus 4.2 months and was also significantly greater for patients who received nanoliposomal irinotecan with 5-FU/leucovorin compared with patients who received 5-FU/leucovorin without irinotecan ($P = .042$). Grade 3 or 4 adverse events that occurred most frequently with this regimen were neutropenia (27%), fatigue (14%), diarrhea (13%), and vomiting (11%).[69] Irinotecan liposomal injection, combined with 5-FU/leucovorin, was recently approved by the US Food and Drug Administration to be used as second-line treatment following gemcitabine-based therapy in patients with metastatic disease.[69]

The AIO-PK0104 trial also assessed second-line therapy in a randomized crossover trial and found capecitabine to be efficacious after progression on gemcitabine/erlotinib in patients with advanced disease.[70] Gemcitabine/erlotinib followed by second-line capecitabine was compared with a reverse experimental sequence of capecitabine/erlotinib followed by gemcitabine. Two-hundred and seventy-four patients were randomly assigned to first-line treatment with either gemcitabine plus erlotinib or capecitabine plus erlotinib. In case of treatment failure such as progression of disease or toxicity, patients were allocated to second-line treatment with the comparator cytostatic drug without erlotinib. Forty-three patients had locally advanced disease and 231 had metastatic disease. One-hundred and forty (51%) received second-line chemotherapy. Median time to treatment failure after second-line therapy was estimated as 4.2 months in both arms; median overall survival was 6.2 months with gemcitabine/erlotinib followed by capecitabine and 6.9 months with capecitabine/erlotinib followed by gemcitabine, respectively (P = .90). Time to treatment failure for first-line therapy was significantly prolonged with gemcitabine/erlotinib compared with capecitabine/erlotinib (3.2 vs 2.2 months; P = .0034). The investigators concluded that both treatment strategies are feasible and showed comparable efficacy (**Table 5**).

CHEMORADIATION IN LOCALLY ADVANCED DISEASE

Results of 2 early randomized trials comparing up-front chemoradiation with chemotherapy in locally advanced disease were contradictory.[71,72] Three phase II

Table 5
Overall survival data from prospective, randomized trials of chemotherapy in locally advanced or metastatic pancreas cancer

Trial	N	Randomization	Overall Survival (mo)	P	Classification
BAYPAN	104	Gemcitabine/sorafenib or gemcitabine/placebo	9.2 vs 8	.23	Ia
MPACT	861	Gemcitabine plus albumin-bound paclitaxel or gemcitabine alone	8.7 vs 6.6	.0001	Ia
NCIC CTG	569	Gemcitabine + erlotinib or gemcitabine + placebo	6.24 vs 5.91	.038	Ia
CALGB	535	Gemcitabine + bevacizumab or gemcitabine + placebo	5.8 vs 5.9	.95	Ia
Cunningham et al,[58] 2009	533	Gemcitabine + capecitabine or gemcitabine alone	6.2 vs 7.1	.08	Ib
PRODIGE	342	FOLFIRINOX vs gemcitabine in patients with metastatic pancreatic cancer	11.1 vs 6.8	.001	Ia
CONKO-003	160	OFF or 5-FU/LV in patients with advanced pancreatic cancer who progressed on gemcitabine	5.9 vs 3.3	.01	Ia
PANCREOX	108	FOLFOX or infusional 5-FU/LV in patients with advanced pancreatic cancer who progressed on gemcitabine	6.1 vs 9.9	.02	Ib
NAPOLI-1	417	Nanoliposomal irinotecan monotherapy + 5-FU/LV or 5-FU/LV	6.2 vs 4.2	.042	Ib
AIO-PK0104	274	Gemcitabine/erlotinib followed by second-line capecitabine was compared with a reverse experimental sequence of capecitabine/erlotinib followed by gemcitabine	6.2 vs 6.9	.9	Ib

Abbreviation: LV, leucovorin.

trials also assessed the up-front chemoradiation approach in locally advanced pancreatic adenocarcinoma, with median survival rates ranging from 8.2 to 9 months.[73–76]

The phase III randomized ECOG-4201 trial, which assessed gemcitabine compared with gemcitabine plus radiation followed by gemcitabine alone in patients with locally advanced, unresectable pancreatic cancer was closed early because of poor accrual. However, an intention-to-treat analysis of data for the 74 patients enrolled in this study showed that median overall survival was significantly longer in the CRT arm of the study (11.1 months vs 9.2 months; $P = .017$).[77] However, the poor accrual rate decreased its statistical power. There was no difference in progression-free survival, and the CIs for overall survival overlapped between the two groups of patients, leading claims that the results do not achieve the level of evidence required to determine standard of care.

The benefit of chemotherapy versus chemoradiation was also addressed in the phase III Francophone de Cancerologie Digestive (FFCD)/Société Française de. Radiothérapie Oncologie (SFRO) study from France in 2008, in which patients with locally advanced pancreatic cancer were randomly assigned to receive either gemcitabine alone or an intensive induction regimen of chemoradiation with 5-FU plus cisplatin followed by gemcitabine maintenance treatment. Gemcitabine alone was associated with a significantly increased overall survival rate at 1 year compared with chemoradiation (53% vs 32%; $P = .006$).[78] This study was stopped before the planned accrual because an interim analysis revealed that patients in the chemoradiation arm had a lower survival rate. Also, patients in the chemoradiation arm experienced severe toxicity and were more likely to receive a shorter course of maintenance therapy with gemcitabine, suggesting that the observed differences in survival were most likely attributable to the extreme toxicity of this chemoradiation regimen. Thus, the role of up-front chemoradiation in the setting of locally advanced pancreatic cancer is still undefined. If patients present with poorly controlled pain or local invasion with bleeding, then starting with up-front CRT is an option.

Chemoradiation Following Chemotherapy in Locally Advanced Disease

In locally advanced pancreatic cancer, the role of chemoradiotherapy is controversial and the efficacy of erlotinib is unknown. In the international phase III LAP07 RCT, 269 patients with locally advanced pancreatic cancer received chemoradiation with capecitabine following 4 months of induction chemotherapy with either gemcitabine monotherapy or gemcitabine and erlotinib.[79] The goal was to assess whether chemoradiotherapy improves overall survival of patients with locally advanced pancreatic cancer controlled after 4 months of gemcitabine-based induction chemotherapy and to assess the effect of erlotinib on survival. Chemoradiation in this setting provided no survival benefit compared with chemotherapy only ($P = .83$).[79]

In a recent single-arm phase II trial examining stereotactic body radiotherapy (SBRT) following gemcitabine monotherapy in 49 patients with locally advanced pancreatic cancer, this regimen showed low toxicity and favorable freedom from local disease progression.[80] The median overall survival was 13.9 months (95% CI, 10.2–16.7 months). Patients reported a significant improvement in pancreatic pain ($P = .001$) 4 weeks after SBRT. The investigators concluded that fractionated SBRT with gemcitabine results in minimal acute and late gastrointestinal toxicity and that future studies should incorporate SBRT with more aggressive multiagent chemotherapy compared with gemcitabine monotherapy alone (**Table 6**).

Table 6
Overall survival data from prospective, randomized trials of chemoradiation in locally advanced or metastatic pancreas cancer

Trial	N	Randomization	Overall Survival (mo)	P	Classification
ECOG-4201	74	Gemcitabine or gemcitabine + radiation followed by gemcitabine	9.2 vs 11.1	.17	Ib
FFCD-SFRO	119	Gemcitabine alone or chemoradiation with 5-FU + cisplatin followed by gemcitabine maintenance	13 vs 8.6	.03	Ib
LAP07	269	In the second randomization involving patients with progression-free disease after 4 mo, 136 patients received 2 mo of the same chemotherapy (gemcitabine or gemcitabine + erlotinib) and 133 received chemoradiation + capecitabine	16.5 vs 15.2	.83	Ib

REFERENCES

1. Oettle H, Post S, Neuhaus P, et al. Adjuvant chemotherapy with gemcitabine vs observation in patients undergoing curative-intent resection of pancreatic cancer: a randomized controlled trial. JAMA 2007;297(3):267–77.

2. Oettle H, Neuhaus P, Hochhaus A, et al. Adjuvant chemotherapy with gemcitabine and long-term outcomes among patients with resected pancreatic cancer: the CONKO-001 randomized trial. JAMA 2013;310(14):1473–81.

3. Kalser MH, Ellenberg SS. Pancreatic cancer. Adjuvant combined radiation and chemotherapy following curative resection. Arch Surg 1985;120(8):899–903.

4. Rudloff U, Maker AV, Brennan MF, et al. Randomized clinical trials in pancreatic adenocarcinoma. Surg Oncol Clin North Am 2010;19(1):115–50.

5. Smeenk HG, van Eijck CH, Hop WC, et al. Long-term survival and metastatic pattern of pancreatic and periampullary cancer after adjuvant chemoradiation or observation: long-term results of EORTC trial 40891. Ann Surg 2007;246(5):734–40.

6. Neoptolemos JP, Dunn JA, Stocken DD, et al. Adjuvant chemoradiotherapy and chemotherapy in resectable pancreatic cancer: a randomised controlled trial. Lancet 2001;358(9293):1576–85.

7. Neoptolemos JP, Stocken DD, Friess H, et al. A randomized trial of chemoradiotherapy and chemotherapy after resection of pancreatic cancer. N Engl J Med 2004;350(12):1200–10.

8. Regine WF, Winter KA, Abrams RA, et al. Fluorouracil vs gemcitabine chemotherapy before and after fluorouracil-based chemoradiation following resection of pancreatic adenocarcinoma: a randomized controlled trial. JAMA 2008; 299(9):1019–26.

9. Regine WF, Winter KA, Abrams R, et al. Fluorouracil-based chemoradiation with either gemcitabine or fluorouracil chemotherapy after resection of pancreatic adenocarcinoma: 5-year analysis of the U.S. Intergroup/RTOG 9704 phase III trial. Ann Surg Oncol 2011;18(5):1319–26.

10. Abrams RA, Winter KA, Regine WF, et al. Failure to adhere to protocol specified radiation therapy guidelines was associated with decreased survival in RTOG 9704–a phase III trial of adjuvant chemotherapy and chemoradiotherapy for

patients with resected adenocarcinoma of the pancreas. Int J Radiat Oncol Biol Phys 2012;82(2):809–16.

11. Neoptolemos JP, Moore MJ, Cox TF, et al. Effect of adjuvant chemotherapy with fluorouracil plus folinic acid or gemcitabine vs observation on survival in patients with resected periampullary adenocarcinoma: the ESPAC-3 periampullary cancer randomized trial. JAMA 2012;308(2):147–56.

12. Neoptolemos JP, Palmer DH, Ghaneh P, et al. Comparison of adjuvant gemcitabine and capecitabine with gemcitabine monotherapy in patients with resected pancreatic cancer (ESPAC-4): a multicentre, open-label, randomised, phase 3 trial. Lancet 2017;389(10073):1011–24.

13. Uesaka K, Boku N, Fukutomi A, et al. Adjuvant chemotherapy of S-1 versus gemcitabine for resected pancreatic cancer: a phase 3, open-label, randomised, non-inferiority trial (JASPAC 01). Lancet 2016;388(10041):248–57.

14. Van Laethem JL, Hammel P, Mornex F, et al. Adjuvant gemcitabine alone versus gemcitabine-based chemoradiotherapy after curative resection for pancreatic cancer: a randomized EORTC-40013-22012/FFCD-9203/GERCOR phase II study. J Clin Oncol 2010;28(29):4450–6.

15. Schmidt J, Abel U, Debus J, et al. Open-label, multicenter, randomized phase III trial of adjuvant chemoradiation plus interferon alfa-2b versus fluorouracil and folinic acid for patients with resected pancreatic adenocarcinoma. J Clin Oncol 2012;30(33):4077–83.

16. Sinn M, TL, Klaus Gellert, et al. CONKO-005: adjuvant therapy in R0 resected pancreatic cancer patients with gemcitabine plus erlotinib versus gemcitabine for 24 weeks—A prospective randomized phase III study. 2015.

17. Weden S, Klemp M, Gladhaug IP, et al. Long-term follow-up of patients with resected pancreatic cancer following vaccination against mutant K-ras. Int J Cancer 2011;128(5):1120–8.

18. Middleton G, Silcocks P, Cox T, et al. Gemcitabine and capecitabine with or without telomerase peptide vaccine GV1001 in patients with locally advanced or metastatic pancreatic cancer (TeloVac): an open-label, randomised, phase 3 trial. Lancet Oncol 2014;15(8):829–40.

19. Jaffee EM, Hruban RH, Biedrzycki B, et al. Novel allogeneic granulocyte-macrophage colony-stimulating factor-secreting tumor vaccine for pancreatic cancer: a phase I trial of safety and immune activation. J Clin Oncol 2001;19(1):145–56.

20. Lutz E, Yeo CJ, Lillemoe KD, et al. A lethally irradiated allogeneic granulocyte-macrophage colony stimulating factor-secreting tumor vaccine for pancreatic adenocarcinoma. A Phase II trial of safety, efficacy, and immune activation. Ann Surg 2011;253(2):328–35.

21. Galili U, LaTemple DC. Natural anti-Gal antibody as a universal augmenter of autologous tumor vaccine immunogenicity. Immunol Today 1997;18(6):281–5.

22. LaTemple DC, Abrams JT, Zhang SY, et al. Increased immunogenicity of tumor vaccines complexed with anti-Gal: studies in knockout mice for alpha1,3galacto-syltransferase. Cancer Res 1999;59(14):3417–23.

23. Hardacre JM, Mulcahy M, Small W, et al. Addition of algenpantucel-L immunotherapy to standard adjuvant therapy for pancreatic cancer: a phase 2 study. J Gastrointest Surg 2013;17(1):94–100 [discussion: 100–1].

24. Araujo RL, Gaujoux S, Huguet F, et al. Does pre-operative chemoradiation for initially unresectable or borderline resectable pancreatic adenocarcinoma increase post-operative morbidity? A case-matched analysis. HPB (Oxford) 2013;15(8):574–80.

25. Lim KH, Chung E, Khan A, et al. Neoadjuvant therapy of pancreatic cancer: the emerging paradigm? Oncologist 2012;17(2):192–200.
26. Landry J, Catalano PJ, Staley C, et al. Randomized phase II study of gemcitabine plus radiotherapy versus gemcitabine, 5-fluorouracil, and cisplatin followed by radiotherapy and 5-fluorouracil for patients with locally advanced, potentially resectable pancreatic adenocarcinoma. J Surg Oncol 2010;101(7):587–92.
27. Kim EJ, Ben-Josef E, Herman JM, et al. A multi-institutional phase 2 study of neoadjuvant gemcitabine and oxaliplatin with radiation therapy in patients with pancreatic cancer. Cancer 2013;119(15):2692–700.
28. Palmer DH, Stocken DD, Hewitt H, et al. A randomized phase 2 trial of neoadjuvant chemotherapy in resectable pancreatic cancer: gemcitabine alone versus gemcitabine combined with cisplatin. Ann Surg Oncol 2007;14(7):2088–96.
29. Heinrich S, Pestalozzi BC, Schäfer M, et al. Prospective phase II trial of neoadjuvant chemotherapy with gemcitabine and cisplatin for resectable adenocarcinoma of the pancreatic head. J Clin Oncol 2008;26(15):2526–31.
30. Evans DB, Varadhachary GR, Crane CH, et al. Preoperative gemcitabine-based chemoradiation for patients with resectable adenocarcinoma of the pancreatic head. J Clin Oncol 2008;26(21):3496–502.
31. Varadhachary GR, Wolff RA, Crane CH, et al. Preoperative gemcitabine and cisplatin followed by gemcitabine-based chemoradiation for resectable adenocarcinoma of the pancreatic head. J Clin Oncol 2008;26(21):3487–95.
32. Golcher H, Brunner TB, Witzigmann H, et al. Neoadjuvant chemoradiation therapy with gemcitabine/cisplatin and surgery versus immediate surgery in resectable pancreatic cancer: results of the first prospective randomized phase II trial. Strahlenther Onkol 2015;191(1):7–16.
33. Tachezy M, Gebauer F, Petersen C, et al. Sequential neoadjuvant chemoradiotherapy (CRT) followed by curative surgery vs. primary surgery alone for resectable, non-metastasized pancreatic adenocarcinoma: NEOPA- a randomized multicenter phase III study (NCT01900327, DRKS00003893, ISRCTN82191749). BMC Cancer 2014;14:411.
34. Digestivo, G.E.M.d.C., Phase II study open, not randomized to evaluate the efficacy and safety of neoadjuvant treatment with gemcitabine and erlotinib followed by gemcitabine, erlotinib and radiotherapy in patients with resectable pancreatic adenocarcinoma. Available at: https://clinicaltrials.gov/ct2/show/NCT01389440.
35. Poplin E, Wasan H, Rolfe L, et al. Randomized, multicenter, phase II study of CO-101 versus gemcitabine in patients with metastatic pancreatic ductal adenocarcinoma: including a prospective evaluation of the role of hENT1 in gemcitabine or CO-101 sensitivity. J Clin Oncol 2013;31(35):4453–61.
36. Goncalves A, Gilabert M, François E, et al. BAYPAN study: a double-blind phase III randomized trial comparing gemcitabine plus sorafenib and gemcitabine plus placebo in patients with advanced pancreatic cancer. Ann Oncol 2012;23(11):2799–805.
37. Von Hoff DD, Ramanathan RK, Borad MJ, et al. Gemcitabine plus nab-paclitaxel is an active regimen in patients with advanced pancreatic cancer: a phase I/II trial. J Clin Oncol 2011;29(34):4548–54.
38. Von Hoff DD, Ervin T, Arena FP, et al. Increased survival in pancreatic cancer with nab-paclitaxel plus gemcitabine. N Engl J Med 2013;369(18):1691–703.
39. Chiorean EG, Von Hoff DD, Reni M, et al. CA19-9 decrease at 8 weeks as a predictor of overall survival in a randomized phase III trial (MPACT) of weekly nab-paclitaxel plus gemcitabine versus gemcitabine alone in patients with metastatic pancreatic cancer. Ann Oncol 2016;27(4):654–60.

40. Ramanathan RK, Goldstein D, Korn RL, et al. Positron emission tomography response evaluation from a randomized phase III trial of weekly nab-paclitaxel plus gemcitabine versus gemcitabine alone for patients with metastatic adenocarcinoma of the pancreas. Ann Oncol 2016;27(4):648–53.

41. Goldstein D, El-Maraghi RH, Hammel P, et al. nab-Paclitaxel plus gemcitabine for metastatic pancreatic cancer: long-term survival from a phase III trial. J Natl Cancer Inst 2015;107(2) [pii:dju413].

42. Kindler HL, Niedzwiecki D, Hollis D, et al. Gemcitabine plus bevacizumab compared with gemcitabine plus placebo in patients with advanced pancreatic cancer: phase III trial of the Cancer and Leukemia Group B (CALGB 80303). J Clin Oncol 2010;28(22):3617–22.

43. Xiong HQ, Rosenberg A, LoBuglio A, et al. Cetuximab, a monoclonal antibody targeting the epidermal growth factor receptor, in combination with gemcitabine for advanced pancreatic cancer: a multicenter phase II trial. J Clin Oncol 2004; 22(13):2610–6.

44. Moore MJ, Goldstein D, Hamm J, et al. Erlotinib plus gemcitabine compared with gemcitabine alone in patients with advanced pancreatic cancer: a phase III trial of the National Cancer Institute of Canada Clinical Trials Group. J Clin Oncol 2007;25(15):1960–6.

45. Van Cutsem E, Vervenne WL, Bennouna J, et al. Phase III trial of bevacizumab in combination with gemcitabine and erlotinib in patients with metastatic pancreatic cancer. J Clin Oncol 2009;27(13):2231–7.

46. Philip PA, Benedetti J, Corless CL, et al. Phase III study comparing gemcitabine plus cetuximab versus gemcitabine in patients with advanced pancreatic adenocarcinoma: Southwest Oncology Group-directed intergroup trial S0205. J Clin Oncol 2010;28(22):3605–10.

47. Kindler HL, Ioka T, Richel DJ, et al. Axitinib plus gemcitabine versus placebo plus gemcitabine in patients with advanced pancreatic adenocarcinoma: a double-blind randomised phase 3 study. Lancet Oncol 2011;12(3):256–62.

48. Rougier P, Riess H, Manges R, et al. Randomised, placebo-controlled, double-blind, parallel-group phase III study evaluating aflibercept in patients receiving first-line treatment with gemcitabine for metastatic pancreatic cancer. Eur J Cancer 2013;49(12):2633–42.

49. O'Neil BH, Scott AJ, Ma WW, et al. A phase II/III randomized study to compare the efficacy and safety of rigosertib plus gemcitabine versus gemcitabine alone in patients with previously untreated metastatic pancreatic cancer. Ann Oncol 2015;26(9):1923–9.

50. Fuchs CS, Azevedo S, Okusaka T, et al. A phase 3 randomized, double-blind, placebo-controlled trial of ganitumab or placebo in combination with gemcitabine as first-line therapy for metastatic adenocarcinoma of the pancreas: the GAMMA trial. Ann Oncol 2015;26(5):921–7.

51. Bergmann L, Maute L, Heil G, et al. A prospective randomised phase-II trial with gemcitabine versus gemcitabine plus sunitinib in advanced pancreatic cancer: a study of the CESAR Central European Society for Anticancer Drug Research-EWIV. Eur J Cancer 2015;51(1):27–36.

52. Kaufman B, Shapira-Frommer R, Schmutzler RK, et al. Olaparib monotherapy in patients with advanced cancer and a germline BRCA1/2 mutation. J Clin Oncol 2015;33(3):244–50.

53. Domchek SM, Hendifar AE, McWilliams RR, et al. RUCAPANC: an open-label, phase 2 trial of the PARP inhibitor rucaparib in patients with pancreatic cancer

and a known deleterious germline or somatic BRCA mutation. ASCO Meeting Abstracts 2016;34:4110.

54. Kindler HL, LG, Mann H, et al. POLO: A randomized phase III trial of olaparib tablets in patients with metastatic pancreatic cancer (mPC) and a germline BRCA1/2mutation (gBRCAm) who have not progressed following first-line chemotherapy. Meeting Abstracts 2015;35:4149.

55. Colucci G, Giuliani F, Gebbia V, et al. Gemcitabine alone or with cisplatin for the treatment of patients with locally advanced and/or metastatic pancreatic carcinoma: a prospective, randomized phase III study of the Gruppo Oncologia dell'Italia Meridionale. Cancer 2002;94(4):902–10.

56. Colucci G, Labianca R, Di Costanzo F, et al. Randomized phase III trial of gemcitabine plus cisplatin compared with single-agent gemcitabine as first-line treatment of patients with advanced pancreatic cancer: the GIP-1 study. J Clin Oncol 2010;28(10):1645–51.

57. Heinemann V, Quietzsch D, Gieseler F, et al. Randomized phase III trial of gemcitabine plus cisplatin compared with gemcitabine alone in advanced pancreatic cancer. J Clin Oncol 2006;24(24):3946–52.

58. Cunningham D, Chau I, Stocken DD, et al. Phase III randomized comparison of gemcitabine versus gemcitabine plus capecitabine in patients with advanced pancreatic cancer. J Clin Oncol 2009;27(33):5513–8.

59. Herrmann R, Bodoky G, Ruhstaller T, et al. Gemcitabine plus capecitabine compared with gemcitabine alone in advanced pancreatic cancer: a randomized, multicenter, phase III trial of the Swiss Group for Clinical Cancer Research and the Central European Cooperative Oncology Group. J Clin Oncol 2007; 25(16):2212–7.

60. Trouilloud I, Dupont-Gossard AC, Malka D, et al. Fixed-dose rate gemcitabine alone or alternating with FOLFIRI.3 (irinotecan, leucovorin and fluorouracil) in the first-line treatment of patients with metastatic pancreatic adenocarcinoma: an AGEO randomised phase II study (FIRGEM). Eur J Cancer 2014;50(18):3116–24.

61. Sho M, Shimizu A, Yanagimoto H, et al. Multicenter randomized phase II study comparing alternate-day oral therapy using S-1 with the standard regimen as a first-line treatment for patients with locally advanced and metastatic pancreatic cancer: PAN-01 study. Meeting Abstracts 2016;34:4107.

62. Conroy T, Paillot B, François E, et al. Irinotecan plus oxaliplatin and leucovorin-modulated fluorouracil in advanced pancreatic cancer–a Groupe Tumeurs Digestives of the Federation Nationale des Centres de Lutte Contre le Cancer study. J Clin Oncol 2005;23(6):1228–36.

63. Conroy T, Desseigne F, Ychou M, et al. FOLFIRINOX versus gemcitabine for metastatic pancreatic cancer. N Engl J Med 2011;364(19):1817–25.

64. Stein SM, James ES, Deng Y, et al. Final analysis of a phase II study of modified FOLFIRINOX in locally advanced and metastatic pancreatic cancer. Br J Cancer 2016;114(7):737–43.

65. Boeck S, Vehling-Kaiser U, Waldschmidt D, et al. Erlotinib 150 mg daily plus chemotherapy in advanced pancreatic cancer: an interim safety analysis of a multicenter, randomized, cross-over phase III trial of the 'Arbeitsgemeinschaft Internistische Onkologie'. Anticancer Drugs 2010;21(1):94–100.

66. Reni M, Cereda S, Milella M, et al. Maintenance sunitinib or observation in metastatic pancreatic adenocarcinoma: a phase II randomised trial. Eur J Cancer 2013;49(17):3609–15.

67. Oettle H, Riess H, Stieler JM, et al. Second-line oxaliplatin, folinic acid, and fluorouracil versus folinic acid and fluorouracil alone for gemcitabine-refractory

pancreatic cancer: outcomes from the CONKO-003 trial. J Clin Oncol 2014; 32(23):2423–9.

68. Gill S, Yoo-Joung Ko, Cripps MC, et al. PANCREOX: a randomized phase 3 study of 5FU/LV with or without oxaliplatin for second-line advanced pancreatic cancer (APC) in patients (pts) who have received gemcitabine (GEM)-based chemotherapy (CT). ASCO Meeting Abstracts 2014;32:4022.

69. Wang-Gillam A, Li CP, Bodoky G, et al. Nanoliposomal irinotecan with fluorouracil and folinic acid in metastatic pancreatic cancer after previous gemcitabine-based therapy (NAPOLI-1): a global, randomised, open-label, phase 3 trial. Lancet 2016;387(10018):545–57.

70. Heinemann V, Vehling-Kaiser U, Waldschmidt D, et al. Gemcitabine plus erlotinib followed by capecitabine versus capecitabine plus erlotinib followed by gemcitabine in advanced pancreatic cancer: final results of a randomised phase 3 trial of the 'Arbeitsgemeinschaft Internistische Onkologie' (AIO-PK0104). Gut 2013; 62(5):751–9.

71. Klaassen DJ, MacIntyre JM, Catton GE, et al. Treatment of locally unresectable cancer of the stomach and pancreas: a randomized comparison of 5-fluorouracil alone with radiation plus concurrent and maintenance 5-fluorouracil–an Eastern Cooperative Oncology Group study. J Clin Oncol 1985;3(3):373–8.

72. Treatment of locally unresectable carcinoma of the pancreas: comparison of combined-modality therapy (chemotherapy plus radiotherapy) to chemotherapy alone. Gastrointestinal Tumor Study Group. J Natl Cancer Inst 1988;80(10):751–5.

73. Blackstock AW, Tepper JE, Niedwiecki D, et al. Cancer and leukemia group B (CALGB) 89805: phase II chemoradiation trial using gemcitabine in patients with locoregional adenocarcinoma of the pancreas. Int J Gastrointest Cancer 2003;34(2–3):107–16.

74. Brunner TB, Grabenbauer GG, Kastl S, et al. Preoperative chemoradiation in locally advanced pancreatic carcinoma: a phase II study. Onkologie 2000; 23(5):436–42.

75. Macchia G, Valentini V, Mattiucci GC, et al. Preoperative chemoradiation and intra-operative radiotherapy for pancreatic carcinoma. Tumori 2007;93(1):53–60.

76. Thomas CR Jr, Weiden PL, Traverso LW, et al. Concomitant intraarterial cisplatin, intravenous 5-fluorouracil, and split-course radiation therapy for locally advanced unresectable pancreatic adenocarcinoma: a phase II study of the Puget Sound Oncology Consortium (PSOC-703). Am J Clin Oncol 1997;20(2):161–5.

77. Loehrer PJ Sr, Feng Y, Cardenes H, et al. Gemcitabine alone versus gemcitabine plus radiotherapy in patients with locally advanced pancreatic cancer: an Eastern Cooperative Oncology Group trial. J Clin Oncol 2011;29(31):4105–12.

78. Chauffert B, Mornex F, Bonnetain F, et al. Phase III trial comparing intensive induction chemoradiotherapy (60 Gy, infusional 5-FU and intermittent cisplatin) followed by maintenance gemcitabine with gemcitabine alone for locally advanced unresectable pancreatic cancer. Definitive results of the 2000-01 FFCD/SFRO study. Ann Oncol 2008;19(9):1592–9.

79. Hammel P, Huguet F, van Laethem JL, et al. Effect of chemoradiotherapy vs chemotherapy on survival in patients with locally advanced pancreatic cancer controlled after 4 months of gemcitabine with or without erlotinib: the LAP07 randomized clinical trial. JAMA 2016;315(17):1844–53.

80. Herman JM, Chang DT, Goodman KA, et al. Phase 2 multi-institutional trial evaluating gemcitabine and stereotactic body radiotherapy for patients with locally advanced unresectable pancreatic adenocarcinoma. Cancer 2015;121(7): 1128–37.

Future Clinical Trials

Genetically Driven Trials

Igor Astsaturov, MD, PhD

KEYWORDS

- Basket clinical trial • Biomarker • Molecular profiling

KEY POINTS

- Molecular profiling identifies distinct molecular mechanistic classes in major human cancers.
- Therapeutic successes are more likely when matching drugs with biologically relevant cancer mechanisms.
- Molecular profiling of cancers is an essential step in defining therapeutic strategies and clinical trials enrollment.

INTRODUCTION

Rapid incorporation of cost- and time-efficient genomic analysis technologies has been transformative for cancer medicine. Therapy selection on part of treating physicians is progressively shifting from the empirically validated one-size-fits-all chemotherapy or biological agents to tailoring agents to specific molecular features of patients' tumors. It has become even more imperative to identify a drug-amenable mechanism in the setting of clinical trials selection for patients. Again and again, studies have shown that randomly assigned treatments in patients participating in clinical trials are rarely beneficial with response rates less than 5%. Contrastingly, in the matched scenario when a drug is given because of the existence of a mechanism defined by genetic alteration, the likelihood of benefit increases to 20% to 30% range.[1,2] For a physician searching for investigational therapy options, the task of deciphering the actionable cancer mechanism poses an unprecedented challenge previously unknown to cancer medicine. This challenge was nicely formulated by Dr George Sledge[3] in his 2011 American Society for Clinical Oncology (ASCO) presidential address as being "a clinical cancer biologist." In this new reality, we are learning, in real time with the basic science, how cancer is a complex constellation of diseases sharing highly diverse alterations across previously incontestable organ and histologic

Disclosure Statement: The author is a consultant for Caris Life Sciences.
Department of Hematology and Oncology, Fox Chase Cancer Center, 333 Cottman Avenue, Philadelphia, PA 19111, USA
E-mail address: Igor.Astsaturov@fccc.edu

groupings and boundaries. For that reason alone, it has become more common for clinical trials to seek patients based on their tumors' molecular signatures. As a result, molecular profiling is viewed as a critical element in the design and conduct of oncology clinical trials, as it allows investigators to match the biomarkers within an individual's tumor with agents that specifically target those biomarkers. In the context of daily clinical practice, increasing numbers of oncologists are using molecular profiling to obtain insights into the dominant mechanism of their patients' cancers to find appropriate anticancer therapies, either through clinical trials or through off-label use of a growing number of the Food and Drug Administration (FDA)–approved targeted drugs. Here, the author reviews the successes of such matching exercises on the part of clinical trial investigators and on the part of practicing clinicians whose smartness in choosing the right trial for the right patient oftentimes remains unrecognized and does not earn podium applauses.

Targeting the Oncogenic Driver Mechanism

To date, genetic characterization of most human cancers consistently revealed a high level of diversity of oncogenic mechanisms within each site of origin and histologic subtype.[4–6] To complicate matters more, there is a growing appreciation of the existence of multiple genetically distinct clones within the same tumor that can compete for fitness and survival under selective pressures of anticancer therapies.[7] Monitoring these clonal dynamics becomes a major focus of genetic cancer surveillance, which spurred rapid development of noninvasive approaches of DNA sampling from blood,[7] saliva,[8,9] vaginal swabs,[10] and so forth. Despite the branched genetic phylogeny, some of the critical founding oncogenic lesions are shared between the tumor clones. In this context, molecular profiling can be used to uncover the dominant oncogenic mechanism in a tumor and to select therapies that target the oncogenic driver.[11] Although this approach may seem new, it dates back to 1960, when Nowell and Hungerford[12] described the famous Philadelphia chromosome translocation t(8,21) activating the abelson murine leukemia viral oncogene homolog 1 kinase and the malignant transformation in chronic myeloid leukemia. Four decades later, ST1571, later known as imatinib (Gleevec), was used for the first time in humans to suppress the culprit tyrosine kinase and to reverse the cancer process clinically and biologically.[13,14] Since the first validation of the oncogene-targeted therapy with imatinib, it has been appreciated that treating the principal driver oncogene can have a powerful impact. Experimental evidence further suggested that the rapidity of withdrawal of oncogene activity has the greatest impact on the anticancer effect.[15] This finding led to the proposed pulsatile blockade[16] and ideas of synthetic lethality[17] or combination of targeted agents.[18]

The ongoing trials are poised to investigate the efficacy of molecularly targeted treatments for *oncogene-defined* subsets of cancers across different tumor histologies.[19] In addition to the National Cancer Institute (NCI) (United States)–supported Molecular Analysis for Therapy Choice (MATCH) clinical trial, the ASCO launched its own Targeted Agent and Profiling Utilization Registry (TAPUR) trial offering access to the FDA-approved agents to patients with mechanistically relevant and well-defined genetic biomarkers.[20] These efforts require a genomic prescreening study to identify patients whose tumors harbor specific molecular abnormalities that can be matched to the relevant targeted treatments, regardless of tumor histology type. Success of these matching experiments is anxiously awaited. Single-institution pioneering studies[1] have clearly demonstrated that the unmatched cohorts of patients with advanced cancer rarely benefit from these targeted therapies, whereas the patients with a matched drug-to-cancer mutation do substantially better. For clinical practice, it made a random choosing of a phase I trial for patients rather unethical.[2] Despite the expense of finding rare patients with a desired mutation akin to searching a needle in a haystack, the rewarding successful demonstration of targeted drug's activity motivated Pfizer to develop crizotinib, an anaplastic lymphoma kinase and v-ros avian UR2 sarcoma virus oncogene homolog 1 inhibitor for treatment of less than 5% of patients with non–small-cell lung cancer.[21–23] Other examples abound. The tumor suppressor genes *BRCA1*, *BRCA2*, and *PALB2* (partner and localizer of BRCA2), which are implicated in hereditary breast and ovarian cancers, also confer the extreme sensitivity to platinum and mitomycin C that has been observed in patients with pancreatic cancer.[24,25]

Signaling Redundancies, Tumor Clonality, and Escape Routes

Despite similarity of biological mechanisms shared across different cancers, tissue and site of origin do exist. For instance, the success of BRAF inhibitors in V600E-mutated melanoma could not be reproduced in colorectal or tumors of nonmelanoma histologies carrying identical BRAF mutations.[26,27] The phenomenon here is less likely related to the difference in the BRAF biology but rather a more rapid evolution of resistance, for example, in colorectal cancer via epidermal growth factor receptor (EGFR) signaling activation. The reactivation of the mitogen-activated protein kinase (MAPK) pathway is indeed universally seen in resistance to BRAF inhibitors, including in BRAF V600E-mutated melanoma.[28,29] These discoveries prompted various groups of investigators to design colorectal trials that would use multilevel MAPK cascade blockade with BRAF, MEK inhibitors, and EGFR antibodies. The last approach demonstrated some activity.[30]

The earlier example illustrates the commonalities that clearly exist among highly diverse cancers not only in the shared mechanisms of the dominant oncogenic driver but also in the resistance. Clonal tumor heterogeneity poses additional diagnostic and longitudinal genetic surveillance challenges to the design of clinical trials. The rate of discrepancies in human EGFR 2 (HER2) status, for example, in breast cancer biopsied at different time points, can be as high as around 10%.[31] Similar challenges are encountered in gastroesophageal carcinomas in which co-occurrence of HER2, EGFR, and MET amplifications have been reported in the chromosomal instability subset of carcinomas.[4] Even more strikingly, under the selection pressure of a targeted agent, the minority clones will become dominant. These rare clones are now being picked up with a highly sensitive deep next-generation sequencing methodology, such as in the case of preexisting KRAS mutation in colorectal cancer treated with anti-EGFR antibodies.[32]

Rethinking the Clinical Trials Conduct

As the NCI launched the NCI-MATCH trial,[33–35] an ongoing screening effort of 795 samples (according to the interim analysis at http://ecog-acrin.org/nci-match-eay131/interim-analysis) identified 9% mutations matching one of the 10 arms of the study. To a large extent influenced by the study drug/gene menu, finding the matched mutation was as likely as 18% in melanoma, brain tumors, and lymphomas and 13% in colorectal and breast cancers versus no matching in all patients screened so far with pancreatic adenocarcinoma, head and neck, endometrial, and small cell carcinoma. Other tumor types showed 2% to 5% matching rate. With expansion to a total of 24 arms, including options for immunotherapy, fibroblast growth factor receptor 1/2/3 inhibitor, and palbociclib, the range of available options to match will grow significantly to the expected 23%. The lessons learned from this unprecedented exercise are set to influence the future decades of genetically tailored cancer trials and how we think of offering clinical trial opportunities to the patients. One example of the turnaround time increasing from 14 days in the early months of accrual to 36 days later, as the samples flooded the sequencing laboratories, imposes certain restriction on who and when to be recommended to go on such trials. Nevertheless, the study succeeded in 87% of all samples completing the tumor characterization process.

The NCI-MATCH trial represents what is called a basket trial design: multiple arms, evolving drugs portfolio, adaptive protocol flexibility, and dropout of the futile drug-gene combinations. These experiments drastically change the definition of success and target outcomes. A recent SHIVA trial (Molecularly targeted therapy based on tumor molecular profiling vs conventional therapy for advanced cancer)[36] used the ratio of progression-free survival (PFS) on genotype-matched treatment to PFS on genotype-unmatched treatment to assess the efficacy of therapy guided by patients' tumor molecular profiling. This particular estimation of the clinical efficacy was used to compensate for the extreme cohort heterogeneity of tumor types. As all 195 patients were allowed to cross over on progression, the investigators compared the algorithm-based treatment assignment with the physician's choice. The ratio of PFS of algorithm-based treatment selection over the physician choice exceeded 1.3 in 37% of patients who switched to the algorithm-guided treatment arm. Contrastingly, 61% of patients who crossed over from the algorithm arm to the-physician-choice arm exceeded prior PFS by a factor of 1.3.[36] (We are smarter than the computers, are we not?) The selection of PFS ratio in a prespecified percentage of patients when comparing treatment assignment by molecular biomarkers has been first field tested in the pivotal trial by Van Hoff and colleagues.[37] In that study, which used mRNA profiling to guide chemotherapy selection, 27% of patients exceeded the PFS on their last prior therapy by a factor of 2.9 and the overall response rate was 10%.

The outcomes of these novel trials (eg, SHIVA,[36] Signature trial by Novartis[38]) suggest that the lower response rates in the range of 2% to 4% are underestimating the clinical benefit accounted for as prolonged disease stability, which translates to a greater PFS. The Signature trial is particularly worth mentioning as it used uniquely a patient-specific expedited Institutional Review Board approval process and the site initiation process breaking the restrictive administrative thresholds. Its successful execution for the first time demonstrated the flexibility of patient-centered administration of innovative experimental therapy. The author hopes more examples of this approach will follow. The ASCO's TAPUR trial is yet another version of the molecularly tailored therapeutic experiment, as it is run essentially as a tissue-agnostic open registry of the outcomes for the currently FDA-approved agents provided through the network of participating centers.[20] Its set primary end point, the overall response rate or stable disease at 16 weeks, will be prospectively evaluated at the growing number of clinical sites. The study is currently ongoing as it passed the interim futility threshold of clinical benefit in 7 out of 28 participants.

The NCI initiative to define the mechanisms of the exceptional responders[39,40] further emphasizes the critical value of even singular clinical observations. For many patients with rare tumors or rare genetic alterations, the access to innovative therapies or even discovery of their cancer's molecular aberrations can be transformative and results in many years of life gained, as the author and colleagues recently reported in the case of KIT-mutated neuroendocrine carcinoma.[41] The modern matching trials are, at best, covering the cancer proteome that can be drugged, encompassing optimistically around 10% of cancer driver mutations, while leaving the major oncogenes (RAS paralogs, MYC, beta-catenin, mutant TP53, and so forth) practically unattended. We still have a long way to go to call a success.

SUMMARY

The present era of molecularly targeted and immune therapies presents the unprecedented opportunities to transform cancer medicine to clinical cancer biology. This change is difficult and gratifying; it faces enormous regulatory, financial, and administrative challenges. It redefines the clinical evidence with appreciation that each cancer is absolutely unique in its molecular makeup, clonality, patients' demographics, and its perpetual evolution over time. Despite this uniqueness, common biological denominators exist and are defined, not only in the laboratory but also clinically, as oncogenic drivers. Impinging on these principal mechanistic elements is often successful and can be measured prospectively and retrospectively. The value of these rapidly acquired observations reshapes the regulatory and the payer policies making it easier for patients to have access to so much needed treatment options.

REFERENCES

1. Tsimberidou AM, Iskander NG, Hong DS, et al. Personalized medicine in a phase I clinical trials program: the MD Anderson Cancer Center initiative. Clin Cancer Res 2012;18:6373–83. Available at: http://www.ncbi.nlm.nih.gov/pubmed/22966018.
2. Schwaederle M, Zhao M, Lee JJ, et al. Association of biomarker-based treatment strategies with response rates and progression-free survival in refractory malignant neoplasms: a meta-analysis. JAMA Oncol 2016;2:1452–9. Available at: http://www.ncbi.nlm.nih.gov/pubmed/27273579.
3. Sledge GW Jr. The Challenge and Promise of the Genomic Era. Journal of Clinical Oncology 2012;30(2):203–9.
4. Cancer Genome Atlas Research Network. Comprehensive molecular characterization of gastric adenocarcinoma. Nature 2014;513:202–9. Available at: https://www.ncbi.nlm.nih.gov/pubmed/25079317.
5. Kandoth C, McLellan MD, Vandin F, et al. Mutational landscape and significance across 12 major cancer types. Nature 2013;502:333–9. Available at: http://www.ncbi.nlm.nih.gov/pubmed/24132290.
6. Zhang B, Wang J, Wang X, et al. Proteogenomic characterization of human colon and rectal cancer. Nature 2014;513:382–7. Available at: http://www.ncbi.nlm.nih.gov/pubmed/25043054.
7. Murtaza M, Dawson SJ, Tsui DW, et al. Non-invasive analysis of acquired resistance to cancer therapy by sequencing of plasma DNA. Nature 2013;497:108–12. Available at: http://www.ncbi.nlm.nih.gov/pubmed/23563269.
8. Fliss MS, Usadel H, Caballero OL, et al. Facile detection of mitochondrial DNA mutations in tumors and bodily fluids. Science 2000;287:2017–9. Available at: http://www.ncbi.nlm.nih.gov/pubmed/10720328.
9. Wang Y, Springer S, Mulvey CL, et al. Detection of somatic mutations and HPV in the saliva and plasma of patients with head and neck squamous cell carcinomas. Sci Transl Med 2015;7:293ra104. Available at: http://www.ncbi.nlm.nih.gov/pubmed/26109104.
10. Kinde I, Bettegowda C, Wang Y, et al. Evaluation of DNA from the Papanicolaou test to detect ovarian and endometrial cancers. Sci Transl Med 2013;5:167ra4. Available at: http://www.ncbi.nlm.nih.gov/pubmed/23303603.
11. Kris MG, Johnson BE, Berry LD, et al. Using multiplexed assays of oncogenic drivers in lung cancers to select targeted drugs. JAMA 2014;311:1998–2006. Available at: http://www.ncbi.nlm.nih.gov/pubmed/24846037.
12. Nowell PC, Hungerford DA. A minute chromosome in human chronic granulocytic leukemia. Science 1960;132:1497.

13. Druker BJ, Sawyers CL, Kantarjian H, et al. Activity of a specific inhibitor of the BCR-ABL tyrosine kinase in the blast crisis of chronic myeloid leukemia and acute lymphoblastic leukemia with the Philadelphia chromosome. N Engl J Med 2001; 344:1038–42. Available at: http://www.ncbi.nlm.nih.gov/pubmed/11287973.

14. Druker BJ, Talpaz M, Resta DJ, et al. Efficacy and safety of a specific inhibitor of the BCR-ABL tyrosine kinase in chronic myeloid leukemia. N Engl J Med 2001; 344:1031–7. Available at: http://www.ncbi.nlm.nih.gov/pubmed/11287972.

15. Sharma SV, Gajowniczek P, Way IP, et al. A common signaling cascade may underlie "addiction" to the Src, BCR-ABL, and EGF receptor oncogenes. Cancer Cell 2006;10:425–35. Available at: http://www.ncbi.nlm.nih.gov/pubmed/17097564.

16. Shah NP, Kasap C, Weier C, et al. Transient potent BCR-ABL inhibition is sufficient to commit chronic myeloid leukemia cells irreversibly to apoptosis. Cancer Cell 2008;14:485–93. Available at: http://www.ncbi.nlm.nih.gov/pubmed/19061839.

17. Astsaturov I, Ratushny V, Sukhanova A, et al. Synthetic lethal screen of an EGFR-centered network to improve targeted therapies. Sci Signal 2010;3:ra67. Available at: http://www.ncbi.nlm.nih.gov/pubmed/20858866.

18. Sawyers CL. Cancer: mixing cocktails. Nature 2007;449:993–6. Available at: http://www.ncbi.nlm.nih.gov/pubmed/17960228.

19. McNeil C. NCI-MATCH launch highlights new trial design in precision-medicine era. J Natl Cancer Inst 2015;107 [pii:djv193]. Available at: http://www.ncbi.nlm.nih.gov/pubmed/26142446.

20. Markman M. Maurie Markman on the groundbreaking TAPUR trial. Oncology (Williston Park) 2017;31:158–68. Available at: https://www.ncbi.nlm.nih.gov/pubmed/28299751.

21. Shaw AT, Kim DW, Nakagawa K, et al. Crizotinib versus chemotherapy in advanced ALK-positive lung cancer. N Engl J Med 2013;368:2385–94. Available at: http://www.ncbi.nlm.nih.gov/pubmed/23724913.

22. Shaw AT, Ou SH, Bang YJ, et al. Crizotinib in ROS1-rearranged non-small-cell lung cancer. N Engl J Med 2014;371:1963–71. Available at: http://www.ncbi.nlm.nih.gov/pubmed/25264305.

23. Solomon BJ, Mok T, Kim DW, et al. First-line crizotinib versus chemotherapy in ALK-positive lung cancer. N Engl J Med 2014;371:2167–77. Available at: http://www.ncbi.nlm.nih.gov/pubmed/25470694.

24. Chantrill LA, Nagrial AM, Watson C, et al, Australian Pancreatic Cancer Genome Initiative (APGI), Individualized Molecular Pancreatic Cancer Therapy (IMPaCT) Trial Management Committee of the Australasian Gastrointestinal Trials Group (AGITG). Precision medicine for advanced pancreas cancer: the Individualized Molecular Pancreatic Cancer Therapy (IMPaCT) trial. Clin Cancer Res 2015;21:2029–37. Available at: http://www.ncbi.nlm.nih.gov/pubmed/25896973.

25. Kaufman B, Shapira-Frommer R, Schmutzler RK, et al. Olaparib monotherapy in patients with advanced cancer and a germline BRCA1/2 mutation. J Clin Oncol 2015;33:244–50. Available at: http://www.ncbi.nlm.nih.gov/pubmed/25366685.

26. Prahallad A, Sun C, Huang S, et al. Unresponsiveness of colon cancer to BRAF (V600E) inhibition through feedback activation of EGFR. Nature 2012;483:100–3. Available at: http://www.ncbi.nlm.nih.gov/pubmed/22281684.

27. Hyman DM, Puzanov I, Subbiah V, et al. Vemurafenib in multiple nonmelanoma cancers with BRAF V600 mutations. N Engl J Med 2015;373:726–36. Available at: http://www.ncbi.nlm.nih.gov/pubmed/26287849.

28. Kwong LN, Boland GM, Frederick DT, et al. Co-clinical assessment identifies patterns of BRAF inhibitor resistance in melanoma. J Clin Invest 2015;125:1459–70. Available at: http://www.ncbi.nlm.nih.gov/pubmed/25705882.

29. Schreuer M, Jansen Y, Planken S, et al. Combination of dabrafenib plus trameti-nib for BRAF and MEK inhibitor pretreated patients with advanced BRAFV600-mutant melanoma: an open-label, single arm, dual-centre, phase 2 clinical trial. Lancet Oncol 2017;18:464–72. Available at: http://www.ncbi.nlm.nih.gov/pubmed/28268064.

30. Hong DS, Morris VK, El Osta B, et al. Phase IB study of vemurafenib in combina-tion with irinotecan and cetuximab in patients with metastatic colorectal cancer with BRAFV600E mutation. Cancer Discov 2016;6:1352–65. Available at: http://www.ncbi.nlm.nih.gov/pubmed/27729313.

31. Allott EH, Geradts J, Sun X, et al. Intratumoral heterogeneity as a source of discordance in breast cancer biomarker classification. Breast Cancer Res 2016;18:68. Available at: http://www.ncbi.nlm.nih.gov/pubmed/27349894.

32. Misale S, Yaeger R, Hobor S, et al. Emergence of KRAS mutations and acquired resistance to anti-EGFR therapy in colorectal cancer. Nature 2012;486:532–6. Available at: http://www.ncbi.nlm.nih.gov/pubmed/22722830.

33. Lih CJ, Harrington RD, Sims DJ, et al. Analytical validation of the next-generation sequencing assay for a nationwide signal-finding clinical trial: molecular analysis for therapy choice clinical trial. J Mol Diagn 2017;19:313–27. Available at: https://www.ncbi.nlm.nih.gov/pubmed/28188106.

34. Coyne GO, Takebe N, Chen AP. Defining precision: the precision medicine initia-tive trials NCI-MPACT and NCI-MATCH. Curr Probl Cancer 2017 [Epub ahead of print]. Available at: https://www.ncbi.nlm.nih.gov/pubmed/28372823.

35. Colwell J. NCI-MATCH trial draws strong interest. Cancer Discov 2016;6:334. Available at: https://www.ncbi.nlm.nih.gov/pubmed/26896095.

36. Belin L, Kamal M, Mauborgne C, et al. Randomized phase II trial comparing molecularly targeted therapy based on tumor molecular profiling versus conven-tional therapy in patients with refractory cancer: cross-over analysis from the SHIVA trial. Ann Oncol 2017;28:590–6. Available at: https://www.ncbi.nlm.nih.gov/pubmed/27993804.

37. Von Hoff DD, Stephenson JJ Jr, Rosen P, et al. Pilot study using molecular profiling of patients' tumors to find potential targets and select treatments for their refractory cancers. J Clin Oncol 2010;28:4877–83. Available at: https://www.ncbi.nlm.nih.gov/pubmed/20921468.

38. Slosberg ED, Kang B, Beck JT, et al. The signature program, a series of tissue-agnostic, mutation-specific signal finding trials. J Clin Oncol 2014;32. TPS2646-TPS. Available at: http://ascopubs.org/doi/abs/10.1200/jco.2014.32.15_suppl.tps2646.

39. Printz C. NCI launches exceptional responders initiative: researchers will attempt to identify why some patients respond to treatment so much better than others. Cancer 2015;121:803–4. Available at: https://www.ncbi.nlm.nih.gov/pubmed/25739575.

40. Prasad V, Vandross A. Characteristics of exceptional or super responders to can-cer drugs. Mayo Clin Proc 2015;90:1639–49. Available at: https://www.ncbi.nlm.nih.gov/pubmed/26546106.

41. Perkins J, Boland P, Cohen SJ, et al. Successful imatinib therapy for neuroendocrine carcinoma with activating Kit mutation: a case study. J Natl Compr Canc Netw 2014;12:847–52. Available at: http://www.ncbi.nlm.nih.gov/pubmed/24925195.

UNITED STATES POSTAL SERVICE ®

Statement of Ownership, Management, and Circulation
(All Periodicals Publications Except Requester Publications)

1. Publication Title	2. Publication Number	3. Filing Date
SURGICAL ONCOLOGY CLINICS OF NORTH AMERICA	012 – 565	9/18/2017

4. Issue Frequency	5. Number of Issues Published Annually	6. Annual Subscription Price
JAN, APR, JUL, OCT	4	$296.00

7. Complete Mailing Address of Known Office of Publication (Not printer) (Street, city, county, state, and ZIP+4®)

ELSEVIER INC.
230 Park Avenue, Suite 800
New York, NY 10169

Contact Person
STEPHEN R. BUSHING

Telephone (Include area code)
215-239-3688

8. Complete Mailing Address of Headquarters or General Business Office of Publisher (Not printer)

ELSEVIER INC.
230 Park Avenue, Suite 800
New York, NY 10169

9. Full Names and Complete Mailing Addresses of Publisher, Editor, and Managing Editor (Do not leave blank)

Publisher (Name and complete mailing address)

ADRIANNE BRIGIDO, ELSEVIER INC.
1600 JOHN F KENNEDY BLVD. SUITE 1800
PHILADELPHIA, PA 19103-2899

Editor (Name and complete mailing address)

JOHN VASSALLO, ELSEVIER INC.
1600 JOHN F KENNEDY BLVD. SUITE 1800
PHILADELPHIA, PA 19103-2899

Managing Editor (Name and complete mailing address)

PATRICK MANLEY, ELSEVIER INC.
1600 JOHN F KENNEDY BLVD. SUITE 1800
PHILADELPHIA, PA 19103-2899

10. Owner (Do not leave blank. If the publication is owned by a corporation, give the name and address of the corporation immediately followed by the names and addresses of all stockholders owning or holding 1 percent or more of the total amount of stock. If not owned by a corporation, give the names and addresses of the individual owners. If owned by a partnership or other unincorporated firm, give its name and address as well as those of each individual owner. If the publication is published by a nonprofit organization, give its name and address.)

Full Name	Complete Mailing Address
WHOLLY OWNED SUBSIDIARY OF REED/ELSEVIER, US HOLDINGS	1600 JOHN F KENNEDY BLVD. SUITE 1800 PHILADELPHIA, PA 19103-2899

11. Known Bondholders, Mortgagees, and Other Security Holders Owning or Holding 1 Percent or More of Total Amount of Bonds, Mortgages, or Other Securities. If none, check box ☐ None

Full Name	Complete Mailing Address
N/A	

12. Tax Status (For completion by nonprofit organizations authorized to mail at nonprofit rates) (Check one)
The purpose, function, and nonprofit status of this organization and the exempt status for federal income tax purposes:
☒ Has Not Changed During Preceding 12 Months
☐ Has Changed During Preceding 12 Months (Publisher must submit explanation of change with this statement)

13. Publication Title	14. Issue Date for Circulation Data Below
SURGICAL ONCOLOGY CLINICS OF NORTH AMERICA	JULY 2017

PS Form **3526**, July 2014 [Page 1 of 4 (see instructions page 4)] PSN: 7530-01-000-9931 PRIVACY NOTICE: See our privacy policy on www.usps.com

15. Extent and Nature of Circulation			Average No. Copies Each Issue During Preceding 12 Months	No. Copies of Single Issue Published Nearest to Filing Date
a. Total Number of Copies (Net press run)			22	151
b. Paid Circulation (By Mail and Outside the Mail)	(1)	Mailed Outside-County Paid Subscriptions Stated on PS Form 3541 (Include paid distribution above nominal rate, advertiser's proof copies, and exchange copies)	84	72
	(2)	Mailed In-County Paid Subscriptions Stated on PS Form 3541 (Include paid distribution above nominal rate, advertiser's proof copies, and exchange copies)	0	0
	(3)	Paid Distribution Outside the Mails Including Sales Through Dealers and Carriers, Street Vendors, Counter Sales, and Other Paid Distribution Outside USPS®	53	55
	(4)	Paid Distribution by Other Classes of Mail Through the USPS (e.g. First-Class Mail®)	0	0
c. Total Paid Distribution (Sum of 15b (1), (2), (3), and (4))			137	127
d. Free or Nominal Rate Distribution (By Mail and Outside the Mail)	(1)	Free or Nominal Rate Outside-County Copies included on PS Form 3541	39	24
	(2)	Free or Nominal Rate In-County Copies Included on PS Form 3541	0	0
	(3)	Free or Nominal Rate Copies Mailed at Other Classes Through the USPS (e.g. First-Class Mail)	0	0
	(4)	Free or Nominal Rate Distribution Outside the Mail (Carriers or other means)	0	0
e. Total Free or Nominal Rate Distribution (Sum of 15d (1), (2), (3) and (4))			39	24
f. Total Distribution (Sum of 15c and 15e)			176	151
g. Copies not Distributed (See instructions to Publishers #4 (page #3))			46	0
h. Total (Sum of 15f and g)			222	151
i. Percent Paid (15c divided by 15f times 100)			77.84%	84.11%

* If you are claiming electronic copies, go to line 16 on page 3. If you are not claiming electronic copies, skip to line 17 on page 3.

16. Electronic Copy Circulation	Average No. Copies Each Issue During Preceding 12 Months	No. Copies of Single Issue Published Nearest to Filing Date
a. Paid Electronic Copies	0	0
b. Total Paid Print Copies (Line 15c) + Paid Electronic Copies (Line 16a)	137	127
c. Total Print Distribution (Line 15f) + Paid Electronic Copies (Line 16a)	176	151
d. Percent Paid (Both Print & Electronic Copies) (16b divided by 16c × 100)	77.84%	84.11%

☒ I certify that 50% of all my distributed copies (electronic and print) are paid above a nominal price.

17. Publication of Statement of Ownership

☒ If the publication is a general publication, publication of this statement is required. Will be printed in the OCTOBER 2017 issue of this publication. ☐ Publication not required.

18. Signature and Title of Editor, Publisher, Business Manager, or Owner

STEPHEN R. BUSHING - INVENTORY DISTRIBUTION CONTROL MANAGER

Date 9/18/2017

I certify that all information furnished on this form is true and complete. I understand that anyone who furnishes false or misleading information on this form or who omits material or information requested on the form may be subject to criminal sanctions (including fines and imprisonment) and/or civil sanctions (including civil penalties).

PS Form **3526**, July 2014 (Page 2 of 4) PRIVACY NOTICE: See our privacy policy on www.usps.com

Moving?

Make sure your subscription moves with you!

To notify us of your new address, find your **Clinics Account Number** (located on your mailing label above your name), and contact customer service at:

Email: journalscustomerservice-usa@elsevier.com

800-654-2452 (subscribers in the U.S. & Canada)
314-447-8871 (subscribers outside of the U.S. & Canada)

Fax number: 314-447-8029

Elsevier Health Sciences Division
Subscription Customer Service
3251 Riverport Lane
Maryland Heights, MO 63043

*To ensure uninterrupted delivery of your subscription, please notify us at least 4 weeks in advance of move.

Printed and bound by CPI Group (UK) Ltd, Croydon, CR0 4YY

03/10/2024

01040398-0011